"This collection is eye-opening, accessible and pioneering. An invaluable toolkit for anybody interested in criminal justice and mental health."

David Lammy, MP, Shadow Secretary of State for Foreign, Commonwealth and Development Affairs of the United Kingdom

"Justice is a key concept in medical ethics, with respect for justice identified as one of four principles of bioethics. This timely book provides a welcome review of how systemic injustices can affect patients and staff in forensic services. The editors have brought together a range of rich and thoughtful chapters which should make forensic practitioners question themselves about whether their services always act justly; and how forensic services can be more respectful of diversity and justice."

Dr. Gwen Adshead, Consultant Forensic Psychiatrist and Psychotherapist at Broadmoor Hospital, United Kingdom

"An intellectual entertainment was defined by Lord Reith as educating, informing, and entertaining. Science and medicine do not fare well as entertainments, but entertainment and literary criticism do not fare well as nostrums for life-shortening illnesses. In this book, Tomlin and Völlm give fair and equal hearings to both. The reader will benefit from the choice."

Prof. Harry Kennedy, Clinical Professor of Forensic Psychiatry and Executive Clinical Director of National Forensic Mental Health Service in Ireland

Diversity and Marginalisation in Forensic Mental Health Care

This book explores the ways in which diversity and experiences of marginalisation are present in forensic mental health care settings around the globe and suggests ways of moving forward beyond these.

Forensic mental health services provide care for a group of patients who are marginalised in several respects. Many have experienced childhood adversity and abuse, substance use, serious and chronic mental disorders, poor healthcare education or treatment, inadequate educational opportunities, social isolation, and pervasive forms of stigmatisation. On top of these individual experiences of marginalisation, wide diversity exists across patients' socio-demographic, cultural, and clinical characteristics. Chapters in this book discuss these crucial and often sensitive problems, such as working with transgender prisoners, the impact of incarceration for children from non-white backgrounds, cultural and linguistic diversity in forensic settings, and more.

Combining global perspectives, current evidence and case studies, this book will be of interest to patients, carers, practitioners, researchers, and students of forensic mental health.

Jack Tomlin is Lecturer in Criminology at the University of Greenwich, United Kingdom. He has studied, taught, and researched crime and mental health in the United Kingdom, the Netherlands, and Germany.

Birgit Völlm is Professor of Forensic Psychiatry and Director of the Hospital of Forensic Psychiatry at Rostock University Medical Center. She is also Chair of the Forensic Section of the World Psychiatric Association.

International Perspectives on Forensic Mental Health

A Routledge Book Series
Edited by Patricia Zapf
Palo Alto University

The goal of this series is to improve the quality of health care services in forensic and correctional settings by providing a forum for discussing issues and disseminating resources related to policy, administration, clinical practice, and research. The series addresses topics such as mental health law; the organization and administration of forensic and/or correctional services for persons with mental disorders; the development, implementation and evaluation of treatment programs and interventions for individuals in civil and criminal justice settings; the assessment and management of violence risk, including risk for sexual violence and family violence; and staff selection, training, and development in forensic and/or correctional systems. The book series will consider proposals for both monographs and edited works on these and related topics, with special consideration given to proposals that promote evidence-based best practices and that are relevant to international audiences. Workbooks and manuals targeted toward practitioners and reflecting evidence-based practice and intervention will also be considered.

Published Titles

Evaluating Juvenile Transfer and Disposition Law, Science, and Practice
Kirk Heilbrun, David DeMatteo, Christopher King, Sarah Filone

Handbook of Forensic Mental Health Services
Ronald Roesch, Alana N. Cook

A Treatment Manual for Justice Involved Persons with Mental Illness Changing Lives and Changing Outcomes
Robert D. Morgan, Daryl Kroner, Jeremy F. Mills

Forthcoming Titles

Safeguarding Forensic Violence Risk Assessment A Review Across Western Nations
Michiel van der Wolf

Diversity and Marginalisation in Forensic Mental Health Care
Edited by Jack Tomlin and Birgit Völlm

For more information about this series, please visit: www.routledge.com/ International-Perspectives-on-Forensic-Mental-Health/book-series/IPFMF

Diversity and Marginalisation in Forensic Mental Health Care

Edited by Jack Tomlin and Birgit Völlm

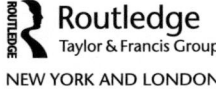

Routledge
Taylor & Francis Group

NEW YORK AND LONDON

Cover image: © Cover Graffiti by Marcel Dietermann

First published 2023
by Routledge
605 Third Avenue, New York, NY 10158

and by Routledge
4 Park Square, Milton Park, Abingdon, Oxon, OX14 4RN

Routledge is an imprint of the Taylor & Francis Group, an informa business

© 2023 selection and editorial matter, Jack Tomlin and Birgit Völlm; individual chapters, the contributors

Library of Congress Cataloging-in-Publication Data
A catalog record for this book has been requested

ISBN: 978-1-032-02711-1 (hbk)
ISBN: 978-1-032-02697-8 (pbk)
ISBN: 978-1-003-18476-8 (ebk)

DOI: 10.4324/9781003184768

Contents

Foreword

The editors begin by setting themselves a formidable task: 'by definition society includes some people and excludes others'. But the modern civil state is ruled by rights and laws that emphasise that no one is excluded. Citizenship itself has never been so open. Implicit therefore is a distinction between the state and society. If this is correct, then they have set themselves another problem since forensic psychiatry is generally practiced in state hospitals and prisons. Modern civil society is diverse in principle and in fact. So when a person or a group is marginalised, one must ask – marginalised from what? It is a pleasure to read a book that tackles these problematic conditions so well.

This book is a wide-ranging and carefully curated collection of chapters. Chapters address different aspects of diversity – some by special groups while others consider broader issues about what marginalisation or exclusion might mean. Groups considered are women, children and adolescents, migrants, first nations peoples, and fathers.

As this is also a book about forensic mental health care, a recurring observation is that being mentally disordered as defined by law, having come before the courts charged with a crime, and being made subject to a forensic treatment order is a double disadvantage, a double stigma which might be regarded as marginalising and would certainly demarcate exclusion from the mainstream of society, by the state's rule of law. For convenience, marginalisation might be used to describe the exclusion of groups as groups; however, the group is defined – typically by some essentialist characterisation such as race, nation, or religion (Said, 2012) though more fundamental categories can also be used – 'woman', 'child', and 'father'.

Being a forensic psychiatric patient could also be one of the end points of a process of alienation. Alienation may be used here as a name for a more personal or individual exclusion from society, which can be an active withdrawal by choice. Either exclusion or withdrawal or both may apply to the individual person. Each of these chapters struggles with formulating the problem of distinguishing between these as a process, status, or choice and between cause and effect. The goal of court orders for forensic psychiatric treatment is to reintegrate into 'society' by facilitating an end to exclusion and marginalisation, case by case, patient by patient, person by person. Forensic psychiatry aims to do this by restoring the forensic patient to full health, where heath is itself a social concept (Lewis, 2013), for example, defined by the WHO (World Health, 2018; Galderisi et al., 2015). This is an obvious source of conflict since many forensic psychiatric patients choose withdrawal and alienation as an active expression of their will and preference. Unfortunately, marginalisation and alienation are often the unforeseen consequences of choices – to refuse treatment that prevents violence, for example (Fazel & Grann, 2004).

Alienation is more commonly understood in economic terms, from Marxism to the Chicago school of social ecology (Faris & Dunham, 1939). Durkheim was able to show that suicide rates could be reliably related to demographic and economic characteristics (Durkheim, 2020). Durkheim interpreted this in terms of social forces and factors of cohesion, belief, and personal exclusion. Faris and Dunham (1939) were able to extend these regularities in populations to mental illness, crime, and economic inequality. Homicide, crimes of violence, and suicide rates can be related to population density, deprivation, and cohesion, with social cohesion predominating (Kennedy et al., 1999). The use of forensic psychiatric beds can be related to measures of social cohesion or lack of cohesion in the same way (Coid et al., 2001; Pierzchniak et al., 1999; O'Neill et al., 2005).

Goffman (2009), studying stigma (spoiled social identity, arguably the same concept as marginalisation or alienation in relation to forensic psychiatry patients), described a holistic picture of the alienated, rule-breaking, violent, and substance misusing person and their associates some of whom may as part of their natural history develop delusions and hallucinations in the context also of social drift. Goffman was also careful to describe the privileged role of the professionals, the psychiatrists, nurses, and probation officers who are valued by their patients or clients precisely because they can recognise and value the human qualities of opposition and defiance, delinquency, rule breaking, and criticism for criticism's sake (Goffman, 2009).

Nothing is more alienating than interpersonal violence. When violence manifests as a dysfunctional way of coping with stresses in social and interpersonal relationships due to some inherent impairment of functional mental capacity arising from a traumatic upbringing, mental illness, or another mental disability, then there is a role for therapeutic interventions to restore or support capacities so that non-violent ways of coping replace violence. Nothing is more likely to repair alienation arising from violence than treatments that are effective in providing alternatives to violence.

Working with the patient who at times is a danger to others is the most consistent challenge in forensic secure hospitals and services. Violence in schools, prisons, and society generally will lead rapidly to exclusion and marginalisation. In some cases, the violent person in an institution is exploited and used by other more deliberative and callous inmates, residents, or patients. In some cases, the violent person dominates those in their vicinity and will in the process destroy any therapeutic milieu (Toch, 1992).

The relationship between diversity and marginalisation is complex. Diversity in its own right should never be pathologised. Social injustices that lead to the marginalisation of any group identified by some essentialism may cause secondary mental health problems, a form of structural violence. Psychiatric services including forensic psychiatric services obviously cannot solve the social injustices that are the root causes of marginalisation. However, the victims of such processes including those who manifest violence have a right to be seen as individuals not as social ciphers or pawns in someone else's political agenda. They have a right to the best medical services for physical health and mental health that is appropriate to their needs. This should be true whether there is a social benefit or not. Social dangerousness most commonly arises in the absence of any essentialist characteristic or characterisation and also in the absence of any mental health problem. Where a mental health problem is found, diagnosing the mental illness, formulating a legally defined mental disorder, and offering effective treatment can be caught in the crossfire of political argument. All too often, the popular libertarian approach to forensic mental health services and all psychiatric services is to deny the reality of severe neurodevelopmental, neurodegenerative, and disabling diseases and illnesses. Schizophrenia shortens life expectancy by on average 16 years (Lomholt et al., 2019). Denials or attacks on psychiatry under these circumstances serve only to deprive the severely mentally ill of the treatments they need to restore autonomy and dignity. Blaming the messenger (Hermenoia, broadly translated as attacking Hermes the messenger of the Gods (Kennedy, 2014)) is a common cultural confusion in modern times.

In the chapters of this book that deal with various special groups broadly described as diversity, there are many associations but few causal explanations. The chapter on fathers in forensic psychiatric services is to be praised for gently recognising that while fathers who are detained in forensic psychiatric secure hospitals may be deprived of their role as a father and their children may be deprived of access to their father, the same fathers may have parenting problems concerning trans-generational parenting behaviours acquired through trauma and neglect that may lead to delinquency through trauma and neglect (Farrington et al., 2009). This subtle recognition of the ambiguity concerning the causation or direction of causation also recognises the potential for therapeutic intervention to disrupt the cycle for the benefit of both father and child.

Chapters on gender, developmental disorders, and other specific categories are similarly therapeutically sophisticated but what of the patients in the mainstream, the person with delusions and hallucinations who acts on these beliefs to harm others, who does not want to be a patient, who does not want to accept any treatment, and who insists on their delusional beliefs as justifiable anger and moral outrage (O'Reilly et al., 2018; O'Reilly et al., 2019). The goal of forensic psychiatry and forensic mental health legislation like all mental health legislation is not to enforce any social norm or to oblige the person to integrate and assimilate into a dominant culture. The goal instead is to alleviate the individual suffering due to tormenting symptoms and incapacitating mental diseases, to restore the person as an individual to the full exercise of their rights, health, and life expectancy within an inclusive rights-based civil society. This should include achieving both self-actualisation as an individual and self-transcendence as a member of a culture and a group (Toch, 2000). A hospital should not be the battlefield for an ideological war. Post-modern jargon is no substitute for scientific medicine, science, or respect for objectiveness (Barish, 2014). Post-modernism and its obfuscations are contradicted by the fact of medical and scientific success (Sokal & Bricmont, 1998). A vital starting point therefore is a conversation in which the scientific clinicians listen carefully to the needs and preferences of all of their patients; however, they may be described, divided, or defined, by themselves or by others. A learning point that emerges from some accounts of the difficulties building cultural awareness into more effective forensic psychiatric services as described in New Zealand is that there must first be a formal model of care to set out goals, pathways, treatments, and evaluation (Kennedy, 2021).

An intellectual entertainment was defined by Lord Reith as educating, informing, and entertaining. Science and medicine do not fare well as entertainments, but entertainment and literary criticism do not fare well as nostrums for life-shortening illnesses. In this book, Tomlin and Völlm give fair and equal hearings to both. The reader will benefit from the choice.

Professor Harry Kennedy
National Forensic Mental Health Service
Portrane Demesne
Portrane
Co. Dublin
K36 FD79

References

Barish, E. (2014). *The double life of Paul de Man*. WW Norton & Company.

Coid, J., Kahtan, N., Cook, A., Gault, S., & Jarman, B. (2001). Predicting admission rates to secure forensic psychiatry services. *Psychological Medicine, 31*, 531.

Durkheim, E. (2020). *Le suicide: Etude de sociologie*. République des Lettres.

Faris, R. E. L., & Dunham, H. W. (1939). *Mental disorders in urban areas: an ecological study of schizophrenia and other psychoses*. The University of Chicago Press.

Farrington, D. P., Ttofi, M. M., & Coid, J. W. (2009). Development of adolescence-limited, late-onset, and persistent offenders from age 8 to age 48. *Aggressive Behavior, 35*, 150–163.

Fazel, S., & Grann, M. (2004). Psychiatric morbidity among homicide offenders: A Swedish population study. *American Journal of Psychiatry, 161*, 2129–2131.

Galderisi, S., Heinz, A., Kastrup, M., Beezhold, J., & Sartorius, N. (2015). Toward a new definition of mental health. *World Psychiatry, 14*, 231.

Goffman, E. (2009). *Stigma: Notes on the management of spoiled identity*. Simon and Schuster.

Kennedy, H. G. (2014, July 25). Blaming the messenger. *Irish Times*, Friday.

Kennedy, H. G. (2021). Models of care in forensic psychiatry. *BJPsych Advances*, 1–14.

Kennedy, H. G., Iveson, R. C., & Hill, O. (1999). Violence, homicide and suicide: strong correlation and wide variation across districts. *British Journal of Psychiatry, 175*, 462–466.

Lewis, A. (2013). *The state of psychiatry (psychology revivals): Essays and addresses*. Taylor & Francis.

Lomholt, L. H., Andersen, D. V., Sejrsgaard-Jacobsen, C., Øzdemir, C. M., Graff, C., Schjerning, O., Jensen, S. E., Straszek, S. P. V., Licht, R. W., Grøntved, S., & Nielsen, R. E. (2019). Mortality rate trends in patients diagnosed with schizophrenia or bipolar disorder: A nationwide study with 20 years of follow-up. *International Journal of Bipolar Disorders, 7*, 6.

O'Neill, C., Kelly, A., Sinclair, H., & Kennedy, H. (2005). Deprivation: Different implications for forensic psychiatric need in urban and rural areas. *Social Psychiatry and Psychiatric Epidemiology, 40*, 551–556.

O'Reilly, K., O'Connell, P., Corvin, A., O'Sullivan, D., Coyle, C., Mullaney, R., O'Flynn, P., Grogan, K., Richter, M., & Kennedy, H. (2018). Moral cognition and homicide amongst forensic patients with schizophrenia and schizoaffective disorder: A cross-sectional cohort study. *Schizophrenia Research, 193*, 468–469.

O'Reilly, K., O'Connell, P., O'Sullivan, D., Corvin, A., Sheerin, J., O'Flynn, P., Donohoe, G., McCarthy, H., Ambrosh, D., O'Donnell, M., Ryan, A., & Kennedy, H. G. (2019). Moral cognition, the missing link between psychotic symptoms and acts of violence: A cross-sectional national forensic cohort study. *BMC Psychiatry, 19*, 408.

Pierzchniak, P., Farnham, F., Taranto, N. D., Bull, D., Gill, H., Bester, P., Mccallum, A., & Kennedy, H. (1999). Assessing the needs of patients in secure settings: A multi-disciplinary approach. *The Journal of Forensic Psychiatry, 10*, 343–354.

Said, E. W. (2012). *Culture and imperialism*. Vintage.

Sokal, A. D., & Bricmont, J. (1998). *Intellectual impostures: Postmodern philosophers' abuse of science*. Profile Books.

Toch, H. (1992). *Violent men: An inquiry into the psychology of violence* (Rev. ed.). American Psychological Association.

Toch, H. (2000). Altruistic activity as correctional treatment. *International Journal of Offender Therapy and Comparative Criminology, 44*, 270–278.

World Health Organization. (2018). *Mental health atlas 2017*. World Health Organization.

Contributors

Jack Tomlin is Lecturer in Criminology at the University of Greenwich, United Kingdom. Prior to this, he was a post-doctoral research fellow at the Department of Forensic Psychiatry at Rostock University Medical Centre, Germany. He studied for an LLB and LLM at Maastricht University in the Netherlands before completing his PhD in forensic mental health at the University of Nottingham, United Kingdom, in 2019. He is on the Editorial Board of the International Journal of Forensic Mental Health and is Review Editor for the Forensic Psychiatry section of Frontiers in Psychiatry. He has a growing body of international peer-reviewed publications and has received funding from German, UK, and EU bodies. His research interests relate to forensic mental health patients' experiences of care, procedural justice and legitimacy, and mental health in the criminal justice system.

Birgit Völlm has been Professor of Forensic Psychiatry and Director of the Hospital of Forensic Psychiatry at the Rostock University Medical Center since September 2018. Before then, she was Professor of Forensic Psychiatry at the University of Nottingham, United Kingdom, and Consultant Forensic Psychiatrist in the enhanced service for personality disorders at Rampton high-secure hospital. Her main research interests include the neurobiology of personality disorders and social cognition, treatment of personality disorders, service development, comparisons between services in different countries, and ethical issues in forensic psychiatric care. Prof Völlm has held national and European grants on long stay, the effectiveness of Individual Placement Support, and Circles of Support and Accountability. She has published nearly 150 scientific papers and book chapters. Prof Völlm was Chair of the Forensic Section of the European Psychiatric Association from 2012 to 2016 and has been Chair of the Forensic Section of the World Psychiatric Association since 2020. Prof Völlm is a regular expert for the Committee for the Prevention of Torture and Inhumane and Degrading Treatment (CPT).

Patrick Bennett is Advanced Nurse Practitioner specialising in Psychiatric Intensive Care Units in Secure Care and Offender Health within the National Health Service (NHS) in Birmingham, United Kingdom. He helped develop policy and practice for two medium-secure unit intensive care services, and his professional interest involves implementing strategies to manage service users with behaviours that challenge staff in a forensic setting.

Jan Bulla, Medical Director of the Clinic for Forensic Psychiatry and Psychotherapy in Reichenau, Germany, is a specialist in psychiatry and psychotherapy with a focus on forensic psychiatry. Jan Bulla has a teaching position at the University of Ulm.

James Cavney is Consultant Forensic Psychiatrist and Deputy Clinical Director of the Auckland Regional Forensic Psychiatry Services – Mason Clinic. He has a background in anthropology and psychology with both clinical and research interests in improving service delivery and clinical outcomes for Maori, New Zealand's indigenous people.

Jessica Collier is an art psychotherapist and clinical supervisor, working with women in the criminal justice system. She has been a visiting lecturer at the University of Hertford-shire and a senior lecturer at Roehampton University. Her published work focuses on art psychotherapy in connection with trauma, violence, and unconscious re-enactments. She is a co-editor of the *International Journal of Forensic Psychotherapy* and co-convenor of the Forensic Arts Therapies Advisory Group.

Beresford Dawkins is Community Development Lead for the NHS Mental Health Foundation Trust in Birmingham, United Kingdom. He is a mature undergraduate student studying at Queens Theology College Birmingham, with specific interest in social justice, Pentecostalism music and mental health. He is working in partnership with community's and statutory organisations to develop equitable access to social care and mental health services since 1981. His life experience, Jamaican heritage, Christian faith, and his role in the community have all influenced his work towards community healing within the context of systemic and institutional colonialism. He presents and produces a local radio show discussing a range of health-related topics broadcasted via new emerging digital networks for the community of Birmingham and the wider West Midland region.

Sophie D'Souza is a researcher with an interest in systemic transformation, risk, and resilience in young people with experience of incarceration and social justice issues. Following Masters degrees from Cambridge and Harvard, she has worked in research, practice, and policy contexts internationally, including in the Department of Mental Health and Substance Use at the World Health Organization. Most recently, Sophie has been working on evaluations of complex health and social programmes, including a trauma-informed cultural transformation programme across the Children and Young People's Secure Estate in England, and a cash transfers project for people experiencing homelessness. She has published research in the area of forensic child and adolescent mental health.

María Isabel Fontao studied psychology at the Universities of Buenos Aires and Ulm. She completed her doctoral studies at the University of Ulm and her psychotherapy training in Tübingen, Germany. She is now academic coordinator for the master´s programme in Forensic Psychology at the University of Konstanz. Her research interests focus on forensic psychology and psychotherapy research. She has published in the areas of psychotherapy, forensic psychiatry, and psychotherapy.

Vivek Furtado is Head of Unit – Mental Health and Wellbeing at the University of Warwick. He is Associate Clinical Professor of Forensic Psychiatry at Warwick Medical School and holds Honorary Consultant Forensic Psychiatry post at Birmingham and Solihull Mental Health NHS Foundation Trust. In addition, he is a visiting forensic psychiatrist at Her Majesty's Prison in Birmingham. He is Expert Advisor to the National Institute of Health and Care Excellence Centre for Guidelines. He has published widely in the field of forensic psychiatry.

Leigh Gale is a Clinical Psychologist working in a regional medium secure unit in Wales, UK. Working predominantly alongside male service users within a trauma and attachment-based framework. Dr Gale has developed a keen interest in exploring the impact of fatherhood on an individual's mental health recovery and future risk of violence.

Christine Haddow is Lecturer in Criminology at Edinburgh Napier University. Her research interests focus on the intersections between mental disorder, violence, and gender identity; ex-military personnel in the criminal justice system; and desistance from crime.

Andrez Harriott is Chief Executive Officer and Founder of 'The Liminality Group'. Andrez is a criminologist and a sociologist and holds a master's degree from the Tavistock and Portman NHS Foundation Trust in Consulting and Leading in Organisations. Following nearly a decade of work within Youth Offending Services as a senior practitioner, he founded The Liminality Group in 2013, which specialises in working with high harm, high vulnerability, and complex children and young adults across the community and secure settings.

Christopher Hartwright is a Consultant Clinical Psychologist and Head of Psychology and Psychological Therapies for Powys Teaching Health. Dr Hartwright has experience as a Consultant Clinical Psychologist and Clinical Lead for the Powys Complex Trauma Service, as a Senior Clinical Tutor for the South Wales Doctoral Programme in Clinical Psychology and working with clients with complex psychological needs within a secure forensic mental health setting.

Clare Holt is Registered and Chartered Clinical Psychologist who, since qualifying in 2011, has specialised in working with adolescents and young adults who are involved with, or at risk of involvement with, the criminal justice system. Clare's clinical experience has included roles in the third sector and statutory services, within both the community and the youth custodial estate. Clare advocates and strives for systemic change that enables services to best meet the needs of the individuals and communities that they serve.

Fiona Houben is Senior Lecturer at Canterbury Christ Church University, Kent, United Kingdom, with a background in the anthropology of health care. Her research with mental health service users has focused on lived experiences of secure psychiatric care, including experiences of parenthood and ageing, with the aim of identifying support needs and improving services.

Antoinette Kavanaugh is Board Certified in Forensic Psychology, is the former clinical director of the Juvenile Justice Division of the Cook County Juvenile Court Clinic, served as a clinical professor at Northwestern University's School of Law for 10 years, is a lecturer at the Feinberg School of Medicine, Northwestern University, Chicago, IL, is an alumnus of the American Psychological Association's Leadership Institute for Women in Psychology, and Fellow for APA's Division 42, Psychologists in Independent Practice. She has authored several peer-reviewed articles and routinely educates lawyers and psychologists on issues related to obtaining and conducting forensic evaluations, adolescent development, and the impact of racism and discrimination on mental health. In private practice since 1999, she has been evaluating juveniles and adults for civil cases, as well as criminal state and federal court cases. Dr. Kavanaugh and Dr. Thomas Grisso co-authored Sentencing Juveniles in Adult Court, which details a developmentally sensitive approach to conducting de facto life or Miller sentencing evaluations.

Kimberly Sham Ku is Senior Forensic Psychologist at a male medium-secure unit in Birmingham, United Kingdom. She is Trinidadian and has knowledge of the Caribbean mental health system along with United Kingdom forensic mental health services. She has been working in forensic services since 2012 across prisons, community and private practice. Her work and interests lie in improving access to services for ethnic minorities and refugees and asylum seekers by creating culturally sensitive psychological practice.

Maria Livanou is Director of BSc Forensic Psychology and Senior Lecturer of Psychology at the School of Law, Social and Behavioural Sciences, Kingston University. Her research interests lie in (forensic) applied health research, mental health policy and practice, children and adolescents with complex needs, multiple vulnerabilities and high-risk presentation, emerging personality disorders, and neurodiversity in forensic mental health settings. She has collaborated with the Department of Health to develop national transition guidelines for young people moving from adolescent secure services to adult hospitals.

Rebecca Lockwood has many years of experience working with individuals with diverse physical, mental health, and personality difficulties in a variety of clinical and research contexts. Within the NHS, she previously worked as Lead Clinical Psychologist at a high secure female prison within the Offender Care CNWL NHS Foundation Trust. She also provides training and supports NHS staff teams working in highly pressured environments and supervises psychologists. Currently, she is Consultant Clinical Psychologist working in the addictions service for CNWL NHS Trust. She has published extensively and presented at national and international conferences on the topics of working with personality disorders, managing self-harm and suicide and eating disorders.

Emma Longfellow is Consultant Forensic Psychologist and Psychology Lead for the National High Secure Learning Disability and Autism Service. She has over 20 years of experience working with intellectual and developmental difficulties across the National Health Service and Her Majesty's Prison and Probation Service. Emma has a particular interest in the cognitive impact of developmental trauma and the role of complex trauma in behaviour that challenges and harms.

Karen Machin works from a perspective of lived experience. She was a member of the research teams for the studies of the experiences of carers in secure care in Scotland and England, alongside Dr. Ridley. She is co-director of With-you Consultancy and supported the development of peer-based approaches in secure care for NHSE/I.

Douglas MacInnes is Professor of Mental Health at Canterbury Christ Church University, Canterbury, United Kingdom. His recent research activity has included examining older people's uses and experiences of forensic mental health services, evaluating a psychological intervention with active collaboration between users, carers, and clinicians, an examination of the social networks of people with long-term mental health service use, the introduction and embedding of peer support workers into a mental health trust, and interventions to support prisoners with mental health needs.

Frances Maclennan is a consultant clinical psychologist. She has worked in prisons and secure units for over 15 years. She is currently working with men in the high secure estate. She is a visiting lecturer at the University of Hertfordshire and at the Institute of Psychiatry. She has a particular interest in personality disorders and trauma presentations in prison. She is a member of the parole board and provides trauma training to professionals working in the criminal justice system. She has published and presented at conferences on a range of topics including trauma and psychological treatments in prison.

Mary O. Madu is Specialty Resident in Forensic Psychiatry at the Victorian Institute of Forensic Mental Health, Australia.

Sarah Markham is Visiting Researcher in the Department of Biostatistics and Health Informatics, Institute of Psychiatry, Psychology and Neuroscience, King's College London. Her main research interests include risk-related practices in secure and forensic psychiatric services, the quality of practice in the First Tier Tribunals for mental health, and the development and application of digital technologies to deliberation in Health Technology Assessment.

Abdullah Mia is Consultant Clinical Psychologist for the NHS at a male medium-secure unit in Birmingham, United Kingdom. He has completed training in group analysis, organisational dynamics, and various therapeutic modalities. He also works in private practice as a therapist, a trainer, and an organisational consultant focusing on equality, diversity, and inclusion consulting to large corporations, universities, and the prison service in the United Kingdom.

Sara Morgan is a Consultant Clinical Psychologist and Head of Psychology for Rushcliffe Independent Hospitals. She is also a Non-Executive Director at Vestige Healthcare. She works with clients who have complex needs both within inpatient secure settings and within residential homes and the community. Dr Morgan has an interest in forensic risk and the impact of risk and mental health on identity; particularly as a father.

Shelagh Musgrave has been Family Carer Peer Support Worker in a forensic unit and a carer expert by experience member of a project team developing a Family and Carer Pathway in a mental health trust. She now works within the museums and galleries sector. She is the primary advocate for her daughter who has long-standing, complex mental health issues. Shelagh is passionate about seeing an improvement in carer engagement as her own experiences have led her to believe that it is essential for professionals to consider, and seek to understand, the impact of the mental ill health of a loved one on families and carers. She believes that this creates a more supportive working partnership that will ultimately better support the service user.

Annette Opitz-Welke works in the Department of Psychiatry and Psychotherapy at the Justizvollzugskrankenhaus Plötzensee in Berlin and at the Institute for Forensic Psychiatry, Charité Medical University of Berlin, Germany.

Janet Parrott is Consultant Forensic Psychiatrist at Oxleas NHSFT, United Kingdom. She has wide experience in forensic mental health services and a current research interest in the experience of older service users in secure mental health settings and how their needs can best be met.

Karen Persaud became a carer adviser and campaigner for Mental Health Services reform in 2016. She works with NHS England Adult Mental Health and The Royal College of Psychiatrists in Rehabilitation and Forensic psychiatry. Her advisory work includes the Community Mental Health Framework, addressing mental health inequalities and crisis care, and as Hon Researcher with NIHR MH PRU. Karen recently joined an NHS Trust as Carer, Families & Friends Involvement Co-ordinator to raise the profile of the importance of this group and embed their involvement across all areas of the service from strategy to front line services.

Julie Ridley is Reader and Co-Director of the Centre for Citizenship and Community at the University of Central Lancashire. She led the research for Support in Mind Scotland assessing carer support for family and friend carers of people across the forensic estate in Scotland and was part of the research team for NHS England that produced a Toolkit for forensic services offering best practice guidelines for working in partnership with carers.

Thomas Ross is an adjunct professor at the University of Ulm, coordinator for the Baden-Württemberg group for process optimisation and quality assurance in forensic psychiatry in Baden-Württemberg, and head of research at the Clinic for Forensic Psychiatry and Psychotherapy Reichenau.

Celia Sadie is a UK-based consultant clinical psychologist who has specialised in working with adolescents. Starting at the Northgate Clinic, then the Brookside Unit, she moved into youth custody as Consultant Lead across HMYOI Cookham Wood, HMYOI Feltham, and Medway STC, becoming the Clinical Lead for SECURE STAIRS. She is now the Director of Care and Wellbeing for Oasis Restore, the United Kingdom's first Secure

School. Her interests and publications focus on developing therapeutic systems, trauma, and systemic change in custodial settings.

Stephane M. Shepherd is Associate Professor of forensic psychology at the Centre for Forensic Behavioural Science, Swinburne University of Technology, Australia. His research explores cross-cultural issues at the intersection of the mental health and criminal justice sectors.

Julia Skelding is a registered learning disability nurse and nurse consultant/trainee Approved Clinician within the learning disability community service at Rotherham, Doncaster, and South Humber NHS Trust, United Kingdom. Julia has 10 years' experience working within the national high secure Learning Disabilities service and was involved in the development of the first high secure LD/ASD ward, she has a special interest in ensuring that the needs of people who have Learning Disabilities and autism are met and is particularly focussed on taking forward the LD/ASD agenda within services. Julia has an MA Autism and is trained in diagnostic assessment. Julia was shortlisted in the 2020 Autism Professionals Awards (National Autistic Society) in the Outstanding Healthcare professional category.

Dawn M. Sutherland is Advanced Nurse Practitioner and Family and Carer Lead for the Secure Care and Offender Health Directorate within the NHS in Birmingham, United Kingdom. She is also Behavioural Family Therapist and is trained to deliver culturally adapted family interventions (CaFI). She has worked in the NHS for 22 years and within secure services for 17 years. Her interests involve ensuring families and carers are supported in navigating the secure mental health system.

Jayne Taylor is Consultant Clinical Psychologist and, currently, Clinical Lead for Adult Psychological Therapies at Pennine Care NHS Foundation Trust. Prior to this, Jayne worked for many years with women within adult forensic services.

Renske Visser is Research Fellow at the University of Surrey. She is Medical Anthropologist interested in ageing, dying, and death. She has conducted research on the meaning of home in later life, parental bereavement in young adulthood, ageing in secure psychiatric settings, and cancer care in prison.

Tammi Walker is Principal of St Cuthbert's Society and Professor of Forensic Psychology at Durham University. She is Chartered Psychologist and Fellow of the British Psychological Society, Registered Senior Fellow with Advance HE, and a mental health nurse by clinical background. Tammi has a visiting position at Manchester University.

Javel Watt is a young entrepreneur, the founder of a clothing label, and a musician. He uses his past experiences, including time in custody, as stepping stones to develop his future, trying to find ways to share his knowledge with the people who deserve and need it most. He was a co-author on the youth custody submission to the Lammy Review (2017) and has advised the Parliamentary sub-committee on Human Rights regarding conditions in prison.

Brittany A. Wells is Licensed Clinical Psychologist with specialisation in psycholegal matters, psychological assessments, and issues of culture and diversity. Dr. Wells serves as Chief Psychologist of the Mental Health Resource Unit at the Law Office of the Cook County Public Defender where she developed and implemented their mental health program. Dr. Wells previously worked in the criminal justice system at the county, state, and federal levels and has nearly 10 years of experience working in hospital settings.

Michelle Wells is a Clinical Psychologist working in South Wales, in the UK. She is currently working in the Forensic Adolescent Consultation and Treatment Service (FACTS) team, which operates across Wales and involves both direct and indirect work. The foundation of such work is focused on viewing behaviour through the lens of trauma and attachment, where the underlying needs of the child are identified and a multi-agency plan is developed to meet such needs accordingly. Dr. Wells has held a longstanding interest in the forensic field, both in terms of research and clinical practice – she has experience of working in forensic inpatient and custodial settings. She is particularly interested in how attachment and trauma can be applied to understanding and formulating offending behaviour, as reflected in the book chapter focused on fatherhood in the forensic inpatient context.

Acknowledgements

The editors would like to thank Dr. Deniz Cerci for his help reviewing several chapters in this book. They would also like to thank Dr. Patricia Zapf and the editorial team at Routledge/ Taylor & Francis for their support in seeing this through to publication. Jack Tomlin would like to thank Kenza El-Madani for her help in thinking about some of the important issues included in the introduction chapter.

Part 1

Introduction

Chapter 1

Marginalisation and diversity in forensic mental health care

An introduction

Jack Tomlin and Birgit Völlm

Introduction

By definition, a society includes some people and excludes others. Inclusion may take the form of citizenship or free passage across national borders. It also involves full participation in social, political, and economic life. Those belonging to the in-group can expect to enjoy social goods like secure housing, quality education and healthcare, access to banking and loans, decent career prospects, and social networks that help navigate the uncertainties of life and provide support in times of need. Exclusion, by contrast, can be seen as the extent to which people cannot avail themselves of such goods. Their status as a full participant in society is reduced; they are marginalised. Marginalised individuals and groups are less likely to enjoy fair legal arrangements and procedures, be encouraged into political and public life, or be given the opportunities to express their individuality and personhood without stigmatisation or prejudice. This book is about a group of people who live at the intersection of multiple marginalised or minority identities: forensic mental health patients. This chapter describes the rationale for this book and locates it within other works seeking to address structural inequalities in criminal justice and mental health.

Forensic mental health, criminal justice, and marginalisation

Forensic mental health care offers treatment to individuals who have committed a criminal offence or have engaged in high-risk behaviours and live with a mental disorder. This mental disorder is often related to the offence for which they were convicted but is not always. In systems like the Netherlands or Germany, a link is required between the offence and a mental disorder present at the time of the offence and affecting the individual's criminal responsibility; in England and Wales, it is required that an individual has a mental disorder that needs treatment at the time of their conviction (Edworthy et al., 2016). Legal systems differ in the way and to whom they provide care; however, common across all systems is that this patient group is one of the most marginalised and excluded.

Patients' backgrounds are likely characterised by childhood adversity and abuse, periods of institutional care, psychiatric treatment, substance abuse, imprisonment, and criminal convictions to name but a few. Placement in forensic services may therefore be seen as the failure of missed opportunities for intervention and support earlier in life – adequate housing and schooling, appropriate parental/caregiver support and supervision, earlier identification and management of mental health needs, or diversion away from traditional criminal justice sanctions. Though the causes of crime and mental disorder are many, complex, and multifaceted, we have a good understanding of what lifestyle factors are predictive of both. For example,

DOI: 10.4324/9781003184768-2

substance use, poverty, deprivation, social exclusion, family rearing practices, low social status, and isolation are associated with both the development of mental disorders and crime (Draine et al., 2002). People who experience a combination of these factors are at higher risk of developing mental disorders or committing crimes. Most of these disproportionately affect marginalised groups and people from minority cultural backgrounds.

The nature and quality of forensic care vary considerably around the world (Roesch et al., 2018). It can be provided in prisons, community settings, or in low-, medium-, and high-security hospitals. In the most developed systems, multi-disciplinary treatment teams work collaboratively to support a patient's complex mental and physical health needs (Haines et al., 2018). These needs are typically chronic and overlapping, with many patients having several diagnoses. The most commonly diagnosed disorders are severe mental illnesses such as psychosis, bipolar disorder, depression, and anxiety disorder; personality disorders like antisocial, narcissistic, or borderline; and substance use disorders. Treatment aims to decrease the risk of future offending by minimising 'risk factors' and maximising 'protective factors', reduce mental health symptoms, and empower patients (de Ruiter & Nicholls, 2011; Kennedy, 2021). This involves a range of individual and group psychotherapies, pharmacological interventions, and social/occupational skills to support recovery in secure care and later in the community. Studies show that people are less likely to reoffend after release from forensic services when compared to prison (Fazel et al., 2016; Igoumenou et al., 2019).

Despite considerable developments in the provision of mental health care for criminal justice-involved persons, outcomes for this group are poor. According to one international review, about one-quarter of men and 20% of women in prisons have an alcohol use disorder, and 30% of men and about half all women in prison have a substance use disorder (Fazel et al., 2017). In another international review, between 3.6 and 3.9% of prison inmates met the diagnostic criteria for psychosis and between 10.2 and 14.1% for depression (Fazel & Seewald, 2012). People diagnosed with serious mental illness are over three times as likely to be victims of violence than their siblings without mental illness (Fazel & Sariaslan, 2021). Forensic patients will biologically 'age' 10–15 years quicker and die earlier than the general population (Merkt et al., 2020; Parrott et al., 2019). There are also numerous indirect harms such as the external and internalised stigma of having a mental health diagnosis and being an offender. These stigmata are highly consequential and have been linked to social exclusion and isolation and pose barriers to housing and work (Mezey et al., 2016). Significant media attention depicts forensic patients as 'monstrous' or 'evil', frustrating efforts to safely reintegrated high-profile patients into the community (Morley & Taylor, 2016).

These outcomes become increasingly distressing when considered alongside marginalised intersectional identities. Psychotic disorders are frequently diagnosed at higher rates in ethnic minority groups in the community (1.5–3 times across most studies; Morgan et al., 2019). A study in Germany found that patients with a migration background were 32% more likely to be ordered into forensic treatment than non-migrants (Bulla et al., 2017). An influential UK inquiry into Black, Asian, and Minority Ethnic (BAME) groups in the criminal justice system found that despite being 14% of the population, BAME individuals made up 25% of prison inmates and 40% of youths in custody (Lammy, 2017). Black men are kept in low-security hospitals longer than their White peers, while the Black Caribbean and Black African patients are more frequently detained under mental health legislation involuntarily (The Mental Health Taskforce, 2016; Wessely, 2018). Women in secure care are more likely to self-harm than men and have more frequently experienced sexual abuse in childhood; they are also processed through the CJS differently, being more likely to be found not guilty by reason of insanity than men (de Vogel & Nicholls, 2016; Krammer et al., 2018). Marginalised patients are triply burdened by their mental disorder(s), their offending history, and their identity as a member of the social out-group.

Qualitative research has found that marginalised groups experience the criminal justice and (forensic) mental health systems differently. Hui and colleagues (2021) interviewed 77 people with mental health needs who identified themselves as having at least one marginalised characteristic. They found evidence of 'institutional injustice', as participants reported having their experiences, voice, and identity discredited by formal care services. Respondents felt unable to articulate their own lived experienced within the frameworks of dominant medical discourses that place primacy on policy or evidence derived from majority or androcentric experiences. This led many to self-edit, moderate, or disengage from services entirely, further perpetuating marginalisation and poor health and social outcomes.

Researchers have suggested that inappropriate or inadequate services that do not match the needs of specific patient groups result in unnecessarily lengthy treatment periods. For deaf patients, for example, the paucity of trained sign language speakers, and methods of communication used by deaf patients that are sometimes misconstrued as aggression are barriers to treatment progression (Wakeland et al., 2019). Interviews with 'older' patients (aged >50 years) report that many feel isolated, have too few age-appropriate activities, do not seek medical help for conditions that they consider would label them as old and vulnerable, and are pessimistic about the future; all of these can hinder successful recovery (di Lorito et al., 2018; Visser et al., 2019). LGBTQI+ inmates describe how heteronormativity and hyper-masculinity in correctional settings discourage them from 'coming out' and participating in prison life for fear of verbal, physical, emotional, or psychological abuse (Carr et al., 2016). This means support services for this group are inadequate as prisons lack an awareness of LGBTQI+ inmates and their needs. These few examples illustrate that marginalised forensic patients can experience prejudiced attitudes, inadequate or unresponsive services, poor understanding of their needs, and epistemic marginalisation and must edit narratives of self.

Why should we examine marginalisation and diversity in forensic mental health care?

It is important to examine marginalisation in forensic mental health care for moral and clinical reasons. There is a moral case to undertake research examining to what extent social inequalities in wider society are reflected in secure care and how placement in these settings may reproduce or worsen these. As already argued, disparities concerning health and economic outcomes experienced by marginalised forensic patients reflect those of the general population. The term 'structural violence' captures this. It refers to the higher levels of poverty, threat of violence, and discrimination experiences by minority social groups, stemming from: 'long-term historical processes that, in predominantly White societies, have systematically marginalized and excluded those from minority groups, creating systematic barriers to education and economic opportunities, to wealth and upward mobility, to living in more prosperous areas, and to positions of power' (Morgan et al., 2019, p. 254).

Whilst treatment of forensic patients is often beneficent, placement in settings away from one's family and work can exacerbate these problems. As forensic care oftentimes represents the port-of-last-call for many people and is one of the most intrusive forms of state intervention, the overrepresentation of people with particular social characteristics in secure settings and their lived experiences during treatment are demonstrative of how society defines and treats its 'in-groups' and 'out-groups': those who receive early primary interventions and those who receive correctional treatment in restrictive settings. As put by Nelson Mandela: 'A nation should not be judged by how it treats its highest citizens, but its lowest ones'.

Patients have constellations of needs, the causes, and prognoses of which can be influenced by intersecting marginalised characteristics. A moral society is one where individuals or groups are not overrepresented in forensic care settings due to these arbitrary socially constructed identities or differential access to social goods across the life course. Such a society would strive to provide equitable care (here meaning the provision of different levels, forms, and intensities of care to achieve equitable outcomes for patients instead of providing the same or equal care for all patients). Interventions that aren't sensitive to traumas experienced by refugees, therapeutic interactions that are not responsive to culturally derived notions of respect or deference, or paternalistic coercive measures that don't acknowledge the gendered histories of sexual abuse experienced by many women patients, may work for some patients but will be ineffective or harmful for others. This reduces the chance for meaningful engagement in care and can reproduce identity or social-economic marginalisation existing prior to admission to secure services. There are thus clear moral and clinical reasons to examine issues of equity, diversity, and marginalisation in forensic mental health.

What is this book trying to achieve?

The middle of the 21st century onwards – a period referred to as *Late Modernity* by some scholars – is characterised by numerous cultural, economic, and political shifts. One of these relates to how human beings as *unique individuals endowed with diverse experiences* are recognised. International human rights instruments following WWII enshrined in law the inviolability of individual dignity. Deinstitutionalisation in psychiatry has foregrounded the autonomy of mental health patients. Post-modernist and social-constructivist scholarship encouraged us to consider the contingency and subjectivity of knowledge claims. Feminists foregrounded the individual experiences of women and children in both social and private spheres, demonstrating the barriers and inequalities women are confronted with. The civil rights movement of the United States which rippled around the world brought into public discourse the racism and prejudices directed at people of colour and minority ethnic groups.

These developments collectively point to a shift away from androcentric knowledge claims and ways of doing, towards a recognition of a collectivity of lived experiences. In the social sciences, methods of knowledge production, or knowledge co-construction, have evolved to reflect this. Patients are more frequently involved in research funding applications, conduct, interpretation, and dissemination (Domecq et al., 2014; Völlm et al., 2017); researchers are encouraged to engage in reflexivity, the act of acknowledging or embracing one's subjectivities in the research process (Haynes, 2012); and methods that reduce power imbalances between the 'researcher' and 'researched' such diary methods, peer-led interviews, photo-elicitation, and lived experience advisory panels are more commonly employed. These demonstrate efforts to present a wider range of epistemic standpoints and reduce the injustices and harms that follow the exclusion of diverse lived experiences from research (Hui et al., 2021).

This book is situated within these developments. By reductively thinking of forensic mental health patients as simply 'mad' or 'bad' – or even some combination of just these two – we obfuscate reality and deny ourselves the chance to critically assess how multiple marginalised characteristics shape the lives of forensic patients and what as scholars, practitioners, commissioners, carers, patients, and ex-patients, we can do about it. This book acknowledges that individuals in forensic settings have multiple identities and backgrounds, the multiplicity of which forms a complex and unique human being with experiences, strengths, and needs. It further holds that the inequitable distribution of social goods through complex, embedded, long-term phenomena described in concepts like structural violence or institutional injustice can be exacerbated in forensic settings unless critical and reflexive practice and research are undertaken cognisant of these intersectional fault lines.

The chapters in this book are ordered into five sections. Section 1 introduces readers to the broader issues of equality, diversity, racism, and marginalisation that underpin many of the experiences described in the following chapters. Section 2 focuses on groups of patients defined by social or demographic characteristics: women patients, transgender patients, youths in custody, foreign national patients in Germany, and patients who are fathers. Section 3 explores groups characterised by clinical characteristics: patients with autism, patients with learning disabilities, young people transitioning into adult services, and long-stay patients. Following this, culturally sensitive care models in New Zealand, the United Kingdom, and Australia are discussed in Section 4. Finally, Section 5 looks at what effective communication with marginalised patient groups and barriers to this can look like. This book aims to highlight the lived experiences and treatment of different marginalised and minority groups, whilst offering readers guidance on how to engage in culturally sensitive treatment and communication.

References

Bulla, J., Hoffmann, K., Querengässer, J., & Ross, T. (2017). Socioeconomic disadvantage and schizophrenia in migrants under mental health detention orders. *International Journal of Social Psychiatry*, *63*(6), 550–558. https://doi.org/10.1177/0020764017716696

Carr, N., Mcalister, S., & Birkbeck, T. S. (2016). Out on the inside: The rights, experiences and needs of LGBT people in prison ESRC knowledge exchange view project neoliberalism and sexual respectability view project. https://doi.org/10.13140/RG.2.1.5055.2082

de Ruiter, C., & Nicholls, T. L. (2011). Protective factors in forensic mental health: A new frontier. *International Journal of Forensic Mental Health*, *10*(3), 160–170. https://doi.org/10.1080/14999013.2011.600602

de Vogel, V., & Nicholls, T. L. (2016). Gender matters: An introduction to the special issues on women and girls. *International Journal of Forensic Mental Health*, *15*(1), 1–25. https://doi.org/10.1080/14999013.2016.1141439

di Lorito, C., Dening, T., & Völlm, B. (2018). Ageing in forensic psychiatric secure settings: The voice of older patients. *Journal of Forensic Psychiatry and Psychology*, *29*(6), 934–960. https://doi.org/10.1080/14789949.2018.1513545

Domecq, J. P., Prutsky, G., Elraiyah, T., Wang, Z., Nabhan, M., Shippee, N., Brito, J. P., Boehmer, K., Hasan, R., Firwana, B., Erwin, P., Eton, D., Sloan, J., Montori, V., Asi, N., Dabrh, A. M. A., & Murad, M. H. (2014). Patient engagement in research: A systematic review. *BMC Health Services Research*, *14*(1), 89. BioMed Central. https://doi.org/10.1186/1472-6963-14-89

Draine, J., Salzer, M. S., Culhane, D. P., & Hadley, T. R. (2002). Role of social disadvantage in crime, joblessness, and homelessness among persons with serious mental illness. *Psychiatric Services*, *53*, 565–573.

Edworthy, R., Sampson, S., & Völlm, B. (2016). Inpatient forensic-psychiatric care: Legal frameworks and service provision in three European countries. *International Journal of Law and Psychiatry*, *47*, 18–27. https://doi.org/10.1016/j.ijlp.2016.02.027

Fazel, S., Fimińska, Z., Cocks, C., & Coid, J. (2016). Patient outcomes following discharge from secure psychiatric hospitals: Systematic review and meta-Analysis. *British Journal of Psychiatry*, *208*(1), 17–25. https://doi.org/10.1192/bjp.bp.114.149997

Fazel, S., & Sariaslan, A. (2021). Victimization in people with severe mental health problems: The need to improve research quality, risk stratification and preventive measures. *World Psychiatry*, *20*(3), 437–438. https://doi.org/10.1002/WPS.20908

Fazel, S., & Seewald, K. (2012). Severe mental illness in 33 588 prisoners worldwide: Systematic review and meta-regression analysis. *The British Journal of Psychiatry*, *200*(5), 364–373. https://doi.org/10.1192/bjp.bp.111.096370

Fazel, S., Yoon, I. A., & Hayes, A. J. (2017). Substance use disorders in prisoners: An updated systematic review and meta-regression analysis in recently incarcerated men and women. https://doi.org/10.1111/add.13877

Haines, A., Perkins, E., Evans, E. A., & McCabe, R. (2018). Multidisciplinary team functioning and decision making within forensic mental health. *Mental Health Review Journal*, *23*(3), 185–196. https://doi.org/10.1108/MHRJ-01-2018-0001

Haynes, K. (2012). Reflexivity in qualitative research. *Qualitative Organizational Research: Core Methods and Current Challenges*, 72–89. https://doi.org/10.4135/9781526435620.N5

Hui, A., Rennick-Egglestone, S., Franklin, D., Walcott, R., Llewellyn-Beardsley, J., Ng, F., Roe, J., Yeo, C., Deakin, E., Brydges, S., Moran, P. P., McGranahan, R., Pollock, K., Thornicroft, G., & Slade, M. (2021, April 4). Institutional injustice: Implications for system transformation emerging from the mental health recovery narratives of people experiencing marginalisation. *PLoS One*, *16*, e0250367. https://doi.org/10.1371/journal.pone.0250367

Igoumenou, A., Kallis, C., Huband, N., Haque, Q., Coid, J. W., & Duggan, C. (2019). Prison vs. hospital for offenders with psychosis; effects on reoffending. *Journal of Forensic Psychiatry and Psychology*, *30*(6), 939–958. https://doi.org/10.1080/14789949.2019.1651381

Kennedy, H. G. (2021). Models of care in forensic psychiatry. *BJPsych Advances*, 1–14. https://doi.org/10.1192/bja.2021.34

Krammer, S., Eisenbarth, H., Fallegger, C., Liebrenz, M., & Klecha, D. (2018). Sociodemographic information, aversive and traumatic events, offence-related characteristics, and mental health of delinquent women in forensic-psychiatric care in Switzerland. *International Journal of Offender Therapy and Comparative Criminology*, *62*(12), 3815–3833. https://doi.org/10.1177/0306624X17749638

Lammy, D. (2017). *The Lammy review: An independent review into the treatment of, and outcomes for, Black, Asian and minority ethnic individuals in the criminal justice system*. https://assets.publishing.service.gov.uk/government/uploads/system/uploads/attachment_data/file/643001/lammy-review-final-report.pdf

The Mental Health Taskforce. (2016). *The five year forward view for mental health*. www.england.nhs.uk/wp-content/uploads/2016/02/Mental-Health-Taskforce-FYFV-final.pdf

Merkt, H., Haesen, S., Meyer, L., Kressig, R. W., Elger, B. S., & Wangmo, T. (2020). Defining an age cut-off for older offenders: A systematic review of literature. *International Journal of Prisoner Health*, *16*(2), 95–116. Emerald Group Publishing Ltd. https://doi.org/10.1108/IJPH-11-2019-0060

Mezey, G., Youngman, H., Kretzschmar, I., & White, S. (2016). Stigma and discrimination in mentally disordered offender patients – a comparison with a non-forensic population. *Journal of Forensic Psychiatry and Psychology*, *27*(4), 517–529. https://doi.org/10.1080/14789949.2016.1172658

Morgan, C., Knowles, G., & Hutchinson, G. (2019). Migration, ethnicity and psychoses: Evidence, models and future directions. *World Psychiatry*, *18*(3), 247–258. https://doi.org/10.1002/wps.20655

Morley, S., & Taylor, P. (2016). 'Cashing in' on curiosity and spectacle: The forensic patient and news media. *Journal of Forensic Psychiatry and Psychology*, *27*(5), 705–721. https://doi.org/10.1080/14789949.2016.1187760

Parrott, J. M., Houben, F. R., Visser, R. C., & MacInnes, D. L. (2019). Mental health and offending in older people: Future directions for research. *Criminal Behaviour and Mental Health*, *29*(4), 218–226. John Wiley and Sons Ltd. https://doi.org/10.1002/cbm.2121

Roesch, R., Cook, A. N., Crocker, A. G., Livingston, J. D., & Leclair, M. C. (2018). Forensic mental health systems internationally. In *Handbook of forensic mental health services* (pp. 3–76). Routledge. https://doi.org/10.4324/9781315627823-2

Visser, R. C., MacInnes, D., Parrott, J., & Houben, F. (2019). Growing older in secure mental health care: The user experience. *Journal of Mental Health*. https://doi.org/10.1080/09638237.2019.1630722

Völlm, B., Foster, S., Bates, P., & Huband, N. (2017). How best to engage users of forensic services in research: Literature review and recommendations. *International Journal of Forensic Mental Health*, *16*(2), 183–195. Routledge. https://doi.org/10.1080/14999013.2016.1255282

Wakeland, E., Rose, J., & Austen, S. (2019). Professionals' experience of deaf offenders with mental health difficulties. *American Annals of the Deaf*, *164*(1), 137–157. https://doi.org/10.1353/aad.2019.0012

Wessely, S. (2018). *Modernising the mental health act: Increasing choice, reducing compulsion*. Final Report of the Independent Review of the Mental Health Act 1983 (Issue December). www.gov.uk/dhsc

Chapter 2

The US Criminal Justice System

The experience of racially marginalised people

Brittany A. Wells and Antoinette Kavanaugh

Introduction

The United States of America is infamous for its world leadership in mass incarceration. Inhabiting only about 5% of the world's population, it holds approximately 25% of the world's prison population (Collier, 2014). While some may assume that a country with such a large prison population must have high crime rates, the story of mass incarceration in the United States is far more complex. In a country where criminologists proposed in the mid-1970s that prisons would soon be obsolete, there has been a methodical increase in the prison population that now sits at approximately 2.3 million people (Alexander, 2012; Davis, 2003; Sawyer & Wagner, 2020).

While many factors have facilitated the increase in the prison population (e.g., mandatory minimums and the prison–industrial complex), one thing is clear about mass incarceration in the United States: racial minorities are incarcerated at alarmingly high rates in comparison to their White counterparts. African Americans are five times more likely to be imprisoned than White people (Nellis, 2016). While African Americans make up only 13% of the US adult population, they make up nearly 40% of the US prison population. Similar patterns exist with the Latino population, which is approximately 15% of the US population and nearly 20% of the prison population (Nellis et al., 2016; Sawyer & Wagner, 2020).

This chapter will take a closer look at the racial disparities, or the overrepresentation of racial minorities, in the US criminal justice system and explore how the country's history of racism and oppression contributes to such disparities. In discussing marginalised populations, this chapter focuses on racial and ethnic minorities, mainly African American and Latinx populations. This chapter will also discuss the experience of marginalised populations within the criminal justice system.

Racism and oppression in the United States: from slavery to mass incarceration

Africans began being taken from Africa and brought to the United States as slaves in 1619. Black people were enslaved for hundreds of years before slavery was abolished with the issuance of the Emancipation Proclamation in 1863 and the ratification of the 13th Amendment in 1865. While the legal slave trade ended, the effects of slavery have carried on into modern society.

Slavery was marked by brutality and gross inhumanity. Slaves were dehumanised and considered three-fifths of a person. They were chained, beaten, and deprived of all human rights. They were branded, raped, and mutilated amongst other monstrosities. There were

DOI: 10.4324/9781003184768-3

rules and laws prohibiting slaves from being taught how to read, marrying, or participating in commerce. In addition to the brutality used to control and enslave Black people, slave owners employed tactics to weaken the psyche of the enslaved and further subjugate them. These tactics included deliberate efforts to dismantle the Black family, diminish the esteem of Black men, and create a caste system amongst slaves that divided people of colour (Weld, 2011). Once slavery ended, these tactics had lingering effects on Black families and the Black community.

The abolishment of slavery came with a noticeable increase in the imprisonment of Black men (Godfrey & Soper, 2018). The 13th Amendment was established to outlaw slavery and involuntary servitude 'except as a punishment for crime whereof the party shall have been duly convicted' (US Const. amend. XIII; DuVernay, 2016). Prisoners were forced to work on chain gangs or leased out to provide labour, which made up for the loss of revenue associated with the end of slavery. The prison business was extremely profitable to state governments, and African Americans were once again legally enslaved. The involuntary servitude of prisoners continued for nearly a century before it was thought to be inhumane and was banned in every state (Roth, 2006), though at the present time, many prisoners are required to work for wages as low as $2 per hour.

With the rise of the Civil Rights Movement in the 1960s, racism in America began to transform. While African Americans were gaining more rights, they were about to be victimised by political campaigns that capitalised on racist ideology. From the War on Crime to the War on Drugs, the United States ignited a political movement that vilified African Americans in the public's eye, militarised the police force, and started the era of mass incarceration (Alexander, 2012; DuVernay, 2016).

Systemic racism and racial disparities in policing in modern America

Systemic racism is the ideology, attitudes, practices, norms, and policies embedded in American society and institutions that values whiteness. It causes racial inequality and the perpetual oppression of Black and Brown people (Feagin, 2006). It is important to note that race is not a biological construct but a social one. People and societies have assigned social meaning to physical characteristics, which fuels systemic racism (National Research Council, 2004). Systemic racism contributes to significant disparities in health outcomes, education, housing, employment or wages, and access to resources, which has had devasting consequences for Black and Brown communities. An area in which there are significant racial disparities and detrimental consequences that contribute to the current state of the criminal justice system is in policing and police contact.

The over-policing of people of colour dates back to slave patrols that existed to catch runaway slaves, deter slave revolts, and psychologically and physically terrorise slaves (Hassett-Walker, 2021). Once slavery ended, slave patrols evolved to become police departments (Durr, 2015). Just as slave patrols terrorised slaves, police continue to terrorise people of colour in the United States. Contact with police is a source of racial trauma for many people of colour. Even contacts that do not result in arrest are associated with increased emotional distress, social stigma, and post-traumatic stress disorder (PTSD) symptoms (Geller et al., 2014; Jackson et al., 2019).

Police encounters with people of colour are often fuelled by the practice of *racial profiling*, relying on ethnic or racial stereotypes to suspect a person of criminal activity. Two examples of racial profiling are 'driving while Black or Brown' and 'stop and frisk'. These practices leave people of colour feeling dehumanised and under siege by the police. *Driving While Black* or *Brown* refers to racial profiling practices in which police stop drivers of colour, particularly males of colour (Lundman & Kaufman, 2003). The stops of African American and Latinx drivers are more likely to result in the police frisking the driver and searching the driver's car (LaFraniere & Lehren, 2015). Stop and frisk is a tactic used by police that allows police to stop people on the street, question, and frisk (or search) them. One of the most infamous uses of the stop and frisk policy was in New York City. In the court ruling regarding the legality of the stops, the court noted 4.4 million stops occurred between 2004 and 2012: only 6% resulted in an arrest; 52% of those stopped were Black, 31% Latinx, and 10% White, while the city population was 23%, 29%, and 33%, respectively, for each group. Officers were more likely to use force when a person of colour was stopped (*Floyd, et al. v. City of New York, et al.*, 2013). While the policy has been ruled unconstitutional, the practice still exists.

Racism observed within policing practices is not only of concern because it results in the disproportionate arrest and incarceration of minorities. It can also lead to the death of Black men and women at the hands of the police. Police killing of Black males has been identified as a public health crisis (Edwards et al., 2019; Alang et al., 2017). While organisations and activist movements are attempting to raise awareness around this issue and seek policy change, minorities continue to be traumatised by this policing practice.

The over-policing of minorities does not begin in adulthood. There are also significant racial disparities in policing within the educational system that reflect individual and systemic racism. For instance, students of colour are disproportionately represented at every level of disciplinary response in the school system (United States Government Accountability Office, 2018). Black students are more likely to be criminalised for their misbehaviours at school (U.S. Department of Education Office for Civil Rights, 2014). While Black students represent just 16% of all students grades K–12 (ages 5–18; traditional primary and secondary schooling in the United States), they represent 31% of students arrested for misbehaviour at school. In contrast, White students represent 50% of the student population and 39% of those arrested for misbehaviours at school (U.S. Department of Education Office for Civil Rights, 2014). Reflecting what is known as the *school to prison pipeline*, youths who have been suspended by age 12 are more likely to be involved in the criminal justice system by age 18 (Novak, 2019).

Inside the US Criminal Justice System: the courtroom and beyond

This section briefly describes racial disparities among the professionals in the courtroom before exploring other aspects of the legal system in which racial inequities are present. In the United States, cases in criminal court include a victim, defendant, attorney representing the state (sometimes called State's Attorney or prosecutor), an attorney for the defence, and a judge who may be an attorney. A judge or jury hears the evidence and renders a verdict of guilty or not guilty. When a guilty verdict is rendered, the judge typically imposes the sentence, the exceptions are capital cases (American Bar Association, n.d.; Office of the United States Attorney, n.d.). While the majority of defendants are people of colour, the vast majority of the attorneys, judges, and jurists are white. In 2020, 86% of attorneys were white, while 5% were African American and 5% were Latinx (American Bar Association, 2020). The overwhelming majority of judges at the state and federal levels are white (American Constitution Society, n.d.; Federal Judicial Center, n.d.). The racial disparity among judges extends to the highest court in the judicial system, the US Supreme Court which has only had three non-white Chief Justices.

Bail

Once a person is charged with a crime, they face a bail hearing to determine if they will be released before trial. A judge determines if the defendant will be held, released on their own recognisance, or released on bail. A cash bail requires the defendant to pay a bond, typically 10% of the bail. At the conclusion of the case, the bond, minus court fees, is returned to the defendant (Ofer, 2017). Approximately 30% of inmates awaiting trial are in jail because they cannot afford bail, and this disproportionally impacts people of colour (Curiel & Matthews II, 2019). Racial disparities exist in who is offered a chance to be released on bail and the amount at which bail is set (Demuth, 2003). For instance, judges incorrectly assume Black defendants pose a higher risk than White defendants if released (Arnold et al., 2018). The impact of pretrial detention on subsequent junctures in the case is great. When the severity of charges is equal, pretrial detention is associated with higher conviction rates and harsher sentences and contributes to racial disparities at these junctures (Donnelly & MacDonald, 2018).

Jury

In America, defendants have a constitutional right to a jury of one's peers. Yet this is rarely the case for people of colour because they are often excluded from serving on a jury (Hoag, 2020). Having a jury of one's peers is of the utmost importance because racially diverse juries are associated with increased quality of the jury deliberation for Black defendants (Peter-Hagene, 2019) and decreased racial disparity in conviction rates (Anwar et al., 2012; Flanagan, 2018).

While excluding a potential jurist from serving on a jury because of the jurist's race is technically unconstitutional (see *Batson v. Kentucky*, 476 US 79 (1986)), the practice continues and results in less racial diverse juries (DeCamp & DeCamp, 2020). Proxies for race such as hairstyle, clothing, place of residence, and racial stereotypes are used to eliminate potential jurors (Berkley Law Death Penalty Clinic, 2020; Equal Justice Initiative, 2010). Based on their lived experiences, it is not surprising that potential jurists mistrust the police and the legal system. Prosecutors frequently cite mistrust as a reason to exclude Black and Latinx jurors (Berkley Law Death Penalty Clinic, 2020). Additionally, millions of African Americans and Latinx citizens are not eligible to serve on a jury because of past convictions or charges of a felony offense (Administrative Office of the U.S. Courts, n.d.; Binnall & Petersen, 2020; Roberts, 2013; Jackson-Gleich, 2021). Excluding perspective jurists of colour results in a less diverse, possibly all-white jury.

Wrongful convictions

Wrongful conviction cases are notorious for racial disparities. According to the National Registry of Exonerees, an innocent Black defendant is nearly seven times more likely to be wrongfully convicted of murder than an innocent White defendant. The likelihood of being falsely convicted of murder is also related to the race of the victim. If the victim is white, an innocent African American defendant is more likely to be wrongfully convicted (Possley & Stephens, 2017). Since 1989, 49.6% of all exonerees are Black (Selby, 2021). Black exonerees make up nearly 70% of all DNA exonerations (Clarke, 2020).

Prisons

While it is crucial to understand that the policing and mass incarceration of racial minorities in the United States is a product of deep-seated racial bias, it is also important to understand the history and inner workings of the US prison system. Once promoted as a rehabilitative system (Cullen, 2013; Nussbaum, 1971), the true history of the US prison system is marked by capitalism. The United States profits from mass incarceration through the privatisation of prisons and immigration detention facilities. The increase in the use of private prisons has been so substantial that it was coined the *prison–industrial complex*. The United States has the world's largest for-profit prison population and is home to some of the largest private prison corporations. These companies bring in billions of dollars in revenue benefiting shareholders while maintaining government support through lobbying groups (Gotsch & Basti, 2018). For-profit prisons advertise that they can provide governments with cost-saving detention solutions, though research has demonstrated little to no cost-savings and poorer quality of confinement (Lundahl et al., 2009; Paynter, 2011).

In addition to the inhumane nature of profiting off prisoners, the treatment of prisoners within the US penal system has come under scrutiny within the past few decades. Prisons, by design, strip individuals of their autonomy. Many incarcerated individuals have limited social and family support because they are incarcerated in facilities located in rural areas far from the urban areas where their families reside (Delaney et al., 2018). Some prisoners experience violent attacks and harassment from other prisoners and correctional officers without much protection from personnel or the law. They may also experience dehumanising disciplinary practices such as solitary confinement. Solitary confinement, also known as segregation or isolation, consists of individuals being held in singular cells for 23 or 24 hours a day with limited or no property, limited lighting, and no human contact. Solitary confinement can have severe psychological consequences including depression, anxiety, psychosis, and suicidality (Metzner & Fellner, 2010). Advocacy organisations and government officials have attempted to bring attention to the detrimental effects of solitary confinement in hopes of limiting the use of such practices.

A final area addressed by advocacy organisations and policy reform within recent decades pertains to the treatment of mentally ill prisoners. In 1955, there was a movement to deinstitutionalise the mentally ill, and many mental hospitals and asylums were shut down (Davis et al., 2012). Prisons soon began to function as state hospitals as more than half of the US prison population suffers from severe mental illness (Delaney et al., 2018). Despite the overwhelming number of mentally ill individuals in the prison system, most facilities are understaffed and unable to adequately meet clients' needs due to overcrowding and cost-saving measures (Daniel, 2007). Efforts to address staffing issues and training deficiencies are slowly taking place across the nation due to litigation and federal mandates.

Re-entering the community

Individuals who are subjected to incarceration within the United States are faced with numerous challenges once released back into the community. After spending many years within the walls of correctional facilities, people frequently become 'institutionalized', meaning that they change and adopt a set of behaviours vital to their survival in institutions (Goffman, 1961; Haney, 2001). Upon their release, they are expected to function within society seamlessly and instantly despite being disconnected from it for extended periods of time. This experience can have significant psychological consequences and can be isolating for the formerly incarcerated, as many fail to understand the trauma endured from being institutionalised. It is important to note that many individuals who are wrongfully convicted and later exonerated suffer a number of additional and unique psychological consequences. For instance, it has been found that exonerees specifically experience symptoms of anxiety, depression, posttraumatic stress disorder, and long-lasting personality changes (Brooks & Greenberg, 2021; Wildeman et al., 2011).

In addition to having to reacclimate to society and freedom, formerly incarcerated individuals are tasked with having to establish their lives. They are typically released without employment, financial resources, health insurance, proper identification, and sometimes housing (Li, 2018). Community and social support in addition to linkage to comprehensive services have been found to be essential to successful reentry (Visher & Travis, 2011). Despite this recommendation, most jails and prisons do not provide people with adequate linkage at the time of their release. There are numerous community and grassroots organisations that aim to assist the formerly incarcerated reintegrate into the community; however, there is limited knowledge of resources and poor continuity of care. Most people have to rely on themselves and their families to get established, which can be daunting due to all the barriers for the formerly incarcerated and limited resources of the racial minorities impacted by the system. For instance, many companies are unwilling to hire people with criminal backgrounds. Even in states where asking applicants about their criminal history is prohibited by the Ban the Box Law, formerly incarcerated individuals continue to have difficulties due to limited work experience and a limited skill set (Holzer et al., 2003). Additionally, individuals convicted of certain offenses are ineligible for certain public assistance and public housing. With all these barriers to successful reentry, the likelihood of reoffending, violating conditions of their parole/probation, and reentering the prison system is greater.

Conclusion

It is important for anyone working within the criminal justice system to have a fundamental knowledge of the history and dynamics of the system at play. With the overrepresentation of racial minorities in the penal system and media outlets that perpetuate racial stereotypes, it is easy for individuals to believe that the system is working as intended: to keep 'criminals' or 'bad people' off the streets. However, this is not accurate, and such viewpoints can harm individuals in need of care within the criminal justice system.

The individuals within the criminal justice system, according to statistics, are disproportionately racial minorities, mainly Black and Latinx. They are frequently victims of racism, discrimination, and racial trauma, which can lead to poorer health outcomes and depleted psychological resources (Farmer et al., 2019; Carter & Pieterse, 2020; Joseph et al., 2020). They are typically indigent and come from communities that have been divested in and undervalued. While the problem of mass incarceration has become a greater concern within the past several decades, the individuals affected by the criminal justice system have been combating the oppression of systemic racism and countless racial disparities including their imprisonment for generations. It is this understanding that will allow those working with incarcerated people to truly humanise them on an individual level while viewing them within the larger macrosystem, thus affecting real change.

References

Administrative Office of the U.S. Courts. (n.d.). *Jury qualifications*. United States Courts. www.uscourts.gov/services-forms/jury-service/juror-qualifications

Alang, S., McAlpine, D., McCreedy, E., & Hardeman, R. (2017). Police brutality and Black health: Setting the agenda for public health scholars. *American Journal of Public Health*, *107*(5), 662–665.

Alexander, M. (2012). *The new Jim Crow: Mass incarceration in the age of color blindness*. The New Press.

American Bar Association. (2020). *ABA profile of the legal profession 2020*. www.americanbar.org/content/dam/aba/administrative/news/2020/07/potlp2020.df.

American Bar Association. (n.d.). *How court works*. www.americanbar.org/groups/public_education/resources/law_related_education_ network/how_courts_work/sentencing/

American Constitution Society. (n.d.). *Diversity of Federal Bench: Current statistics on the gender and racial diversity of the Article III courts*. www.acslaw.org/judicial-nominations/diversity-of-the-federal-bench/.

Anwar, S., Bayer, P., & Hjalmarsson, R. (2012). The impact of jury race in criminal trials. *The Quarterly Journal of Economics*, *127*(2), 1017–1055.

Arnold, D., Dobbie, W., & Yang, C. S. (2018). Racial bias in bail decisions. *The Quarterly Journal of Economics*, *133*(4), 1885–1932.

Berkley Law Death Penalty Clinic. (2020). *Whitewashing the jury box: How California perpetuates the discriminatory exclusion of Black and Latinx jurors*. www.law.berkeley.edu/wp-content/uploads/2020/06/Whitewashing-the-JuryBox.pdf.

Binnall, J. M., & Petersen, N. (2020). Building biased jurors: Exposing the circularity of the inherent bias rationale for felon-juror exclusion. *Psychiatry, Psychology, and Law*, *27*(1), 110–125. doi:10.1080/13218719.2019.1687047

Brooks, S. K., & Greenberg, N. (2021). Psychological impact of being wrongfully accused of criminal offences: A systematic literature review. *Medicine, Science and the Law*, *61*(1), 44–54.

Carter, R. T., & Pieterse, A. L. (2020). *Measuring the effects of racism: Guidelines for the assessment and treatment of race-based traumatic stress injury*. Columbia University Press.

Clarke, M. (2020). Racism and wrongful convictions. *Criminal Legal News*. www.criminallegalnews.org/news/2020/may/15/racism-and-wrongful-convictions/

Collier, L. (2014, October). Incarceration nation. *Monitor on Psychology*, *45*(9). www.apa.org/monitor/2014/10/incarceration

Cullen, F. (2013). Rehabilitation: Beyond nothing works. *Crime and Justice*, *42*(1), 299–376. doi:10.1086/670395

Curiel, F., & Matthews II, J. (2019, November 30). Criminal justice debt problems. *American Bar Association*. www.americanbar.org/groups/crsj/publications/human_rights_magazine_home/economic-justice/criminal-justice-debt-problems/

Daniel, A. E. (2007). Care of the mentally ill in prisons: Challenges and solutions. *Journal of the American Academy of Psychiatry and the Law*, *35*(4), 406–410.

Davis, A. (2003). *Are prisons obsolete?* Seven Stories Press.

Davis, L., Fulginiti, A., Kriegel, L., & Brekke, J. S. (2012). Deinstitutionalization? Where have all the people gone? *Current Psychiatry Reports*, *14*(3), 259–269. https://doi-org.tcsedsystem.idm.oclc.org/10.1007/s11920-012-0271-1

DeCamp, W., & DeCamp, E. (2020). It's still about race: Peremptory challenge use on black prospective jurors. *Journal of Research in Crime and Delinquency*, *57*(1), 3–30.

Delaney, R., Subramanian, R., Shames, A., & Turner, N. (2018). Reimagining prison web report. *Vera*. www.vera.org/reimagining-prison-web-report

Demuth, S. (2003). Racial and ethnic differences in pretrial release decisions and outcomes: A comparison of Hispanic, Black, and White felony arrestees. *Criminology*, *41*(3), 873–908.

Donnelly, E. A., & MacDonald, J. M. (2018). The downstream effects of bail and pretrial detention on racial disparities in incarceration. *Journal of Criminal Law & Criminology*, *108*(4), 775–814.

Durr, M. (2015). What is the difference between Slave Patrols and modern day policing? Institutional violence in a community of color. *Critical Sociology*, *41*(6), 873–879. https://doi.org/10.1177/0896920515594766

DuVernay, A. (Director). (2016). 13th [Film]. Forward Movement, Howard Barish, & Kandoo Films.

Edwards, F., Esposito, M., & Lee, H. (2019). Risk of being killed by police use of force in the United States by age, race-ethnicity, and sex. *Proceedings of the National Academy of Sciences*, *116*(34), 16793–16798. doi:10.1073/pnas.1821204116

Equal Justice Initiative. (2010, August). *Illegal racial discrimination in jury selection: A continuing legacy*. https://eji.org/wp-content/uploads/2019/10/illegal-racial discrimination-in-jury-selection.pdf

Farmer, H. R., Wray, L. A., & Thomas, J. R. (2019). Do race and everyday discrimination predict mortality risk? Evidence from the health and retirement study. *Gerontology and Geriatric Medicine*, *5*, 2333721419855665.

Feagin, J. (2006). *Systemic racism: A theory of oppression*. ProQuest Ebook Central. https://ebookcentral.proquest.com

Federal Judicial Center. (n.d.). *Demography of article III Judges, 1789–2020*. www.fjc.gov/history/exhibits/graphs-and-maps/race-and-ethnicity

Flanagan, F. X. (2018). Race, gender, and juries: Evidence from North Carolina. *The Journal of Law and Economics*, *61*(2), 189–214.

Floyd et. al. v. City of N.Y. et al, 959 F. Supp. 2d 540 (S.D.N.Y. 2013).

Geller, A., Fagan, J., Tyler, T., & Link, B. G. (2014). Aggressive policing and the mental health of young urban men. *American Journal of Public Health, 104*(12), 2321–2327.

Godfrey, B., & Soper, S. (2018). Prison records from 1800s Georgia show mass incarceration's racially charged beginnings. *The Conversation.* https://theconversation.com/prison records-from-1800s-georgia-show-mass-incarcerations-racially-charged-beginnings 96612.

Goffman, E. (1961). *Asylums: Essays on the social situations of mental patients and other inmates.* Doubleday (Anchor).

Gotsch, K., & Basti, V. (2018). Capitalizing on mass incarceration: U.S. growth in private prisons. *The Sentencing Project.* www.sentencingproject.org/wp content/uploads/2018/07/Capitalizing-on-Mass-Incarcer ation.pdf

Haney, C. (2001). The psychological impact of incarceration: Implications for post-prison adjustment. *U.S. Department of Health and Human Services.* https://aspe.hhs.gov/system/files/pdf/75001/Haney.pdf

Hassett-Walker, C. (2021). How you start is how you finish? The slave patrol and Jim Crow origins of policing. *American Bar Association.* www.americanbar.org/groups/crsj/publications/human_rights_magazine_home/ civil-rights-reimagining-policing/how-you-start-is-how-you-finish/

Hoag, A. (2020). An unbroken thread: African American exclusion from jury service, past and present. *Louisiana Law Review.* https://digitalcommons.law.lsu.edu/cgi/viewcontent.cgi?article=6814&context=lalrev

Holzer, H. J., Raphael, S., & Stoll, M. A. (2003). Employment barriers facing ex-offenders. *Urban Institute Reentry Roundtable*, 1–23.

Jackson-Gleich, G. (2021). Rigging the jury: How each state reduces jury diversity by excluding people with criminal records. *Prison Policy Initiative.* www.prisonpolicy.org/reports/juryexclusion.html

Jackson, D. B., Fahmy, C., Vaughn, M. G., & Testa, A. (2019). Police stops among at-risk youth: Repercussions for mental health. *Journal of Adolescent Health, 65*(5), 627–632.

Joseph, N. T., Peterson, L. M., Gordon, H., & Kamarck, T. W. (2020). The double burden of racial discrimination in daily-life moments: Increases in negative emotions and depletion of psychosocial resources among emerging adult African Americans. *Cultural Diversity & Ethnic Minority Psychology.* https://doi. org/10.1037/cdp0000337

LaFraniere, S., & Lehren, A. (2015, October). The disproportionate risks of driving while Black. *The New York Times.* www.nytimes.com/2015/10/25/us/racial-disparity-traffic stops-driving-black.html

Li, M. (2018). From prisons to communities: Confronting re-entry challenges and social inequality. *American Psychological Association.* www.apa.org/pi/ses/resources/indicator/2018/03/prisons-to-communities

Lundahl, B., Kunz, C., Brownell, C., Harris, N., & Van Vleet, R. (2009). Prison privatization: A meta-analysis of cost effectiveness and quality of confinement indicators. *Research on Social Work Practice, 19*, 383–395.

Lundman, R. J., & Kaufman, R. L. (2003). Driving while black: Effects of race, ethnicity, and gender on citizen self-reports of traffic stops and police actions. *Criminology, 41*(1), 195–220.

Metzner, J. L., & Fellner, J. (2010). Solitary confinement and mental illness in U.S. prisons: A challenge for medical ethics. *Journal of the American Academy of Psychiatry and the Law, 38*(1), 104–108.

National Research Council. (2004). *Measuring racial discrimination.* The National Academies Press. https:// doi.org/10.17226/10887

Nellis, A. (2016). The color of justice: Racial and ethnic disparity in state prisons. *The Sentencing Project.* www.sentencingproject.org/wp-content/uploads/2016/06/The-Color-of-Justice-Racial-and-Ethnic-Disparity-in-State-Prisons.pdf

Nellis, A., Greene, J., & Mauer, M. (2016). Reducing racial disparity in the criminal justice system: A manual for practitioners and policymakers. *The Sentencing Project.* www.sentencingproject.org/wp-content/ uploads/2016/01/Reducing-Racial-Disparity-in-the-Criminal-Justice-System-A-Manual-for-Practi tioners-and-Policymakers.pdf

Novak, A. (2019). The school-to-prison pipeline: An examination of the association between suspension and justice system involvement. *Criminal Justice and Behavior, 46*(8), 1165–1180. https://doi. org/10.1177/0093854819846917

Nussbaum, A. (1971). The rehabilitation myth. *The American Scholar, 40*(4), 674–676. www.jstor.org/ stable/41209909

Ofer, U. (2017, December 11). We can't end mass incarceration without ending money bail. *American Civil Liberties Union.* www.aclu.org/blog/smart-justice/we-cant-end-mass-incarceration-without-ending-money-bail

Office of the United States Attorney. (n.d.). *Justice 101.* www.justice.gov/usao/justice-101/sentencing

Paynter, B. (2011). Cells for sale: Understand prison costs & savings. *Policy Matters Ohio*. www.policymat tersohio.org/pdf/CellsForSale2011.pdf

Peter-Hagene, L. (2019). Jurors' cognitive depletion and performance during jury deliberation as a function of jury diversity and defendant race. *Law and Human Behavior, 43*(3), 232.

Possley, M., & Stephens, K. (2017, March 7). *Race and wrongful convictions in the United States* (S. R. Gross, Ed.). National Registry of Exonerations. www.law.umich.edu/special/exoneration/Documents/Race_ and_Wrongful_Convictions.pdf

Roberts, A. (2013). Casual ostracism: Jury exclusion on the basis of criminal convictions. *Minnesota Law Review, 98*, 592.

Roth, M. (2006). *Prisons and prison systems: A global encyclopedia*. Greenwood Publishing Group.

Sawyer, W., & Wagner, P. (2020). Mass incarceration: The whole pie 2020. *Prison Policy Initiative*. www.pris onpolicy.org/factsheets/pie2020_allimages.pdf

Selby, D. (2021, February 5). 8 facts you should know about racial injustice in the criminal legal system. *Innocence Project*. https://innocenceproject.org/facts-racial-discrimination-justice-system-wrongful-conviction-black-history-month/

Stanford Encyclopedia of Philosophy. (2019). *Implicit bias*. https://plato.stanford.edu/entries/implicit-bias/

United States Government Accountability Office. (2018, March). *K-12 education: Discipline disparities for Black students, boys, and students with disabilities*. www.gao.gov/assets/gao-18-258.pdf

U.S. Const. amend. XIII.

U.S. Department of Education Office for Civil Rights. (2014, March). *School discipline, restraint, & seclusion highlights*. https://www2.ed.gov/about/offices/list/ocr/docs/crdc-discipline-snapshot.pdf

Visher, C. A., & Travis, J. (2011). Life on the outside: Returning home after incarceration. *The Prison Journal, 91*(3 supplemental), 102S–119S. https://doi.org/10.1177/0032885511415228

Weld, T. D. (2011). *American slavery as it is: Testimony of a thousand witnesses: Vol. DocSouth Books ed*. University of North Carolina at Chapel Hill Library.

Wildeman, J., Costelloe, M., & Schehr, R. (2011). Experiencing wrongful and unlawful conviction. *Journal of Offender Rehabilitation, 50*(7), 411–432. https://doi org.tcsedsystem.idm.oclc.org/10.1080/10509674.2 011.603033

Part 2

Marginalised and diverse social characteristics

Chapter 3

Intersectional inequalities and women in secure settings

Jayne Taylor and Tammi Walker

Background

In 2006, Baroness Corston was commissioned by the UK Home Office to examine what could be done to avoid women with particular vulnerabilities being imprisoned. This work was prompted by the deaths of six women at HMP Styal. The end publication was a *Review of Women with Particular Vulnerabilities in the Criminal Justice System* (2007), and it identified three categories of vulnerabilities for women related to:

- Domestic circumstances such as domestic violence, childcare issues, and being a single parent
- Personal circumstances such as mental illness, low self-esteem, eating disorders, and substance misuse
- Socio-economic factors such as poverty, isolation, and employment.

The Corston review made 43 recommendations and concluded in favour of 'radical' reforms to be instituted to the criminal management and disposal of women offenders and prisoners. The main recommendations included the following:

- Community penalties should be the norm for women offenders.
- A 10-year timetable should be put in place to reduce the capacity of the women's prison estate.
- Spending on women's prisons should be redirected to funding a national network of community-based programmes for women who offend or are at risk of offending.
- Greater use should be made of community sentences.
- Drug rehabilitation programmes and resettlement support for short-sentenced prisoners should be sufficient to generate confidence in noncustodial sentences.
- Support should be put in place for women in the criminal justice system who have experienced domestic or sexual violence or who have been involved in prostitution.

Reflecting on this review today, it would appear that there has been a lack of substantial change in England and Wales since 2007. This is supported by the latest statistics published by the Ministry of Justice, which report that women prisoners in England and Wales decreased from 3,812 in October 2019 to 3,257 in October 2020 (Ministry of Justice, 2020). Although this movement is in the right direction, it is not as substantial as anticipated in the Corston review.

DOI: 10.4324/9781003184768-5

Many women remanded into custody do not go on to receive a custodial sentence. In 2016, 60% of women remanded by the Magistrates' Court and 41% by the Crown Court did not receive a custodial sentence (Prison Reform Trust, 2017). Most women entering prison to serve a sentence (80%) have committed a non-violent offence (Prison Reform Trust, 2017). At the same time, women's experience of custody shows little sign of improvement. The incidence of self-harm in English and Welsh prisons has continued to increase and remains much higher for women – 3,207 per 1,000 prisoners (an increase of 11% in the number of incidents from the previous 12 months) compared to a rate of 661 incidents per 1,000 prisoners in male establishments in the 12 months to March 2020 (with incidents up 11% from the previous 12 months) (Ministry of Justice, 2020).

Although women are more likely to be released on temporary licence (ROTL) than men, the proportion of women in prison receiving ROTL decreased by 40% between 2007 and 2017 compared to an 18% decrease for men over the same period (Prison Reform Trust, 2020). Although women account for less than 5% of the prison population, research by the Prison Reform Trust in December 2018 showed recall numbers for women had increased by 131% in 2017, compared with 22% for men, with more than 1,700 women returned to jail in England and Wales in 2017.

Progress since the Corston report

The lack of implementation of the recommendations of the Corston review has been the subject of many UK reviews since 2007. Hine (2019) highlights several of these. The first, undertaken by the Social Exclusion Task Force of the Cabinet Office in 2009, which although noted as important progress, also emphasised the ongoing high numbers of imprisoned women and the cost relative to community sentences. For example, on average, it costs 12 times more to send a woman to prison than to put her on a probation or community service order (Social Exclusion Task Force, 2009, p. 20). Evidence presented to the Justice Committee in 2012 (House of Commons Justice Committee, 2013a, 2013b) highlighted the lack of progress in implementing the recommendations of the Corston report and identified a lack of a government strategy for imprisoned women. This was despite the Ministry of Justice having published a guide on working with women offenders in March of that year (Ministry of Justice, 2013).

Hine (2019) emphasises that the year of 2017 marked the tenth anniversary of the publication of the Corston report and that the several reviews of progress since its publication indicated they were all disappointed with the lack of improvement. The national UK charity Women in Prison conducted a detailed review of each recommendation in the Corston report (Women in Prison, 2017). This work concluded that just two of the 43 original recommendations had been fully implemented, twelve were assessed as having made no progress, and the remainder had made some progress but still needed much work.

The UK 2018 Female Offender Strategy

In 2018, the Ministry of Justice published the Female Offender Strategy, which aimed to reduce the overall number of women in prison and have fewer women imprisoned for short periods. The Strategy came at a time when there was a substantial agreement on the limited progress made since Corston and recognised how the lack of access to supportive community services, safe accommodation, and substance misuse contributed to women being recalled. It has three strategic priorities: earlier intervention, community-based solutions, and making custody effective and decent as possible for imprisoned women. The Strategy is wide ranging and comprehensive and promises an ambitious programme of work. However, Hine (2019) notes how the Strategy identified many of the themes and recommendations of the Corston report, but that it only referred to it directly just once in the whole publication.

Since its inception two years ago, the Strategy has made some good progress. There has been £5.1 million Strategy funding in 30 different women's services across England and Wales, helping to sustain and enhance existing services, fill gaps in provision, and provide properties for new women's centres. Other achievements include the publication of a new Women's Policy Framework (2018b) that provides guidance to prison and probation staff on a range of practices, for example, how to deliver gender-informed services to women offenders; rolling-out new training for staff; and implementing the recommendations of Lord Farmer's review (2019) into family and other relational ties for women offenders.

It must be noted that the Strategy is not without limitations. Much is made of the need to encourage courts not to use short custodial sentences and to deliver more community sentences instead; however, there appears to be no detailed discussion of direct involvement with judges and magistrates. Rather, the focus is on the improvement of pre-sentence reports written by the probation service, requiring them to 'capture the complexity of an offender's circumstances' (Ministry of Justice, 2018a, p. 19). The strategy does not acknowledge the ways in which policy requirements have led to a more standardised production of reports rather than the individualised approach that Corston promoted.

Finally, and importantly, the notion of 'vulnerabilities' that the Strategy highlights mutates into 'risk' within its proposals, in much the same way in which 'criminogenic need' evolved into 'risk' within policies for the supervision of offenders more generally. The strategy does not acknowledge that many women with 'vulnerabilities' do not come into contact with the criminal justice system, though it does address women 'at risk' of becoming involved. Many women with vulnerabilities are, however, in contact with mainstream services (Social Exclusion Task Force, 2009; HMIP, 2016). Hine (2019) argues that if these services functioned in a more coordinated and effective way, there would be less need for specific services for women offenders and fewer women in the criminal justice system.

Predictive factors

Despite some of the disappointment regarding the longer-term impact of the Corston recommendations, it nonetheless highlighted important vulnerability factors that may contribute to offending in women and sparked significant discussion on the pathways into violence in women which differ from those of men. There are a number of areas in which the perpetration of violence differs in men and women. For example, women are more likely to commit violence within the domestic sphere where intimate partners and family members tend to be the targets of that violence. Quite often this violence occurs within the context of dependency, whereas male violence occurs within the context of competition. We also know that women tend to internalise violence more in the form of self-harm, which we will discuss later in this chapter. For example, Hawton et al. (2013) found that self-harm rates were ten times higher in women in prison than men.

In discussing vulnerability factors, socio-economic factors are considered to play a significant role. The Office for National Statistics (2018) found that women living in households with an income of less than £10,000 per year were four times more likely to have experienced partner abuse in the last 12 months than women living in a household with an annual income of £50,000 or more. It is widely acknowledged that poverty can significantly restrict the options of women living in relationships where they experience intimate partner violence (IPV). The causal mechanisms underpinning the relationship between poverty and being a victim of IPV are multifactorial and complex. Women's lack of financial independence can delay the ability to leave a partner and they may have child-caring responsibilities in the home which may limit the opportunity for employment. There may also be reduced social networks. Morris (2009) notes that violence in households is not haphazard but rather reflects particular patterns of gender dynamics that are already deeply embedded in society.

Gender power dynamics may contribute to a woman becoming a victim of IPV irrespective of wealth – the inherent power imbalance of relationships between men and women may result in situations where women are disproportionately reliant on the validation of 'the other' and the ability to see the self without reference to 'the other' is diminished. Thus, self-esteem, mastery, and agency may all be compromised. This is demonstrated in the literature. Schaefer et al. (2016) found that victimisation was an independent risk factor for violent behaviour in women. In these circumstances, violence is seen to be a solution through the perceived absence of choices.

Evidence for the role of prior victimisation has emerged from a number of areas. In a study focusing on IPV perpetrated by military veterans who were women, Portnoy et al. (2020) found that Military Sexual Assault directly related to later perpetration and victimisation. The authors conclude that IPV perpetration in women veterans may be related to their own IPV victimisation.

Obviously, only a minority of women with a history of IPV perpetrate violence towards others. Understanding pathways to violence is central to developing our support for women who have experienced victimisation.

The developing evidence base on adverse childhood experiences (ACEs) provides a promising approach to the study of vulnerabilities. Motz et al. (2020) note that women are 50% more likely than men to have experienced five or more ACEs. They note that the invisible trauma of women is overlooked in sentencing and placement, yet this can be re-enacted in custody. They argue that powerful intergenerational factors perpetuate cycles of re-offending and trauma re-enactment. In a meta-analysis examining the association between childhood maltreatment and perpetration of violence in adulthood in women, Augsburger et al. (2019) found a small but significant positive association between exposure to childhood maltreatment and a range of aggressive behaviours. Specific types of childhood maltreatment were not found to differ in their effects, demonstrating the importance of emotional abuse and neglect in contributing to pathways to later aggression. Swan et al. (2005) found that the experience of abuse in childhood, subsequent PTSD, and anger were associated with the later commission of IPV in women.

This is also supported by work looking at the relationship between self-harm and violence. Kottler et al. (2018) examined the co-incidence of violence and self-harm in a large sample of women whilst in prison. Although most of the sample were found not to have engaged in either behaviour, there was significant overlap between those that had self-harmed and were violent towards others, which the authors argue suggests that the two behaviours are more closely related than previously thought. In this sense, violence, both directed towards others and the self, can be seen as the manifestation of intense and unbearable affect.

Unsurprisingly, attachment processes have also been considered a predisposing factor in the study of violence in women. In part, this is not only due to the commission of violence in women largely within the context of close relationships but also because there is a significant body of research that has examined the role of attachment in violence committed by men.

One such approach has focused on the role of insecure attachment and fears of abandonment. Insecure attachment and unresolved trauma may lead to unstable working models of self. When triggered, such as by fear of abandonment, there is a fear for survival and also what this means for the perception of self.

Bélanger et al. (2015) conducted a study examining the attachment styles of both partners within the context of IPV. They found that relationship dyads characterised by an avoidant attachment style in male partners and an anxious attachment style in women were associated with the perpetration of IPV by women. It is argued that the demand–withdraw communication pattern could underpin this where anxiety regarding abandonment may be triggered when the partner is experienced as rejecting or withdrawing. The cycle becomes self-perpetuating as a greater need for reassurance results in greater withdrawal which in turn triggers further anxiety. This was supported by Orcutt et al. (2005), who found that women with anxious attachment styles were more likely to assault partners.

Self-harm

Self-harm is a challenge for the criminal justice system due to its associations with physical injury, psychology co-morbidity, and increased lifetime suicide risk (Hawton et al., 2013). The conceptualisation and definition of what has been characterised as 'self-harm' remain problematic, and Walker and Towl (2016) note how issues of confusion continue to remain by the use of multiple definitions. It is clear though that individuals may self-harm either with or without any intention to kill themselves.

Her Majesty's Prison and Probation Service (HMPPS) (as stated in Prison Service Instructions 64/2011) in the United Kingdom defines self-harm as 'any act where a prisoner deliberately harms themselves irrespective of the method, intent or severity of any injury'. This definition focuses on the behaviour, rather than on what the individual intended to achieve by engaging in the behaviour. When attempting to gather accurate statistics on self-harm, in both prison and community samples, the methods have been criticised due to difficulties in identifying and classifying what behaviours are self-harming and when self-harm is different from a suicide attempt (Powis, 2002). Further, the motivations for engaging in self-harming behaviours are very complex, and individuals who have no experience of self-harm may find it an intensely confusing behaviour (Walker & Towl, 2016).

Studies of self-harm in prison populations in the United Kingdom are limited, and until 1997, the focus for reporting self-harm incidents in the prison population was on 'attempted suicide', but the problem with this approach was that prisoner intent was frequently unknown (Ministry of Justice, 2013). From 1997, all self-harm incidents had to be reported, and this led to an increase in reported incidents in the prison population. Further, in 2002, a self-harm monitoring form was introduced based on the F213 'Injuries to Inmate' form (Ministry of Justice, 2013). As a result, reporting of self-harm incidents improved further throughout 2003. The Ministry of Justice has now omitted self-harm statistics before 2004 from publications because they were considerably underreported compared with current standards.

Since 2004, prisons in England and Wales have used the Assessment, Care in Custody and Teamwork (ACCT) procedure. This is a prisoner-centred, proactive, flexible care-planning arrangement that promotes the intensive case management of high-risk individuals (HM Prison Service, 2001). The ACCT scheme has been subject to a number of evaluations (Rickford & Edgar, 2005; Harris, 2015). Logan and Taylor (2019) argue that, in general, the ACCT procedure appears to be a useful way of managing the risk of self-harm and suicide. However, the implementation of the ACCT procedure is not thought to be complete in all cases, for example, not everyone at risk is subject to ACCT (Pratt, 2016).

Methods of self-harm are heterogeneous. Hawton et al. (2013) found in an analysis of prisons in England and Wales between 2004 and 2009 that the most common methods of self-harm for both sexes are cutting and scratching; for imprisoned women, the next most frequent method used is self-strangulation. The use of ligature has been an area of concern across the wider prison estate among in-prison suicides (Marzano et al., 2016), due to its associated high rate of lethality and the availability of ligature points within prison design.

A suggested reason why women in prison are thought to be particularly at risk of self-harm is that many are vulnerable and disempowered *before* they were imprisoned; it has been proposed that being in custody compounds this vulnerability and disempowers women further (Logan & Taylor, 2019; Harris, 2015). The majority of women in prison have extensive traumatic victimisation histories, including childhood abuse, IPV, and violence from non-intimates (Walker & Towl, 2016). Women in prison are far more likely to have experienced sexual and domestic violence than the general female population. Evidence indicates that between 50% and 80% of imprisoned women have experienced domestic and/or sexual abuse (Walker & Towl, 2016). Imprisoned women often describe episodes of *poly-victimisation* (multiple trauma) throughout their life, including chronic and severe abuse. Many women in prison are therefore victims as well as perpetrators.

Logan and Taylor (2019) illustrate that during their imprisonment, women are more likely to be separated from those for whom they have a primary caregiving role (e.g., their children), resulting in their dependents being put into care and future contact being jeopardised (e.g., Corston, 2007). Remand status, substance withdrawal, prior incarceration, negative experiences of imprisonment (e.g., bullying), as well as poor social support have been found to be relevant risk factors for women (e.g., Walker & Towl, 2016). Long-term vulnerabilities are often cited as primary reasons for self-harming, whereas prison-related variables such as transfers are commonly described as proximal or triggering factors.

There is limited research to contextualise factors underpinning the disproportionate rate of self-harm among women offenders (Kenning et al., 2010; Walker & Towl, 2016), and attempting to understand the motivations and context preceding acts of self-harm among this group is important in the delivery of effective interventions. In order to address this, the second author undertook a project with colleagues entitled The Women Offenders Repeat Self-Harm Intervention Pilot II (WORSHIP II) (Walker et al., 2017). WORSHIP II was a randomised controlled trial (RCT) conducted from 2012 to 2015 in three female prisons in England and aimed to reduce their thoughts and actions of self-harm, and suicide risk. Women between the ages of 18 and 65 years were considered eligible if they were currently on an ACCT or have been on one recently, had committed an act of self-harm in the last month, were in the prison establishment for a minimum of six weeks to complete the intervention sessions, and were not receiving any other therapeutic intervention while in prison. After giving written consent, a range of baseline assessments were completed, and following the completion of these, women were randomly assigned to treatment conditions.

Women in the intervention group were offered four-eight sessions of psychodynamic interpersonal therapy (PIT). The therapy, developed by Hobson (1985), entailed identifying and helping to resolve interpersonal therapy difficulties, which cause or exacerbate psychological distress (Walker et al., 2017). In this study, the PIT manual was modified for prison use, but the empirical status of PIT is well established and there are high-quality efficacy and effectiveness studies of PIT (Walker et al., 2017). In working with women who have repeatedly self-injured, the first task is to understand the circumstances that precipitated the episode. Importance is assigned to exploring feelings and bringing these into the here and now. Problems, which have precipitated the self-harm, are studied and linked to feelings, problems, and relationships.

Although the therapy work in WORSHIP II was brief, issues that arose between the therapist and the women were actively explored and linked to important relationships in her life. Sessions were offered weekly in the prison setting, lasted 50 minutes, and were delivered by a psychiatrist, a mental health nurse, an occupational therapist, or a psychologist. Treatment fidelity and adherence were ensured by weekly supervision, digital recording of interviews, and the use of a standardised rating scale (Walker et al., 2017).

Women who were randomised to the 'treatment as usual' arm received an Active Control (AC) session that consisted of being taken out of their cells and engaging in activities such as card games with a researcher. The AC participants had four sessions that occurred weekly and lasted 50 minutes. No personal support was undertaken, and women were aware that they could not talk about emotional topics. The second author (TW) monitored and provided supervision for those involved in these sessions. A small sample of women from both groups ($n = 20$) were followed up at three and six months to examine the feasibility of this process and assess adherence, acceptability, and ongoing skill usage of the intervention.

A total of 76 (PIT, 31; AC, 45) women completed baseline and post-therapy and 20 (PIT, 13; AC, 7) at follow-up. The primary outcome measure was the total score on the Beck Scale for Suicidal Ideation (Beck et al., 1985) since the strength of suicidal ideation is an important predictor of completed suicide. The findings suggested that PIT and AC reduced thoughts of suicide, self-harm, self-harm repetition, as well as self-harm severity post-therapy. The qualitative reports indicated that women in the PIT group continued to use skills learnt and PIT may reduce both the number and severity of events during the intervention (Walker & Towl, 2016). To date, this is the only study that has provided evidence that a modified brief intervention for repeat self-harm can be delivered to women in prison; however, it must be noted that WORSHIP II did not illustrate that the PIT intervention is better than the AC: both reduced behavioural outcomes of self-harm repetition and severity.

Conclusion

Sabri and Granger (2018) make the point that the effects of victimisation or gender-based violence are even more profound for those women who face the effects of multiple characteristics that are marginalising. Intersectionality of factors such as race, socioeconomic status, and gender impacts the outcome following trauma due to the experience of multiple stressors related to one's position in society.

A report in 2017 by Women in Prison on Double Disadvantage demonstrated that BAME women were at an additional disadvantage due to ethnicity, citing further discrimination from courts through to custody, relative to the general experience of white women. When women are violent towards others, there is often a further process of marginalisation as there remains a tendency for society to view this behaviour as a counter to societal expectations of women with little acknowledgement of the antecedents to this. By default, these women are further marginalised as society struggles to explain this behaviour. However, it is only by examining the pathways to violent or self-harming behaviour that we can begin to understand how this can be avoided and address the significant disadvantage that many women face.

References

Augsburger, M., Basler, K., & Maercker, A. (2019). Is there a female cycle of violence after exposure to childhood maltreatment? A meta-analysis. *Psychological Medicine, 49*(11), 1776–1786.

Beck, A., Steer, R., Kovacs, M., & Garrison, B. (1985). Hopelessness and eventual suicide: A 10-year prospective study of patients hospitalized with suicidal ideation. *American Journal of Psychiatry, 142*, 559–563.

Bélanger, C., Mathieu, C., Dugal, C., & Courchesne, C. (2015). The impact of attachment on intimate partner violence perpetrated by women. *American Journal of Family Therapy, 43*(5), 441–453.

Corston, J. (2007). *The Corston report: A review of women with particular vulnerabilities in the criminal justice system.* Home Office.

Harris, T. (2015). *Changing prisons, saving lives: Report of the independent review into self-inflicted deaths in custody of 18–24-year olds.* Her Majesty's Stationery Office.

Hawton, K., Linsell, L., Adeniji, T., Sariaslan, S., & Fazel, S. (2013). Self-harm in prisons in England and Wales: An epidemiological study of prevalence, risk factors, clustering, and subsequent suicide. *The Lancet.* www.thelancet.com. Published online September 16, 2013. http://dx.doi.org/10.1016/S0140-6736(13)62571–4

Hine, J. (2019). Women and criminal justice: Where are we now? *British Journal of Community Justice, 15*(1), 5–18.

HM Prison Service. (2001). *Prevention of suicide and self-harm in the prison service: An internal review.* HM Prison Service.

HMIP. (2016). *A thematic inspection of the provision and quality of services in the community for women who offend.* HM Inspectorate of Probation.

Hobson, R. F. (1985). *Forms of feeling: The heart of psychotherapy.* Routledge.

House of Commons Justice Committee. (2013a). *Women offenders: After the Corston report: Volume I report.* House of Commons.

House of Commons Justice Committee. (2013b). *Women offenders: After the Corston report: Volume II Additional written evidence.* House of Commons.

Kenning, C., Cooper, J., Short, V., Shaw, J., Abel, K., & Chew-Graham, C. (2010). Prison staff and women prisoner's views on self-injury: Their implications for service delivery and development: A qualitative study. *Criminal Behaviour and Mental Health, 20*(4), 274–284.

Kottler, C., Smith, J. G., & Bartlett, A. (2018). Patterns of violence and self-harm in women prisoners: Characteristics, co-incidence and clinical significance. *Journal of Forensic Psychiatry & Psychology, 29*(4), 617–634.

Logan, C., & Taylor, J. (2019). Managing suicide and self-harm. In D. Polaschek, A. Day, & C. Hollin (Eds.), *International handbook of correctional psychology* (pp. 224–245). Wiley.

Marzano, L., Hawton, K., & Rivlin, A. (2016). Prevention of suicidal behavior in prisons *Crisis, 37*, 323–334.

Ministry of Justice. (2013). *Strategic objectives for female offenders.* Ministry of Justice.

Ministry of Justice. (2018). *Female offender strategy.* Ministry of Justice.

Ministry of Justice. (2018b). *Women's policy framework.* Ministry of Justice.

Ministry of Justice. (2019). *The importance of strengthening female offenders family and other relationships to prevent reoffending and reduce intergenerational crime by Lord Farmer.* Ministry of Justice.

Ministry of Justice. (2020). *Her Majesty's prison and probation service offender equalities annual report 2019/20.* Ministry of Justice.

Morris, A. (2009). Gendered dynamics of abuse and violence in families: Considering the abusive household gender regime. *Child Abuse Review, 18*(I), 414–427.

Motz, A., Dennis, M., & Aiyegbusi, A. (2020). *Invisible trauma: Women, difference and the criminal justice system.* Routledge.

Office for National Statistics. (2018). *Domestic abuse: Findings from the Crime Survey for England and Wales: Year ending March 2018.* Office for National Statistics.

Orcutt, H. K., Garcia, M., & Pickett, S. M. (2005). Female-perpetrated intimate partner violence and romantic attachment style in a college student. *Sample Violence and Victims, 20*(3), 287–302.

Portnoy, G. A., Relyea, M. R., Street, A. E., Haskell, S. G., & Iverson, K. M. (2020). A longitudinal analysis of women Veterans' partner violence perpetration: The roles of interpersonal trauma and posttraumatic stress symptoms. *Journal of Family Violence, 35*(4), 361–372.

Powis, B. (2002). *Offenders' risk of serious harm: A literature review.* Home Office Research, Development and Statistics Directorate.

Pratt, D. (Ed.). (2016). *The prevention of suicide in prison: Cognitive behavioural approaches.* Routledge.

Prison Reform Trust. (2017). *Why focus on reducing women's imprisonment?* Prison Reform Trust.

Prison Reform Trust. (2020). *Working it out: Improving employment opportunities for women with criminal convictions.* Prison Reform Trust.

Rickford, D., & Edgar, K. (2005). *Troubled inside: Responding to the mental health needs of men in prison.* Prison Reform Trust, UK.

Sabri, B., & Granger, D. A. (2018). Gender-based violence and trauma in marginalized populations of women: Role of biological embedding and toxic stress. *Health Care for Women International, 39*(9), 1038–1055.18p.

Schaefer, R., Broadbent, M., & Bruce, M. (2016). Violent typologies among women in-patients with severe mental illness. *Social Psychiatry & Psychiatric Epidemiology, 51*(1), 1615–1622.

Social Exclusion Task Force. (2009). *Short study on women offenders.* Cabinet Office.

Swan, S. C., Gambone, L. J., Fields, A. M., Sullivan, T. P., & Snow, D. L. (2005). Women who use violence in intimate relationships: The role of anger, victimization, and symptoms of posttraumatic stress and depression. *Violence and Victims, 20*, 267–285.

Walker, T., Shaw, J., Turpin, C., Reid, C., & Abel, K. (2017). The WORSHIP II study: A pilot of psychodynamic interpersonal therapy with women offenders who self-harm. *Journal of Forensic Psychiatry and Psychology, 28*, 158–171.

Walker, T., & Towl, G. (2016). *Preventing self-injury and suicide in women's prisons.* Waterside Press.

Women in Prison. (2017). The Corston report 10 years on: How far have we come on the road to reform for women affected by the criminal justice system? www.mappingthemaze.org.uk/wp-content/uploads/2017/08/corston-report-10-years-on.pdf

Chapter 4

Transitional spaces
Working with transgender prisoners in the United Kingdom

Jessica Collier, Rebecca Lockwood, and Frances Maclennan

Introduction

This chapter describes some of the challenges and complex issues that emerge for transgender people in prison. It has been written by three colleagues, all of whom have worked clinically in this area. Whilst we share some views, it is important to note that we also hold differing opinions. This capacity to consider more than one position simultaneously allows for a multifaceted clinical perspective. One area of consensus is that the questions, implications, issues, and complexities this chapter presents are considerable. There is no simple answer to managing transgender people within the criminal justice system, and this is particularly complex when their offending is of a sexual and/or violent nature. Throughout this chapter, we have tried to present some of the challenges, confusion, and uncertainty that we have experienced working in this field, the importance of acknowledging what we do not know, sharing what is recommended in terms of physical and mental health care for this population and the necessity for further research, discussion, ongoing curiosity, and professional humility.

Social context

Histories of abuse, neglect, and trauma are extremely common within the prison population. The emergence and development of criminality can be understood as a re-enactment of early childhood trauma (Widom, 1989). Men and women in prison are usually already a group of people who are profoundly disadvantaged. Prison populations are characterised by a range of markers including poor literacy, low levels of education, economic deprivation, poor physical health outcomes, and under-employment (Prison Reform Trust, 2021). These are in addition to systemic prejudices including racism, sexism, homophobia, and transphobia among many others. Over half of the female prison populations have been emotionally, physically, or sexually abused (Prison Reform Trust, 2017). Some people in prison have suffered extremely high levels of trauma which have often continued throughout childhood into adulthood.

Transgender people include individuals who identify in a variety of ways. These gender identities may be fluid and shift over time or be constant and unchanging. They include, but are not limited to, people who identify as trans, transgender, genderqueer, gender nonbinary, transsexual, cross dresser, male to female (MTF), female to male (FTM), gender bender, trans man, trans woman, two-spirit, and many others (APA, 2015). For the purposes of this chapter, we will use the single term transgender, though we acknowledge that this choice may not represent the wide experiences of this diverse group of people.

DOI: 10.4324/9781003184768-6

Transgender populations in prison

It is difficult to estimate precisely how many serving prisoners in England and Wales are transgender. This is partly because Her Majesty's Prison and Probation Service (HMPPS) did not, until the release of the Prison Service Instructions (PSI) in 2017, collect data on the gender identity of prisoners but also because, even if these data were collected, those who are gender non-conforming are less likely to disclose their status, often due to safety concerns within the prison. With recent PSI publications, we now have a better-detailed guide on the care and management of individuals identifying as transgender within the prison population.

The numbers of transgender individuals held in the adult prison estate are low, approximately 1.6 transgender prisoners reported per 1,000 prisoners in custody (PSI, 2020). The best estimate of the general population is that around 200,000–500,000 people in the United Kingdom identify as transgender (Government Equalities Office, 2018). In a snapshot data collection held in 2018 by the HMPPS (MoJ, 2018), there were 139 prisoners currently living in, or presenting as, a gender different from their sex assigned at birth and who had sat on a Local Transgender Case Board. There were 42 transgender prisoners in women's prisons. When asked about the gender they identified as, 22 identified as female, 17 as male, and three did not provide a response. There were 97 transgender prisoners in men's prisons. When asked about the gender they identified as, 92 identified as female, two as male, and three did not provide a response. Emerging HMPPS equality data suggest that most transgender individuals in custody do not seek legal recognition of the gender with which they identify and request to be located in a prison which matches their assigned sex at birth.

In recent years, there have been numerous research reports which indicate that people who are transgender in the criminal justice system have higher rates of mental health problems, self-harm, and suicide (Bashford et al., 2018). In December 2015, following two high profile deaths from the suicide of transgender women held in male prisons, Parliament launched a review of the treatment of transgender people in prison, probation services, and the youth justice system. The most recent guidance, released in 2020, is The Care and Management of Individuals who are Transgender (Transgender Policy Framework; HMPPS, 2020). Included in the scope of this framework are those who identify as transgender but do not seek to acquire a new gender. These include individuals who identify as intersex, non-binary, gender fluid, and transvestite who will be managed in accordance with their legally recognised gender. This Policy Framework is intended to provide staff with clear direction in the support and safe management of transgender individuals in their care, including managing risks both to and from transgender individuals, and enabling risk to be managed when an individual is placed in a prison which is different from that of their legal gender or where a Gender Recognition Certification (GRC) has been obtained.

The guidance for the treatment and care of transgender people in prison has moved significantly away from the previous approach, which focused only on transgender people who had obtained a GRC or had a diagnosis of gender dysphoria. The emphasis has moved towards a more socially informed, flexible definition of transgender, based on self-identification. A balanced approach must be adopted when making the allocation, care, and management decisions relating to transgender individuals, balancing the risks and well-being of the individual with the risks or impact on well-being that the person may present to others, particularly in custodial and residential settings. Structured risk assessments (through Complex Case Boards) are required before a person is allocated or transferred to a part of the estate which does not match their sex assigned at birth.

Safety and risk considerations should be paramount when making decisions about the care and management of transgender individuals. The implementation of a robust decision-making process, by way of Local and Complex Transgender Case Boards, takes account of risks to all prisoners and young people in custody and residents on approved premises, to staff, as well as risks presented to the individual. Assessment of risk is based on valid evidenced factors that relate to that individual. All individuals in the care of HMPPS who disclose they are transgender must have an initial Local Case Board which reviews the care and management of the prisoner. The Local Transgender Case Board must be convened within 14 calendar days of reception into custody or arrival on approved premises. Local Case Boards do not have the authority to agree with a transfer to a part of the opposite gender estate; only centrally managed Complex Case Boards can authorise this. These occur when management decisions are required to be made on behalf of the entire prison or estate and are chaired by a Prison Group Director.

Nevertheless, prisons and policies do not and cannot always protect people within their care. Individuals held in custody have been raped (Starchild, 1990) and rates of self-harm and suicide are high. Prison healthcare departments may be under-resourced and can be overwhelmed with complex cases who need more specialist input than services are able to deliver. In addition, the prison regime itself may contribute to further traumatisation (Kahr, 2020**)**.

In regard to healthcare practices, prisons have a duty of care to deliver comparable services in custody as those available in the community to all prisoners, including those diagnosed with gender dysphoria. Thus, access to counselling, pre-operative and post-operative care, and continued access to hormone treatment and to a consultant specialising in gender dysphoria must be made available.

Transgender sex offenders and unconscious or conscious prejudice

The provision of care to people in prison invites outrage (Kahr, 2020), and this is arguably more so when the care offered is for transgender women who have histories of violent or sexual offending and who are being held within the female prison estate. Whilst recent years have seen an increase in representation of gender diverse people in the media (Barker, 2017), transphobia and homophobia remain pervasive. In June 2019, the BBC reported that transphobic hate crimes had risen by 81% (BBC, 2019). Within the forensic context, which can be seen as historically punitive and holding a patriarchal, binary, perspective of society, progressive multifaceted theories of gender struggle to be accepted.

The, often uninformed, response to transgender prisoners can oversimplify their complex needs. Care may be understood as solely the need to meet their physical needs such as hormone treatment, speech and language therapy, and so on. Whilst it is vital that these needs are addressed, it is also important to acknowledge that a solely medical or material approach will not meet such complex needs. Individuals who have a diagnosis of borderline personality disorder (BPD) are by definition people who are likely to self-harm (Reichl & Kaess, 2021) and may find symbolic thinking difficult or impossible. Concrete answers to their psychic pain, ambivalence, and their fragile identities may be misconstrued, and medication or surgery sought as a solution. This is not to suggest that gender-diverse individuals are more likely than the cis population to have a diagnosis of BPD, although it is estimated that approximately 20% of women in prison attract this diagnosis (Fossey & Black, 2010). Neither does this suggest that transgendered women prisoners must be invulnerable to mental health issues and adverse childhoods. Rather, we wish to think deeply about the experiences that are specific to the forensic population as a whole. In this population, the likelihood of 'action' being taken without due consideration, as happens when violence is committed, needs to be contemplated from a forensic perspective. For example, as a potential enactment: that is an unconscious repetition in the presence of an event from the past, or offence paralleling: unconscious behaviour that may mirror the crime for which the individual is imprisoned. A humanistic and non-prejudicial stance that values freedom of identity and self-expression is also essential.

Personality disordered patients and prisoners have often suffered abuse at the hands of their carers when young and may 'repeat an abusive relationship when they encounter care in later life' (Hinshelwood, 2002). Hinshelwood describes the complexity of caring for people with severe personality disorder and notes that 'the pressures on the staff are complex, caught between control and redemption. Without being fully conscious of these complicated demands, the staff are confronted with the patient's "unreadable" requests for help' (Hinshelwood, 2002).

A further reason as to why the care for transgender prisoners has caused such a challenge may be associated with the notion that transgender identity may be thought of as a powerful tool of activism (Lemma, 2018). Indeed 'trans' has become a central 'cultural site' (Valentine, 2007). Within the prison environment, there is little space for acts of activism and such an expression may be experienced unconsciously, or consciously, as an attack or a threat. It is therefore responded to harshly and punitively rather than understood.

Additional complexity is raised by prisoners who may wish to modify their bodies in line with their gender identity. This may present a threat to those around them because the modification of the body impacts upon a reality that we all have to 'share' (Lemma, 2018). Ideas that it is a privilege to entertain thoughts of non-binary identity conflict with the idea that prisoners should not be allowed such 'luxury'. Indeed, narratives of outrage and fury are commonplace in the media when prisoners are permitted only meagre channels of expression.

The language, narrative, and discourse around forensic patients and environments are laden with fear, danger, and anxiety. The open discussion around gender identity has become inhibited, and this may be related to there being significant repercussions for 'getting it wrong'. The inhibition of the conversation has prevented exploration of the issues and restricts the potential for psychological space to be made to think about the key issues.

It is essential that the different requirements and difficulties faced by individuals in prison who identify as transgender must not be confused with individuals who use the concept of gender diversity as a means of evading justice or committing further offences. In the memorably straightforward words of Britain's longest-serving transgender prisoner Sarah Jane Baker, 'If some pervert should wear a frock to invade a woman's space to commit an offence, that doesn't make them transgender, it makes them a pervert' (Abraham, 2019).

Statistics published by the BBC suggest that you are far more likely to be sexually assaulted in custody *as* a transgender prisoner than *by* a transgender prisoner (Shaw, 2020). Writer Rebecca Solnit, writing in the Guardian newspaper, points out that transwomen are not a threat to ciswomen but rather suggests the danger comes from 'straight men and patriarchy . . . where the lion's share of violence against women comes from, as rape and domestic violence and harassment and murder' (Solnit, 2020). This is important to remember in the context of the female prison estate where many men work, including officers with keys to the women's cells, and where sexual abuse of female prisoners by staff has been reported. This includes the evidence of a transgender woman who alleged, according to The Special Rapporteur on Torture to the Human Rights Council (United Nations, 2001) cited in the Commission for Sex in Prison (Howard League for Penal Reform, 2014), that 'she had been subject to sexual assaults, harassment, intimidation and bullying from male prison staff'. The report also stressed that 'It should not be assumed that just because prisoners do not report abuse by prison staff, abuse is not happening'.

Carol Hay, Associate Professor in the Department of Philosophy at the University of Massachusetts Lowell, writing an opinion piece in the *New York Times*, suggests that widespread misinformation and prejudice, inside and outside the criminal justice system, reinforce ideas that 'Trans people . . . are seen as "make-believers" – cheap counterfeits, pathetically attempting to be something they couldn't possibly actually be' (Hay, 2019). Such ideas, in addition to the socially accepted demonisation and hatred of sex offenders, make sex offenders who self-identify as transwomen, a group who are particularly vulnerable to marginalisation and prejudice, unlikely to have their complex needs met. This is problematic not only at an ethical level but also in terms of access to treatment. The level of psychological complexity may justify and reinforce the idea that such offenders 'just cannot be helped'. Stein contends that such 'bias becomes an excuse for not investigating the possibility that the clinician's withdrawal from the treatment is a function of the counter-transferential rage, terror, hate or boredom rather than a cool assessment of the patient's amenability to treatment' (Stein, 2011, p. 510). Indeed, as Glasser points out, the therapist may 'unwittingly be taking on the role of the neglectful caretakers in the violent patient's past' (Glasser, 1998).

Judith Butler, the American philosopher and gender theorist, suggests in her seminal feminist work Gender Trouble (Butler, 1990) that identity categories are not only descriptive but normative and exclusionary. Prison, by its very nature, is an exclusionary environment, and care should be taken not to exclude individuals further on the basis of their gender identity. Debbie Hayton, a transgender activist who views biological sex as unchangeable, but gender identity as variable, has suggested the importance of risk assessing transgender prisoners prior to placing them in the male or female estate based on their offending history rather than their gender identity. While she herself has not been through the criminal justice system, she asserts that if such circumstances arose, she would 'prefer to be assessed according to my risk profile than for my transgender status' (Hayton, 2019).

Nevertheless, there are many opposing views on this issue. The placement of transgender individuals in prison is complex and remains in contention as is highlighted by the work of the Prisoners' Advice Service (2021) who write that 'Transgender prisoners face a number of serious obstacles to being able to live in their acquired gender in prison. Whilst already struggling to come to terms with his, or her, own identity, being allocated to a prison which does not match his, or her, gender identity is the most traumatic'.

Clinical vignette: 'They Don't See Who I Really Am'

We now present a composite clinical vignette. This case is not based on a single individual but is formulated from a number of prisoners or residents in forensic institutions so as to preserve anonymity. It considers the complexity and impact that being incarcerated may have on individuals who do not conform to societal 'norms', specifically through their gender identity and personality traits.

Sacha was a mixed-race transwoman who had a long forensic history and had spent much of her adult life in prison, in the male estate, and in secure hospitals. Her offending included acquisitive crimes in the context of alcohol addiction, and importantly for this vignette, violent and sexual offences. Sacha had a GRC and was compliant with her hormone therapy.

Sacha would act out concretely and impulsively to perceived unfairness. She experienced feelings of external persecution and emotional isolation which left her highly distressed. The impact she seemed to have on the professionals working with her evoked a range of emotions, including sympathy and frustration, care, and fear, and left the team split in regard to what would 'work' to help her (Main, 1957). These might all have indicated that her history of trauma and resulting personality development was as significant in thinking about her safe progress through prison as her gender identity. It is also important to note that Sacha's feeling of being unseen, or misunderstood, may have related not only to her gender identity or any personality difficulties, but also to the reality of her being mixed race, and thus subject to additional discrimination within the institutional racism of the criminal justice system and wider society. These intersections of gender, mental health, and race must be kept in mind to ensure prisoners are not unduly pathologised.

To support Sacha, she was offered an art psychotherapy assessment, initially to understand if the making and discussion of visual art might offer a way of working with her that might feel less persecutory and provide a 'transitional space' (Winnicott, 1951) in which to explore her identity without a defined task. Art psychotherapy is a form of psychotherapy that recognises the use of art media as an important mode of communication (British Association of Art Therapists, 2021). In forensic settings, the overall aim of the treatment is to enable an individual to better understand the meaning of their offence and risk so as to support change and progress on a personal level through the use of art materials in a safe and challenging environment. One of the strengths of art psychotherapy is the way in which actual visual images emerge in the therapeutic relationship. These may offer insight into the unconscious elements of the patient's thinking, and, importantly, support them in recognising their own agency and identity.

In most populations, but perhaps in forensic populations especially, a frequently used defence mechanism to survive often traumatic life experiences is denial. The minimising of harm done to, or committed by, victims and perpetrators is common. Abusive partners and families are idealised so as to avoid the painful reality of abuse and neglect, and the experience of violence is regarded as a useful life lesson on the road to independence. In art psychotherapy, once an image has been created, it cannot be repudiated. Thus, perceptions that may arise from the work can only be denied if the image is destroyed, an action which may be thought about as concrete denial and/or offence paralleling. For Sacha, seeing different elements of her identity in the images she made may have helped challenge her perception – not one that was entirely unfounded – that 'others don't see who I really am'.

When Sacha and the art psychotherapist first met, Sacha was ambivalent. She felt she was not being listened to and said she would be lodging a complaint with her solicitor about the poor quality of care she felt she was receiving. An especially common response from individuals with personality disorder traits is to feel angry and disappointed, as the individual attempts to manage feelings of grief by transforming them into feelings of grievance (Taylor, 2012). Nevertheless, the art psychotherapist encouraged her to attend the next meeting and calmly returned as scheduled.

The following week, Sacha was ready to meet and made an abstract painting of an oblong shape that resembled a disconnected limb. Sacha had a long history of self-harm and would violently mutilate herself in response to feeling neglected or abused by those charged with her care. She would cut herself deeply and had once, when much younger and residing in a psychiatric intensive care unit, severed her arm at the elbow, causing permanent damage to the tendons and leaving a visible weakness.

This artwork seemed descriptive of Sacha's experience on many levels. On seeing Sacha's image, the art psychotherapist's first thought was of 'transgender broken arm syndrome' (Payton, 2015). This is a phenomenon whereby healthcare professionals conflate physical or mental health issues with an individual's gender identity, therefore assuming all medical problems are a consequence of being trans. 'You go in with a broken arm and they go, "But what about your hormones?"' (Savage, 2019). This propensity to focus on transgender people's gender identity as a risk factor, rather than trauma, offending history, and personality traits, which might be prioritised in the cis population, is discriminatory and may stem from the same social attitude that asserts that transgressing gender norms is of primary concern.

Sacha herself described the image as representing her isolation and self-harm in response to feeling misunderstood and unable to trust anyone. These feelings originated, Sacha said, from her childhood experience of being moved from foster home to foster home, where she was frequently sexually and emotionally abused, and eventually being discharged from the care system without any support. The image could also be understood as a metaphor for the emotional fragmentation that may be experienced by women in prison who have personality disorders arising from traumatic histories and manage through violent self-harm (Collier, 2015). The disconnected, limb-like, oblong, isolated on its own in the middle of the page, might also visually depict the pain, anger, and violence of Sacha's 'broken' internal experience.

During the sessions, Sacha made many paintings, including abstract self-portraits, using shapes and colours to depict what seemed like different 'parts' of her personality; as if evidencing her existence as a 'whole' yet fragmented person. The images were bold and bright, with very little detail on the foregrounded form, but many different, smaller shapes in the background. This prompted discussion about the chaos she had always felt surrounded by, the years of moving around the care system, and the possibility of hiding behind all the disorder. She gave all of these vibrant images away to staff and prisoners, as if symbolically enacting her childhood of being passed around. Sacha said she found the sessions useful as a means to express herself, and her image making, indirectly, led to a discussion about her use of self-harm and violence as related to her confused sense of identity as a child; leaving her feeling neglected and misunderstood – a pattern begun in the multiple foster homes and continually replicated in prison and in all her relationships.

Sacha spoke often about wanting to be accepted as a woman and how important this was for her. She wanted people to see how she felt inside and to 'see who I really am'. Sacha was distressed when people used the wrong pronouns. Indeed, it often seemed that the semantics of Sacha's preferred pronouns were imbued with unconscious, and conscious, prejudice as staff and peers would stumble or manifestly hesitate when calling Sacha 'she'. This carelessness, whether ill-intentioned or not, raised questions for the art psychotherapist about Sacha's own feelings about women and the sexual offences she had committed while identifying as male. If Sacha could not herself be accepted as a woman, perhaps she felt unconsciously compelled to destroy what is female by taking violent control of a woman and humiliating her? While this potential unconscious motivation for Sacha's violence against women could not be substantiated, and so was not explicitly discussed, it might be a helpful idea for clinicians to consider when thinking about the misogyny that is central to patriarchal societies and which Karen Horney formulated as 'womb envy' and its systemic consequences in her seminal paper, The Flight from Womanhood (Horney, 1926). Commonly, we are able to repudiate that which we cannot have through projective identification, unconsciously forcing our own feelings of hatred, vulnerability, and so on into those we identify with or envy. Theoretically then, we can hypothesise that if Sacha's personality structure allowed for less flexible and symbolic defences, her response might be to destroy what she envied, as well as want to be accepted as the very thing she wanted to annihilate.

Sacha was transferred to another prison in the female estate just a few months after beginning art psychotherapy. She had been assessed as a woman, and her risk was deemed acceptable for the location. Sacha was ecstatic, feeling she had at last been acknowledged as female by the prison authorities. Having used her image making to express ideas and stimulate conversations about the expectations she has had as a transwoman, mostly feeling disappointed and let down, she used the final meeting to reflect on how she felt about finally being 'heard'.

Sacha moved on after only twelve art psychotherapy sessions. Her final image showed her signature self-portrait, made from abstract, coloured shapes. This time, however, she had marked features on the central form, creating a face – and thus perhaps presenting a more defined identity; a recognisably human figure, looking directly out of the paper, confronting the viewer, prepared to be seen and accepted.

In the sessions, Sacha did not have time enough to think deeply about her feelings towards women and about being a woman herself. Instead, with only three months to work in art psychotherapy before she was transferred, she explored her sense of self in relation to how others see her. Initially disconnected and damaged, then hectic and distracted; and finally, a more identifiable depiction of an individual emerged. 'Images can hold and contain difficult contradictory emotions, feelings and actions that cannot always be described verbally' (Collier, 2015, p. 16). Given the importance of working through identity for any individual in distress, the opportunity art psychotherapy offers to focus on self-expression in a visual form suggests it is an especially promising intervention for transgender individuals exploring their identity.

Conclusion

It is evident that in order for transgender prisoners to be given equivalent care to the cis-gendered population within prisons and communities, a number of changes need to occur. Healthcare within the prison setting needs clear guidance around the roles and responsibilities of staff for the physical and psychological support of transgendered prisoners. Many of the needs identified by service users are likely to be the responsibility of the prison itself, but healthcare holds responsibility for the emotional support of transgender prisoners and needs to understand the requirements of staff, such as General Practitioners, in the essential pathway of care they have (GMC, 2020; RCGP, 2019). This is also likely to require additional funding and resources.

On an institutional level, all relevant prison and healthcare staff should hold a shared understanding of the policies, guidance, and pathways of care for transgender prisoners (NHS England, 2017; WPATH, 2012; DOH, 2008). Effective and transparent communication is essential, and staff should be encouraged to meet regularly, ideally in professional forums enabling quality assurance of care, and in regular reflexive groups, facilitated by informed professionals, where issues around unconscious bias and difficult emotional responses can be safely processed. Because of the difficulties of arranging and accessing appointments at GICs with existing prisoners, there is a clear need for additional funding for transgender specialists in forensic settings. This would include: access to a gender identity specialist clinician to give a diagnosis of gender dysphoria; plan the ongoing assessment process and address medication needs; a specialist counsellor or clinical psychologist to offer limited sessions for support around transgender related issues; improved access to the additional services offered by GICs; and importantly, access to emotional support for additional mental health or personality difficulties that may exist alongside issues relating directly to their gender identity. Keeping staff informed and aware will require ongoing training, covering the roles and responsibilities of professionals and an improved understanding of transgender-specific requirements, including the wider social context and how this may impact relationships and attitudes within the prison. This should be organised in collaboration with service users so their voices and opinions are heard, and to ensure that consultations are not superficial exercises designed, consciously or unconsciously, to satisfy the institution's mandatory diversity training requirements.

In conclusion, the provision of safe and impartial care for prisoners who identify as transgender is a complex area involving physical, practical, sociological, and psychological considerations. Support for this group will require ongoing audits, reviews, education, and experiential learning. As described earlier, transgender identity covers a wide diversity of human experience, and healthcare teams aiming to provide good quality care must also reflect this continuum of difference and knowledge. It is essential when working with marginalisation and difference that multi-disciplinary teams working with individuals should be just that: genuinely diverse collections of professions and people who can offer a number of divergent perspectives supporting change and progress and incorporating multiple views, ranging from psychiatry, psychology, psychotherapy, and arts psychotherapies to probation, prison staff, and service users.

In this chapter, we aimed to demonstrate that different points of view, professional and lived experience, and the acknowledgement of sometimes opposing ideas can result in cohesive and multifaceted consensus. We hope to see these attitudes integrated into the treatment of prisoners who identify as transgender in the future and, in doing so, offer humane and non-prejudicial care.

References

Abraham, A. (2019). *What's it like to be trans in the UK prison system?* www.dazeddigital.com/life-culture/article/46703/1/what-its-like-to-be-transgender-in-the-uk-prison-system

American Psychiatric Association. (2015). Guidelines for psychological practice with transgender and gender non conforming people. *American Psychologist*, 832–864.

Barker, J. M. (2017). *BACP good practice: Gender, sexual, and relationship diversity (GSRD).* British Association for Counselling and Psychotherapy.

Bashford, J., Hasan, S., Marriott, C., & Patel, P. (2018). *Inside gender identity.* Quality Network for Prison Mental Health Services. www.ciellp.net/inside-gender-identity

BBC. (2019). *Transgender hate crimes recorded by police go up 81%.* BBC News. https://www.bbc.co.uk/news/av/uk-england-48785711

British Association of Art Therapists. (2021). www.baat.org.

Butler, J. (1990). *Gender Trouble.* Routledge.

Collier, J. (2015). 3 Man unlock: Out of sight, out of mind: Art psychotherapy with a woman with severe and dangerous personality disorder in prison: *Psychoanalytic Psychotherapy, 29*(3), 243–261.

Fossey, M., & Black, G. (2010). *Under the radar: Women with borderline personality disorder in prison.* Centre for Mental Health. www.ohrn.nhs.uk/resource/policy/UndertheRadar.pdf

GMC. (2020). *Advice for doctors supporting transgender patients.* General Medical Council. www.gmc-uk.org/news/26555.asp

General Medical Council. (2020). *Prescribing guidance.* www.gmc-uk.org/guidance/ethical_guidance/28859.asp

Glasser, M. (1998). On violence: A preliminary communication. *International Journal of Psychoanalysis, 79,* 887–902.

Government Equalities Office. (2018). *Trans people in the UK.* Retrieved January 11, 2021, from https://assets.publishing.service.gov.uk/government/uploads/system/uploads/attachment_data/file/721642/GEO-LGBT-factsheet.pdf

Guidance for GPs, other clinicians and health professionals on the care of gender variant people. (2008). Transgender wellbeing and healthcare: Department of Health NHS.

Guide to consultation: Specialised gender identity services for adults. Specialised commissioning, NHS England. 2017.

Hay, C. (2019). Who counts as a woman? *The New York Times.* www.nytimes.com/2019/04/01/opinion/trans-women-feminism.html

Hayton, D. (2019). Are transgender prison wings the answer? *Centre for crime and justice studies.* www.crimeandjustice.org.uk/resources/are-transgender-prison-wings-answer

Hinshelwood, R. D. (2002). Abusive help—helping abuse: The psychodynamic impact of severe personality disorder on caring institutions. *Criminal Behaviour and Mental Health, 12*(S2), S20–S30.

HMPPS. (2020). *The care and management of individuals who are transgender.* Her Majesty's Prison and Probation Service.

Horney, K. (1926). The flight from womanhood: The masculinity-complex in women, as viewed by men and by women. *International Journal of Psycho-Analysis, 7,* 324–339.

Howard League for Penal Reform. (2014). *Coercive sex in prison. Briefing Paper 3.* Howard League for Penal Reform. https://howardleague.org/wp-content/uploads/2016/03/Coercive-sex-in-prison.pdf

Kahr, B. (2020). *Dangerous lunatics: Trauma, criminality and forensic psychotherapy.* Confer Books.

Lemma, A. (2018). Trans-itory identities: Some psychoanalytic reflections on transgender identities. *The International Journal of Psychoanalysis, 99*(5), 1089–1106.

Main, T. (1957). The ailment. *The British Journal of Medical Psychology, 39*(2), 129–145.

MoJ. (2018). *Her majesty's prison and probation service offender equalities annual report 2017/18.* Ministry of Justice.

Payton, N. (2015). Feature: The dangers of trans broken arm syndrome. *Pink News.* www.pinknews. co.uk/2015/07/09/feature-the-dangers-of-trans-broken-arm-syndrome/

Prison Reform Trust. (2017). *Why focus on reducing women's imprisonment?* www.prisonreformtrust.org.uk/ Portals/0/Documents/Women/whywomen.pdf

Prison Reform Trust. (2021). *Bromley briefings prison factfile Winter 2021.* www.prisonreformtrust.org.uk/ Portals/0/Documents/Bromley%20Briefings/Winter%202021%20Factfile%20final.pdf

Prison Service Instructions. (2017/2020). *Review on the care and management of transgender offenders.* Policy and guidance for prison and probation professionals in England and Wales. Her Majesty's Prison and Probation Service and Ministry of Justice.

Prisoners' Advice Service. (2021). *Prisoners who are LGBT+.* Retrieved January 10, 2021, from www.prison ersadvice.org.uk/information/prisoners-who-are-lgbt/

Reichl, C., & Kaess, M. (2021). Self-harm in the context of borderline personality disorder. *Current Opinion in Psychology, 37,* 139–144. https://boris.unibe.ch/153008/1/1-s2.0-S2352250X21000014-main.pdf

Royal College of General Practitioners. (2019). www.rcgp.org.uk/policy/rcgp-policy-areas/transgender-care.aspx

Savage, R. (2019). British government accused of 'mishandling' trans healthcare. *Reuters.* https://uk.reuters. com/article/us-britain-lgbt-health/british-government-accused-of-mishandling-trans-healthcare-idUSKCN1OX1LY

Shaw, D. (2020). Eleven transgender inmates sexually assaulted in male prisons last year. *BBC News.* Published May 21, 2020. Https://www.bbc.co.uk/news/uk-52748117

Solnit, R. (2020). Trans women pose no threat to cis women, but we pose a threat to them if we make them outcasts. *The Guardian.* www.theguardian.com/commentisfree/2020/aug/10/trans-rights-feminist-letter-rebecca-solnit

Standards of Care for the Health of Transsexual, Transgender, and Gender-Nonconforming People. The World Professional Association for Transgender Health. Version 7.2012. WPATH guidelines. www.wpath. org/publications/soc

Starchild, A. (1990). Rape of youth in prisons and juvenile facilities. *Journal of Psychohistory, 18,* 145–150.

Stein, A. (2011). The sex monster: Dissociation as parallel process in the response to sex offenders. *Contemporary Psychoanalysis, 47*(4).

Taylor, C. (2012). Complaints as a tool for bullying. In J. Adlam, A. Aiyegbusi, & P. Kleinot (Eds.), *The therapeutic milieu under fire: Security and insecurity in forensic mental health.* Jessica Kingsley Publishers.

United Nations General Assembly. (2001). Fifty-sixth session item 132(a): Report of the Special Rapporteur on the question of torture and other cruel, inhuman or degrading treatment or punishment, 3 July 2001, A/56/156, para.23. United Nations. www.un.org/documents/ga/docs/56/a56156.pdf

Valentine, D. (2007). *Imagining transgender: An ethnography of a category.* Duke Press.

Widom, C. S. (1989). The cycle of violence. *Science* (80), 244, 160–166.

Winnicott, D. W. (1951). Transitional objects and transitional phenomena in collected papers: Through paediatrics to psycho-analysis (1984) (pp. 229–242). Karnac.

Chapter 5

Children in custody

The context and impact of incarceration

*Celia Sadie, Clare Holt, Andrez Harriott,
Sophie D'Souza, and Javel Watt*

Introduction

This chapter describes youth custody in England and Wales, examining what it means to spend crucially formative periods of your life incarcerated, and goes on to explore reforms and developments. We write this chapter from perspectives of lived experience: one author having been incarcerated for several years of his adolescence, and others, as practitioners and researchers. While we cannot eliminate our blind spots or unconscious biases, our intention, by co-writing as a diverse group, is to open respectful, informed, and useful discussions that illuminate a deeper understanding of youth custody and mental health. In becoming aware of the ways in which custody affects and marginalises children, readers might be better placed to support its transformation.

Locating incarcerated young people at the centre of the discussion, we take an exploratory perspective on the concept, ethics, operation, and value of imprisoning children. We draw attention to paradoxes and injustices and explore ways in which incarceration inevitably affects individual development. At the same time, we acknowledge the enormous efforts of many of those working within these systems to do good and provide effective care. We highlight the complex challenges of doing good in the context of powerful social, political, and psychological factors implicated in the protection of the public and the 'reform' or 'rehabilitation' of children and adolescents who have done harm. Furthermore, we discuss race and crime within the youth justice system, issues of labelling, and the use of language and acknowledge the lag in responsiveness to their needs among academics, practitioners, and services.

Our focus is on boys (aged 12–18), given their predominance in these settings, but this in no way detracts from the obvious truth that incarcerated girls' developmental vulnerabilities and needs also deserve space and exploration (see Goodfellow, 2017).

The secure system

The secure youth estate in the United Kingdom has struggled, from its inception, to reconcile the competing objectives of a system expected both to *punish* and *care* for children who break the law. The 20th-century penal project has included the establishment of approved schools, reformatories, detention centres, young offender institutions, youth custody centres, and the 'borstal'. The Crime and Prevention Act 1908 recognised the differences in the needs of children and adults by diverting children to borstals instead of prisons. As the penal system responded to changing social perceptions of youth and criminality, borstals became Youth Custody Centres and were later incorporated into a wider network of Young Offenders' Institutions (YOIs).

DOI: 10.4324/9781003184768-7

The three legal frameworks used to detain children in England and Wales are the Mental Health Act 1983 (as amended in 2007), which can place them in a psychiatric hospital; s. 25 of the Children Act 1989, which can place them in a Secure Children's Home (SCH); or under the youth justice system, on remand or serving a sentence, in an SCH, Secure Training Centre (STC), or a YOI (Hales et al., 2016).

The response to children who break the law shifted significantly during the early 1990s following high profile cases, notably the killing of James Bulger by two 10-year-old boys, and rising public concerns around youths involved in anti-social behaviour. The establishment of the current youth justice system in 1998 sought to provide a strategic response that would check and resolve youth crime with swift and coordinated action. The Crime and Disorder Act 1998 required all local authorities to provide localised multidisciplinary teams including at least one youth justice specialist, a police officer, a social worker, an education officer, a probation officer, and a clinician. These various professionals had historically fulfilled disparate roles but were now encouraged to work in partnership within a Youth Offending Team (Ministry of Justice, 2018).

Current secure provisions for children in England and Wales include 60 secure hospitals (a mixture of high dependency units, psychiatric intensive care units, and low-and medium-secure units) and 19 SCHs, small facilities (ranging between seven and 38 beds), with the highest staff to child ratios. They accommodate children aged 10–17, including girls, and children with identified emotional and neurodevelopmental difficulties.

Only one of the three STCs remains open at the time of writing. STCs, run by private sector organisations, were built to accommodate between 60 and 80 boys and girls aged 12–17, with lower staff-to-child ratios than SCHs. In recent years, two have been closed due to safeguarding and operational failings. There are four YOIs in England, three in Scotland, and one, which is held by the private sector, in Wales. With the lowest staff-to-child ratios, the YOIs accommodate boys aged 15–18, holding between 118 and 336 children. Between 2018 and 2019, 73% of children in custody were housed within YOIs, 17% in STCs, and 10% in SCHs (Beard, 2020). The current youth justice system has remained in this form for more than two decades.

Who are the children in custody and why are they there?

Between April 2018 and March 2019, there were, on average, 859 children in custody, in England and Wales. Compared with the statistics for 2008–9, this reflects a 70% reduction over ten years (YJB, 2011). This was further reduced during the COVID-19 pandemic, with 554 children in youth custody settings in June 2021 (YCS, 2021). Ninety-seven per cent of children in custody in the United Kingdom are boys, and while theoretically children as young as 10 could be placed in custody,[1] 95% are 15–17. Of those, 28% are on remand (awaiting sentencing) and 72% are serving sentences or have been recalled for breaching the terms of licences in the community (YJB, 2020).

Children in custody are increasingly there on remand for, or sentenced for, violent offences. In the year ending March 2019, this group of offences accounted for 51% of the youth custody population. A growing proportion is children serving 'life' sentences for murder. English law maintains that children aged 10 and over can be held responsible for criminal behaviour (the lowest threshold in Europe), a harmful anachronistic assumption of adult capacities that ignores the reality of immature adolescent neurobiology, leading to the highest number of 'child lifers' in Europe, where 22 out of 28 countries have abolished life imprisonment for children (Scott, 2017). Discouragingly, the average minimum tariff for mandatory life sentences also continues to rise, from 12.5 years in 2003 to 21.1 years in 2013 (Crewe et al.,

2020). These children face profound 'biographical ruptures', undergoing a deep existential shock (ibid., p. 17) in the face of detention, possibly, for life.

The narrowing population of children in custody are, unsurprisingly, more likely to present with high-risk behaviours and high levels of harm to self and others. Almost without exception, children placed in custody have experienced multiple forms of disadvantage and needs that span many domains (Harrington et al., 2005). They are more likely to have experienced social and school exclusion and poverty (Paton et al., 2009), to have been designated a Child in Need,[2] exposed to high levels of childhood maltreatment (Moore et al., 2013) and intergenerational experiences of violence. Looked-after children are over-represented in custody, and three-quarters have lived with someone other than a parent (Healthcare Commission, 2007). Given this context of instability and fractured care in their early years, children in contact with the youth justice system are three times more likely to show mental health difficulties than their non-offending peers, particularly depressive difficulties and PTSD (Day et al., 2008; Erwin et al., 2000). Learning, neurodevelopmental, and speech and language difficulties are highly prevalent (Hughes & Chitsabesan, 2015). These labels, despite their uses, inadequately represent the complex consequences of multiple and interacting forms of adversity. What we see, in practice, are children who have adapted to systems that precariously situate them in high-risk conditions, showing unmet needs that custodial environments are not designed to address.

Children of colour in the youth justice system

Despite the overall reduction in numbers, children of colour are increasingly overrepresented. In the year ending March 2019, Black children were four times as likely to be arrested than White children (YJB, 2020). Current data indicate that 51.9% of children in custody are from 'BAME' groups (YJB, 2020), up from 14% in 2009–10, in contrast to their making up only 18% of the general population in this age group (YJB, 2011). While the number of children who are first-time entrants to custody (FTEs) from a Black background has decreased since 2009, the proportion they comprise of all child FTEs has doubled, from 8% to 16%. The disproportionate numbers of incarcerated children from non-dominant ethnic groups have continued to rise steadily in recent years despite the recommendations Member of Parliament David Lammy (2017) and his forerunners made for identifying and reducing the operation of systemic racism in the criminal justice system. Once in custody, 'BAME' children are less likely than White children to be recorded as having health, educational or mental health problems, suggesting unidentified and therefore unmet needs (Lammy, 2017). White children are more likely to be assessed as having mental health concerns (75%, compared with Asian 50%, Black 57%, Mixed 70%, and Other 65%), while Black children are assessed as being at a comparatively high or very high risk of serious harm (White 29.9%, Asian 33.1%, Black 50.4%, Mixed 38.6%, and Other 35.6%) (YJB, 2021, p. 21). It is vital that we interrogate how Black children are held in mind in these systems, and whether the mental health assessments, services, and behavioural change interventions currently provided address their needs.

Black children in the youth justice system suffer the impact of limitations in knowledge surrounding their lived experiences and are criminalised by a system that decontextualises them and sees them as culpable in their exploitation (Firmin, 2020). Glynn (2014) suggests that in custody, Black males' experiences are underpinned by a sense of their own invisibility in oppressive, predominantly White-governed systems that appear 'colour-blind', unable to recognise and validate Black experiences, tending to adultify and demonise them as undeserving (Fasching-Varner et al., 2014). Under such pressures, Black people may construct a code of silence as a way of protecting themselves from harm. Indeed, it is our experience that Black boys can be extremely cautious in relation to statutory services and practitioners, drawing on personal experiences of racism, brutality, and intergenerational messaging.

Box 1   Kai – A case study

'Kai' is a 16-year-old boy whose father is Black Caribbean and whose mother is White British. He grew up in south London but has spent much of his adolescence in care placements, and two periods in STCs, serving short sentences for possession of Class A drugs and of bladed articles. He is currently serving a sentence for GBH (Grievous Bodily Harm). Kai's mother was 15 when he was born and has been in a series of abusive relationships. Between them, she and his father have 12 children and Kai feels he has always had either to fight for attention or to fend for himself. Kai's older brother is serving a life sentence for murder. When Kai was 11, he was taken into care and placed in a foster placement in Suffolk. He had experienced racism at school in London but living with a White family who were unfamiliar with his culture, in a predominantly White community, it took on a new character, and he felt alienated. He was lonely, angry, and missed his mother and siblings. Kai ran away repeatedly, and his links with peers from his local area in London were strengthened. He became involved in 'county lines' drug dealing and witnessed adults using drugs, physical and sexual violence, and sometimes had nowhere to stay and slept rough. He was frequently stopped and searched, arrested, and moved between placements. Kai developed a tough, monosyllabic manner with adults, masking his vulnerability and sadness. Two of his close friends were murdered, and Kai witnessed one of the deaths. In custody, Kai is playful and warm with his peers and shows talent in maths and in music production, where he expresses himself lyrically. With staff, he is involved in frequent altercations and experiences authority as threatening and oppressive, an experience reinforced by frequent sanctions. He attends offending behaviour programmes when offered but says he 'knows this stuff and none of it makes any difference'.

What is it like in custody?

The process for allocating children to a custodial placement is governed by the Youth Custody Service (YCS) which uses particular criteria to determine where a child should live, including age, perceived level of 'risk' and 'vulnerability', and past presentation in custody. Most children in custody in the United Kingdom are in YOIs (74%, according to the most recent census; Hales et al., 2016); hence, much of the following depicts most closely the experiences of boys in YOIs. The reader is reminded that the following description primarily refers to a child's experience at a fairly typical YOI in 2020.

Leaving court, the child, alongside adult prisoners, is transported in prison vans, to the designated secure setting. The vans are subdivided into locked cubicles; seats are made of hard plastic, with no seatbelts, and the child must brace himself to stay seated. They can be in these vans for many hours, as they tour several prisons dropping people off. There are no toilets, so the child is given a bag to urinate into. When he arrives, he is assessed in the YOI reception and asked a series of questions about his health and any risks he may pose to himself or others. He is told to undress, in the presence of prison officers, and is searched, including sitting in a 'BOSS' (body orifice security scanner) chair. He exchanges his belongings for prison clothes.

The boy is then taken to the Induction unit, where he is locked in a single cell which may include a built-in shower as well as a toilet and sink. Apart from a chair, furniture (a bed frame and a desk), is nailed down. There is a barred window that opens slightly, and usually a telephone and a TV, a light, and a cell bell for alerting officers in case of emergency. The walls are sometimes freshly painted but are often covered in graffiti, some of which may be frightening or violent. The child is given £2 credit to use via a pin on his cell landline phone, to pre-authorised numbers, and can call various organisations for free (e.g., Childline, Barnardo's, and The Howard League). Typically, he will be surrounded by loud noise, such as shouting and banging on doors as he arrives, continuing overnight and beyond. Clanking metal doors, jangling keys, and other cell bells may be constant.

During the following week, he is locked in his cell between approximately 7 pm and 8 am, though often from earlier (4.30 pm) if there are too few staff. He will have time out of his cell for fresh air (45 minutes minimum per day), meetings, and initial assessments. Once his induction period finishes and he is moved to an ordinary landing (wing or unit), he will attend Education for up to 27 hours a week. Staffing levels permitting, he may also have time out of his cell 'on association' (with other children), 'dining out' (eating communally), on 'exercise' (in what is usually a concrete yard, overlooked by cells), or visiting the gym or sports pitches. He may also attend offending behaviour programmes (usually, manualised cognitive-behavioural group courses), 1:1 or small group sessions with mental health professionals, youth workers, or other agencies.

He can make calls to authorised numbers for 20 minutes at a time, four times a day, at a far greater cost than in the community. He can buy phone credit, food, and toiletries weekly, paying with money sent into his prison account, and will order meals a week in advance from a small selection. During his time in custody, he will have regular meetings with a Caseworker (often a prison officer), who liaises with his family and external agencies regarding his welfare, his sentence plan, and release arrangements. As he nears release, he may be able to leave the prison on 'ROTL' (Release On Temporary Licence). He may be strip-searched, on his return. Sometimes, his cell will be 'spun' – searched thoroughly, often without regard for how he has arranged his few possessions, if he is suspected of making weapons, taking drugs, or keeping a mobile phone. He may see authorised relatives or friends in small groups, as often as weekly, once he is sentenced. This will take place in a communal setting, for up to two hours. Physical contact is prevented, beyond a brief hug.

Contact with other children is highly restricted, with the child placed on a given landing in the context of known gang associations or enmities, balanced with the availability of space. He may only be escorted around the site alone or with others thought to be unlikely to fight with him. Fights take place daily, sometimes several times a day, and are broken up by officers trained in restraint techniques, once a requisite number of staff have been summoned by means of a prison-wide alarm system. He will never be alone with another child, or anywhere he cannot be watched.

Maturity, selfhood, self-regulation, and interactions with others

Psychological maturity can be understood as an intermittent state, developing throughout the whole lifespan, which becomes evident in the capacity to face reality (Stokoe, 2020). Dmitrieva et al. (2012) describe the development of key aspects of adolescent maturity, 'temperance', 'perspective', and 'responsibility', all of which require a safe and facilitative environment for their development and stability. Loving, protective relationships in which the child is understood to be a child, and therefore in the midst of a developmental process, are essential. Maturation, furthermore, depends on rich and varied learning experiences attuned to the child's level of development, fostering his or her potential (what Vygotsky, 1978 called the 'zone of proximal development', p86). These opportunities are obstructed by the conditions of custody, through limiting experiences and relationships, disrupting sources of stability, and generating states of mind in which a child cannot develop. In their longitudinal study of adolescent development across a range of secure facilities, Dmitrieva et al. (2012) noted that the development of psychological maturity was particularly disrupted among those completing short sentences, though they found differential effects across settings and for varying lengths of time in custody. Notably, they found that children who perceived their settings as 'unsafe' became less able to curb impulsive and aggressive behaviour. As Crewe et al. (2020, p. 307) suggest, incarceration likely fosters a kind of 'contextual' maturity, enabling survival in relation to the demands of prison, but not necessarily beyond its walls.

The concept of 'biographical rupture' (Crewe et al., 2020) provides a valuable way of understanding the impact of incarceration on one's sense of self in youth. We often notice that children in custody lack a coherent narrative of their life experiences; but beyond this, it is clear that incarceration – particularly when it is long-term, or indeterminate – poses an overwhelming ontological threat: *Who am I, if this is happening? Who can I be, now? What happens to my relationships, my hopes and plans?* As Gooch (2019, p. 81) points out, 'juvenile prisoners . . . by virtue of the Children Act 1989, are still children, but are held within a very "adult" prison environment where they are defined first and foremost as a "prisoner"'. The various agencies working within these settings may also have divergent ideas about what they are there to do, and their success may be measured by metrics that directly conflict with each other's operation (e.g., number of hours in educational provision vs. number of contacts with mental health providers). Each organisation and its members will be responding to underlying anxieties in relation to the task (i.e., *Will I be hurt, or destroyed, in the course of my work? Will I be unable to change these children's lives?*) and acting accordingly. The design and architecture of the setting exert a powerful unconscious influence over behaviour (Hancock & Jewkes, 2011), privileging some activities, making others impossible, creating a sense of safety and hope, or bleakness, deprivation, neglect, and oppression. The children and staff exist in a social ecology in which rapidly shifting political narratives and media representations of prison, and of children who commit criminal acts, and their expression in the funding, initiatives, evaluation, and governance, profoundly shape how the tasks of custody are conceptualised and enacted.

This apparent battle of priorities and ownership is mirrored in the adolescent child's own internal process as they negotiate rapid biopsychosocial change. Adolescence has been defined as the process of taking possession of the adult sexual body (Laufer, 1975). This requires a series of often painful adjustments. Opportunities for children to ask adults they trust about what is happening to them, physically, or about sexual relationships, are severely limited in custodial settings (Howard League, 2006). Questioning and experimenting run the risk of public ridicule or a pathologising or punitive response from staff or peers. Being denied the opportunity to work through adolescent sexual anxieties and maturation through having sexual experiences is likely to damage and inhibit development (Steinberg et al., 2004). In their 2015 report, the Howard League suggests that experiencing deprivation and victimisation in custody in adolescence might raise the risk of later sexual violence, given research on heightened levels of adult sexual offending among those exposed to physical violence in childhood.

Opportunities for learning to tolerate and make sense of difficult feelings and experiences are more limited than they would be in the community. The pull of the peer group acquires immense power and meaning during this period. We might suggest that optimal conditions might include a wide variety of female and male peers, access to many forms of cultural stimulation and activity, and prosocial parental, caregiving, or educational oversight. Incarceration, in contrast, places 'remarkable limits on emotional and experiential possibilities' (Crewe et al., 2020). Crewe (2011) describes the 'tightness' of the custodial environment as a way in which the power of the prison might 'wrap them up, smother them and incite them to conduct themselves in particular ways' (p. 522). Given the search for identity and certainty characteristic of adolescence, we should not be surprised that gang affiliations flourish in prison settings and that radicalisation is a serious concern (Campelo et al., 2018). Peer relationships provide the means, alongside adult guidance, of developing social maturity and an increasingly coherent and conscious sense of identity but are difficult to establish without privacy or the freedom to associate with each other under the ever-present possibility of being 'shipped' (transferred to another prison) or moved cell or wing. Activities with peers are more limited in scope and variety than in the community and lack the freedom to enable play, creativity, spontaneity, or joint action: one compelling source of excitement and catharsis remains the ever-present possibility of a fight between themselves or with custodial staff.

Relationships with authority figures – prison officers, teachers, psychologists, and other professionals – assume particular significance in the absence of parents. These operate within systems of responsibility and activity that define their obligations and the character of their relationships. The freedom to access multiple people, to choose from a range of role models, confidants, sources of help, activities, or to have a choice about how and when you make those contacts, is vastly reduced. Furthermore, despite their best intentions, all those working in these environments are identifiable, to young people within them, as part of these systems; if not actively collusive, nevertheless complicit with the process of their incarceration.

Reform in youth custody

In England, there is a major move to change the culture and practices of secure settings for children, reinforced by the wider promotion of trauma-informed care across health and justice settings, and the evidence-based 'Child First' approach (Case & Browning, 2021). A new framework for integrated care, SECURE STAIRS (an acronym summarising a set of principles for trauma-informed, evidence-based, whole-system, relational practice), is being implemented across the youth secure estate (KPMG, 2016). Funding is increased, to expand mental health and custodial staffing and support systemic change. Collaborative formulations, in which children are given support to voice their own narratives of their life experiences, alongside key members of staff who know them well, are a cornerstone of the framework. Training introduces the idea that officers can provide a form of therapeutic parenting (Rose, 2014; Taylor et al., 2018), built on the principle that all behaviour is relational, has meaning, and deserves to be understood. This is difficult: for the most part, children are in custody against their will and often approach staff with hostility and suspicion (Gormally & Deuchar, 2012; Howerton et al., 2007). In turn, staff (often, themselves, traumatised through the experience of the work) may have developed ways of coping that involve distancing themselves from children and their stories (Bloom, 2010).

SECURE STAIRS involves supporting staff, through regular 1:1 supervisory meetings and group reflective practice, to make sense of children's behaviour through attending to the impact it has on them individually, within teams, and organisationally (Sadie & Stokoe, 2020). The framework aims to develop and sustain a culture of benign enquiry throughout the hierarchies of these establishments, encouraging staff at all levels to welcome the expression of anxiety as a source of information about the work, approaching problems and difficulties with curiosity and a willingness to adapt, and nurturing opportunities for reflective discussion. Outcomes are broadly defined, including reducing violence and distress among children, staff sickness and burnout, and, ultimately, reoffending and further harm to the public and cost to the system. An independent evaluation of the SECURE STAIRS Framework runs until 2021 (D'Souza et al., 2021). Complementary youth justice reforms include the expansion of enrichment and educational activities, the professionalisation of the workforce by means of a funded foundation degree in Youth Justice, the creation of specialist Youth Justice Worker posts, and training and support for officers to provide 1:1 guidance informed by motivational interviewing techniques (Rollnick & Miller, 1995).

Beyond SECURE STAIRS, the inception of the first 'Secure School', due to open in 2023, marks the culmination of the recommendations of the 2016 Taylor Review, a report commissioned by the UK government in the context of widespread acknowledgement of the failings of the existing youth custody estate. Lord Taylor was starkly critical of the state of the youth secure estate and proposed an alternative: small, therapeutic residential schools, geographically spread, offering a richer and more individualised form of care. The first, 'Oasis Restore', aims to offer the least restrictive and most aspirational environment possible, designed with the needs and choices of children in mind, drawing on research in adolescent neurobiology and psychology, and best practice in education and health settings. The operating model, in development at the time of writing, is intended to reflect an ethos of 'relentless love' (Chalke, 2020) whereby difficulty and challenge will be expected and embraced by a reflective system that can hold the child in mind and continue to provide care and containment under pressure, while simultaneously working with families, local communities, and agencies towards wider system change.

Sustainable alternatives to incarceration are difficult to envisage but remain a worthy goal. However, well-intentioned, efforts to reform the youth custody estate may only reinforce its continuing existence, making conditions more palatable and diverting attention from systemic injustices. There are numerous examples internationally of predominantly welfare-based and less punitive systems (such as those in Spain, Germany, the Netherlands, Croatia, and Scandinavia) that house and care for children who would, in the United Kingdom, be criminalised.

Conclusion

The history of youth custody in England and Wales reflects changing social and political trends in how we conceptualise children, criminality, and rehabilitation. In recent years, we have seen a disturbing trend towards longer sentences, and the increasing criminalisation and oppression of children of colour. While efforts to reduce the number of children in custody have shown success, the conditions inside, and high rates of recidivism on release, have continued to raise concern. It is too early to tell whether SECURE STAIRS and similar attempts to develop therapeutic conditions can overcome systemic resistance to change, and Secure Schools will need to be freed from the strictures of the systems that have gone before them in order to provide something genuinely different and effective.

Children do not choose to enter into custody, although some see it as an inevitable part of their future life story. Nevertheless, few, if any enter with their own 'rehabilitation' as a goal, but more, perhaps, with the hope that they will survive intact and avoid harm. Establishments designed to care for them must acknowledge this fundamental disjuncture between the 'task' of their inhabitants and the tasks defined by their carers and find some common ground through the development of genuine, trusting relationships. Before this can happen, however, the onus is on the carers, and the stakeholders they represent, to resolve the splits and clashes between them if a common goal – humane, developmentally sensitive, culturally meaningful care, in as free and stimulating an environment as possible – can be realised. Here, we come up against the fundamental issue: the love, hate, and indifference we feel as a society for children who do harm or break rules. Until we reach some consensus as a society around our moral obligations, our hopes for 'offenders' and the means by which we intend to achieve them, the various players within these systems will continue to carry the weight of what society projects onto them, and any attempt to make progress will be wrecked by this conflict.

Finally, those working at the level of policy in these systems must urgently consider the impact of interrupting children's developmental trajectories with the imposition of custody: 'at a time when adolescents require experiences that promote the development of responsible autonomy and competent interpersonal relationships . . . current methods of punishment, such as incarceration in a secure facility, all but preclude the facilitation of psychosocial development' (Steinberg et al., 2004, p. 7). Emerging interventions, based on what we now know about neurological and psychosocial development in adolescence, bring some hope to the work with children in custody, particularly where they create organisational change. Their success will be limited by the constraints of the environments in which they are embedded and the systems with which they interact, which in turn are determined by the values that inform policy and funding at the highest levels. While the systems are different, there is much we can learn from international models. Instilling a culture and system which actively diverts children from custody into social welfare (Storgaard, 2005) brings up different challenges but signifies a set of values to which the United Kingdom could aspire. Fundamentally, we must ask ourselves, and our leaders, what we hope to achieve by incarcerating children.

Notes

1. The minimum age of criminal responsibility in England and Wales is 10 years.
2. Under s.17 of the Children's Act (1989), a Child in Need is defined as a child who is unlikely to achieve or maintain a reasonable level of health or development, or whose health and development is likely to be significantly or further impaired, without the provision of services from the Local Authority, or who has a disability.

References

Beard, J. (2020). *Youth custody*. House of Commons Library Briefing Paper no 8557.

Bloom, S. L. (2010). Trauma-organized systems and parallel process. *Managing Trauma in the Workplace – Supporting Workers and the Organisation*, 139–153.

Campelo, N., Oppetit, A., Neau, F., Cohen, D., & Bronsard, G. (2018). Who are the European youths willing to engage in radicalisation? A multidisciplinary review of their psychological and social profiles. *European Psychiatry: The Journal of the Association of European Psychiatrists*, *52*, 1–14. https://doi.org/10.1016/j.eurpsy.2018.03.001

Case, S., & Browning, A. (2021). *Child first justice: The research evidence-base [Full report]* (Version 1). Loughborough University. https://hdl.handle.net/2134/14152040.v1 ([])

Chalke, S. (2020, December 7). *Relentless Love – the soft option?* Presentation at the Royal College of Psychiatry Adolescent Forensic Psychiatry Special Interest Group Conference, Minimum Age of Criminal Responsibility.

Crewe, B. (2011). Depth, weight, tightness: Revisiting the pains of imprisonment. *Punishment & Society*, *13*(5), 509–529.

Crewe, B., Hulley, S., & Wright, S. (2020). *Life imprisonment from young adulthood*. Palgrave Macmillan.

Day, C., Hibbert, P., & Cadman, S. (2008). *A literature review into children abused and/or neglected prior custody*. Youth Justice Board.

Dmitrieva, J., Monahan, K. C., Cauffman, E., & Steinberg, L. (2012). Arrested development: The effects of incarceration on the development of maturity. *Development and Psychopathology*, *24*(3), 1073–1090. doi:10.1017/S0954579412000545

D'Souza, S., Lane, R., Jacob, J., Livanou, M., Riches, W., Rogers, A., . . . Edbrooke-Childs, J. (2021). Realist process evaluation of the implementation and impact of an organisational cultural transformation programme in the children and young people's secure estate (CYPSE) in England: Study protocol. *BMJ Open*, *11*(5), e045680.

Erwin, B. A., Newman, E., McMackin, R. A., Morrissey, C., & Kaloupek, D. G. (2000). PTSD, malevolent environment, and criminality among criminally involved male adolescents. *Criminal Justice and Behavior*, *27*(2), 196–215.

Fasching-Varner, K., Reynolds, R., Albert, K., & Martin, L. (2014). *Trayvon Martin, race, and American justice*. Sense.

Firmin, C. (2020). Contextual Safeguarding and Child Protection. Routledge.

Glynn, M. (2014). *Black men, invisibility, and desistance from crime: Towards a critical race theory from crime.* Routledge.

Gooch, K. (2019). 'Kidulthood': Ethnography, juvenile prison violence and the transition from boys to men. *Criminology & Criminal Justice, 19*(1), 80–97.

Goodfellow, P. (2017). Outnumbered, locked up and over-looked? *The Griffins Society.* www.thegriffinssociety.org/outnumbered-locked-and-overlooked-use-penal-custody-girls-england-wales

Gormally, S., & Deuchar, R. (2012). Somewhere between distrust and dependence: Young people, the police and anti-social behaviour management within marginalised communities. *International Journal on School Disaffection, 9*(1).

Hales, H., Warner, L., Smith, J., & Bartlett, A. (2016). *Census of young people in secure settings on 14 September 2016: Characteristics, needs and pathways of care.* NHS. www.england.nhs.uk/publication/secure-settings-for-young-people-a-national-scoping-exercise/

Hancock, P., & Jewkes, Y. (2011). Architectures of incarceration: The spatial pains of imprisonment. *Punishment & Society, 13*(5), 611–629. doi:10.1177/1462474511422171

Harrington, R., Bailey, S., Chitsabesan, P., Kroll, L., Macdonald, W., Sneider, S., . . ., & Barrett, B. (2005). *Mental health needs and effectiveness of provision for young offenders in custody and in the community.* Youth Justice Board.

Healthcare Commission. (2007). *Count me in 2006: Results of the 2006 national census of inpatients in mental health and learning disability services in England and Wales.* Commission for Healthcare, Audit and Inspection.

Howard League. (2006). *Healthy sexual development of children in prison.* Briefing Paper 4. Retrieved September 15, 2021, from https://howardleague.org/wp-content/uploads/2016/03/Healthy-sexual-development-of-children-in-prison.pdf

Howerton, A., Byng, R., Campbell, J., Hess, D., Owens, C., & Aitken, P. (2007). Understanding help seeking behaviour among male offenders: Qualitative interview study. *BMJ, 334*(7588), 303.

Hughes, N., & Chitsabesan, P. (2015). *Supporting young people with neurodevelopmental impairment.* Centre for Crime and Justice Studies.

KPMG. (2016). *Health and justice CAMHS transformation workstream report.* www.england.nhs.uk/midlands/wp-content/uploads/sites/46/2019/05/health-and-justice-camhs-transformation-workstream-report.pdf

Lammy, D. (2017). *The Lammy review: An independent review into the treatment of, and outcomes for, Black, Asian and minority ethnic individuals in the criminal justice system.* Criminal Justice.

Laufer, M., & Laufer, M. E. (1975). *Adolescence and developmental breakdown: A psychoanalytic view.* Yale University Press.

Ministry of Justice. (2018). *Secure schools.* www.gov.uk/government/collections/secure-schools

Moore, E., Gaskin, C., & Indig, D. (2013). Childhood maltreatment and post-traumatic stress disorder among incarcerated young offenders. *Child Abuse & Neglect, 37*(10), 861–870.

Paton, J., Crouch, W., & Camic, P. (2009). Young offenders' experiences of traumatic life events: A qualitative investigation. *Clinical Child Psychology and Psychiatry, 14*(1), 43–62.

Rollnick, S., & Miller, W. R. (1995). What is motivational interviewing? *Behavioural and Cognitive Psychotherapy, 23*(4), 325–334. doi:10.1017/S135246580001643X

Rose, J. (2014). It's the stories that are important. In J. Rose (Ed.), *Working with young people in secure accommodation: From chaos to culture* (2nd ed., pp. 75–89). Routledge. ISBN:9780415843225.

Sadie, C., & Stokoe, P. (2020, March). Creating therapeutic environments in youth custody: The SECURE STAIRS programme. *Monitor*, 20–23.

Scott, D. (2017). www.thejusticegap.com/prison-means-life-child-lifers-pains-imprisonment/

Steinberg, L., Chung, H. L., & Little, M. (2004). Re-entry of young offenders from the justice system: A developmental perspective. *Youth Violence and Juvenile Justice, 2*(1), 21. doi:10.1177/1541204003260045

Stokoe, P. (2020). *The curiosity drive.* Phoenix.

Storgaard, A. (2005). Juvenile justice in Scandinavia. *Journal of Scandinavian Studies in Criminology and Crime Prevention, 5*(2), 188–204.

Taylor, J., Shostak, L., Rogers, A., & Mitchell, P. (2018). Rethinking mental health provision in the secure estate for children and young people: A framework for integrated care (SECURE STAIRS). *Safer Communities, 17*(4), 193–201.isolation

Vygotsky, L. S. (1978). *Mind in society: The development of higher psychological processes.* Harvard University Press.

Youth Custody Service. (2021, August). *Youth custody report*. www.gov.uk/government/statistics/youth-custody-data

Youth Justice Board. (2019). *Girls and offending – patterns, perceptions and interventions*. Retrieved November 23, 2020, from https://assets.publishing.service.gov.uk/government/uploads/system/uploads/attachment_data/file/354833/yjb-girls-offending.pdf

Youth Justice Board. (2021). *Ethnic disproportionality in remand and sentencing in the youth justice system: Analysis of administrative data*. Retrieved September 15, 2021, from https://assets.publishing.service.gov.uk/government/uploads/system/uploads/attachment_data/file/952483/Ethnic_disproportionality_in_remand_and_sentencing_in_the_youth_justice_system.pdf

Youth Justice Board/Ministry of Justice. (2011). *Youth justice statistics, 2009–10*. Retrieved September 15, 2021, from https://assets.publishing.service.gov.uk/government/uploads/system/uploads/attachment_data/file/279886/yjb-annual-workload-data-0910.pdf

Youth Justice Board/Ministry of Justice. (2020). *Youth justice statistics 2018/19: England and Wales*. Ministry of Justice. www.gov.uk/government/collections/youth-justicestatistics.

Chapter 6

Ethnic minority forensic patients in the German Federal State of Baden-Württemberg

Thomas Ross, María Isabel Fontao, Annette Opitz-Welke, and Jan Bulla

Ethnicity, ethnic minority, and migration

Ethnicity refers to the quality or fact of belonging to a population group made up of people who share a common cultural background or descent. Ethnic minorities are groups of people who differ in terms of descent, language, sanctuaries and sacrifices, or (inherited) customs from the majority population of the countries they live in (Oxford Dictionaries, 2021). According to the International Organization for Migration (IOT), a migrant is

> any person who is moving or has moved across an international border or within a state away from his/her habitual place of residence, regardless of (a) the person's legal status, (b) whether the movement is voluntary or involuntary, (c) what the causes for the movement are or (d) what the length of the stay is.
>
> (International Organization for Migration, 2021)

Migrants may or may not be members of ethnic minority groups, and individuals belonging to an ethnic minority group may or may not have migrated.

Research on ethnic minorities has focused on demographic, economic, social, and health outcomes across ethnic groups and generations. Commonly, conclusions are drawn as to the extent of integration and exclusion of different ethnic groups in their host countries (Pyper, 2021). Scientific publications on the mental health of individuals belonging to ethnic minorities are abundant and fast evolving (Barnett et al., 2019; Cook et al., 2018; de Freitas et al., 2018; Henry et al., 2020; Tortelli et al., 2018). Another line of research examines the relationships between ethnic minority status and crime, focusing on possible causes for the over-representation of ethnic minorities in the criminal justice system (Boon et al., 2019; Gase et al., 2016; Lammy, 2017; Mercado-Crespo & Mbah, 2012; Webb et al., 2015). Some studies investigated the complex relationships between ethnic minority status and/or migration, mental health, and crime (Acevedo et al., 2019; Denzel et al., 2016).

Ethnic minority migrants in Germany and the state of Baden-Württemberg

In Germany, about a quarter of the population (26%) has a migration background. This includes immigrant and non-immigrant foreigners (12%), naturalised individuals, and (late) repatriates (also called ethnic German re-settlers who returned to the country of their German ancestors to live there permanently), as well as first-degree descendants of all the aforementioned groups. Among the regions of origin, Africa, and especially North, West, and

DOI: 10.4324/9781003184768-8

East Africa, ethnic minorities are becoming more frequent (German Federal Statistical Office, 2021). Ongoing crises such as civil wars, dictatorships, poverty, extreme climate conditions, and rapid population growth are the main reasons for migration from sub-Saharan regions. In North Africa, people suffer particularly from high unemployment, persecution of minorities, and various forms of abuse (Idemudia & Boehnke, 2020; Schraven et al., 2019).

Baden-Württemberg is one of the 16 German federal states representing roughly 13% of the German population. In 2019, it had the fourth-highest share of individuals with migration background of all German states (34%), and between January and November 2018, almost 26% of asylum applications came from sub-Saharan regions (State Statistical Office Baden-Württemberg, 2019).

Ethnic minority migrants in forensic treatment in Baden-Württemberg

Baden-Württemberg runs one of the most comprehensive forensic databases in Germany, providing legal, clinical, and treatment outcome information on all forensic patients (approximately 1.700 individuals per annum). In relation to other migrant groups, ethnic minority patients such as sub-Saharan and North Africans are still relatively few in total numbers, but in recent years, their increase in Baden-Württemberg's forensic psychiatric facilities has been notable (2015: $n = 33$; 2019: $n = 73$; + 221%; Working group process optimisation and quality assurance, 2019; Ross et al., 2020). Yet, it remains unclear which factors are responsible for the sharp increase in patient numbers from Africa and other economically and socially disadvantaged regions. Focusing on variables that might be able to explain this development, our research group started a series of interrelated analyses on ethnic minority patients with migration experiences in 2017.

Bulla and colleagues investigated the relationship between country of origin, the likelihood (hazard) of being assigned to court-ordered forensic psychiatric treatment, and the proportion of those diagnosed with a schizophrenia spectrum disorder (Bulla et al., 2017). The data from the Baden-Württemberg documentation system were compared with the federal population statistics and correlated with the Human Development Index (HDI[1]; United Nations Development Programme, 2020a) and Inequality-Adjusted Human Development Index IHDI[2]; United Nations Development Programme, 2020b) and Multidimensional Poverty Indices (MPI[3]; United Nations Development Programme, 2020b). For Baden-Württemberg residents with migration background, the risk ratio (RR) of receiving a forensic psychiatric hospital order may be considerably higher in comparison to persons without migration background. There was a highly significant correlation between HDIs of the countries of origin and RRs for detention in a forensic psychiatric hospital. The proportion of schizophrenia diagnoses also correlated significantly with the HDI. In contrast, the MPI country rankings were not associated with schizophrenia diagnoses. For sub-Saharan African countries, for whose citizens the risk of becoming a forensic patient in Baden-Württemberg, the RR was the highest at RR = 6.13 (implying this group was approximately six times more likely to receive a forensic treatment order than residents of Baden-Württemberg without a migration background). At the same time, their IHDI was the lowest (0.34), followed by the North African regions with an IHDI of 0.47 and an RR of 2.11. A migrant background was inherently associated with an increased risk of forensic placement, but the magnitude of this risk varied considerably among countries of origin. The main limitations of this study are that these data cannot be controlled for prevalence rates of disorders, possible misdiagnosis, or offending in the general population because national or state-wide data for comparison are not available.

Further research showed that subgroups of forensic patients with migration backgrounds in Baden-Württemberg may differ from each other in various clinical aspects. Bulla et al. (2018a) examined forensic patients with mental disorders and migration backgrounds sentenced to unlimited detention (according to section 63 of the German Criminal Code[4]). Ninety per cent of patients from the Balkans, North Africa, Near-East [Orient], and sub-Sahara Africa had been diagnosed with schizophrenia spectrum disorders, whereas other migrant groups showed a much larger diagnostic spectrum.

Using a larger database than Bulla et al. (2017), a recent German study by Bergmann et al. (2021) examined core analysed characteristics of forensic patients from North and sub-Saharan Africa ($n = 71$). This may offer a deeper understanding of the explanatory factors for the high admission rates to the forensic court-ordered treatment of this ethnic minority subgroup. Compared to individuals in forensic treatment from Western Europe ($n = 73$) and Kazakhstan ($n = 32$), the African group had significantly poorer professional qualifications and a higher rate of homeless individuals at the time of the index offence; the proportion of ICD-10 F20.0 diagnoses in the African patient group was significantly higher than in both comparison groups. Regarding psychiatric diagnoses in the lifetime and criminal history, age at first offence, and substance-related disorders, no differences between the three groups with different migration backgrounds were found. Post-migration factors associated with social disadvantage were discussed as contributors to higher rates of schizophrenia diagnosis rates in some migrant subgroups or ethnic minorities (for related results from Germany, see also Jocher et al., 2021).

Discussion

The number of ethnic minority patients (especially from Africa) undergoing forensic treatment in Baden-Württemberg has been increasing for years. Most of these patients were diagnosed with schizophrenia spectrum disorders. The main lines of explanation derived from scientific findings relate to a) relationships between migration, ethnic minority status, and mental health risk factors and b) the association between schizophrenia and violence.

Migration, ethnic minority status, and mental health risk factors

Ethnic minorities face a range of factors with a negative impact on mental health. A comprehensive dynamic model of risks to the health of migrants by Matlin et al. (2018) described factors before the migration process (e.g., socioeconomic status and education level, specific health conditions, conflict, natural disasters, and other traumatic events), factors occurring during travel (e.g., modes of travel and border crossing, sexual and other violence, detention and other traumatic events, unsanitary conditions, and overcrowding), and factors that show up at transit and the destination (e.g., adaptation to new life, surroundings, and culture, uncertain legal status, social exclusion, cultural, linguistic, and legal barriers to access health services). Idemudia and Boehnke (2020) investigated the psychosocial experiences of roughly 3,500 African migrants in six countries (Germany, France, Italy, Spain, Netherlands, and United Kingdom). The legal status of migrants predicted a range of factors associated with poor mental health (e.g., somatic complaints, anxiety/insomnia, social dysfunction, and depression). Post-migration stress predicted mental health problems and, surprisingly, lower levels of post-traumatic stress disorder (PTSD). Pre-migration stress was associated with PTSD.

The literature also points to the importance of overt or subtle racism and discrimination. Discrimination and racism include poor treatment and verbal and or physical attacks and sometimes systematic marginalisation and discrimination in healthcare, academia, employment, courts, or other law employment agencies (Kleider-Offutt et al., 2017; Behr, 2017; Kutateladze et al., 2014). Racial profiling, i.e., the targeting of ethnic minorities by police officers, contradicts anti-discrimination rules (Boysen, 2020). However, depending on race/ethnic background and appearance, African individuals may be more likely than others to be profiled as a criminal. Racism and perceived discrimination are related to poorer mental and physical health outcomes (Paradies et al., 2015; Pearce et al., 2019).

Migrants and ethnic minorities may also experience social disadvantages, which can be understood as long-lasting effects of racism and discrimination. Immigrant and ethnic minority children are frequently placed in low-ability groups early in their education. For youths and adults, access to the labour market, which is a key factor for integration in the host country, can be impaired. In Germany, progress has been made in recent years in the school system, vocational qualifications, and integration into the labour market. Nonetheless, individuals with a migration background still experience disadvantages: foreign children are more than twice as likely to leave school without a lower secondary school certificate, and the unemployment rate of people with a migration background is higher compared with individuals without a migration background (Harte et al., 2016).

Social and economic disadvantages have been directly linked to a higher prevalence of psychosis. Living in densely populated and socially fragmented neighbourhoods, broken homes, perceived discrimination, and exposure to physical threats and violence, among others, tend to increase the risk of developing schizophrenia or related psychotic disorders (Morgan et al., 2019; Radua et al., 2018).

Schizophrenia and violence

Mental health problems and severe mental disorders among ethnic minorities do not sufficiently explain the rise in admissions of this group to forensic facilities. Because of the high proportion of ICD-10 F20.0 diagnoses ('Schizophrenia, schizotypal, delusional, and other non-mood psychotic disorders') in the African patient group (Bergmann et al., 2021), our knowledge about schizophrenia and its association with violence may help elucidate this phenomenon. High risk for violence in people with schizophrenia seems to be mediated by comorbid substance abuse, and the risk of individuals with comorbidity is similar to that of individuals diagnosed with only substance abuse (Whiting et al., 2021). Additional risk factors for violence in relation to schizophrenia are comorbid substance abuse, hostility, and non-compliance to medication (Witt et al., 2013). With regard to psychopathological risk factors, Coid et al. (2016) suggested that only paranoid ideation is associated with violent acts.

Studies in the general population proposed a dose–response model for the emergence of mental disorders. Childhood adversity, e.g., family conflict and financial strain in childhood, is associated with the risk of impaired physical and mental health and social functioning problems in adulthood (Santini et al., 2021). High odds of schizophrenia in ethnic minority and migrant populations (particularly in Black ethnic groups) compared with ethnic majority groups are a consistent finding (e.g., Halvorsrud et al., 2019). Similar results from Germany have been reported by Mitjans et al. (2019) and Begemann et al. (2020). Based on these findings, our main argument is that ethnic minorities in Baden-Württemberg have an increased risk of being diagnosed with schizophrenia and hence also of showing violent behaviour, which is why they are more often referred to treatment in forensic psychiatric institutions. A direct link between some psychosocial stressors, (antisocial) traits, and violence might theoretically also account for the association between migration background and crime. However, this explanation does not hold, since a severe mental health disorder is a *sine qua non* condition for being assigned to forensic psychiatric treatment.

Prevention, care, and aftercare

General recommendations for the treatment of forensic psychiatric patients apply also to forensic patients with migration background. Moreover, the literature on migrant or ethnic minority patients underlines the importance of specific therapeutic strategies and interventions as well as close coordination between different support and care facilities in all phases of treatment.

Primary prevention

Ideally, primary prevention takes effect when the various stressors or risk factors for mental health during and after the migration (see the section titled: 'Migration, ethnic minority status and mental health risk factors') are effectively addressed. To this purpose, coordinated international and national policy action at different administrative levels are needed to prevent or reduce exposure to risk factors (combating social exclusion, improved policies on individual and institutional discrimination, reducing barriers to labour market participation, etc.) and to facilitate access to health care and other material, social, and cultural goods (promote inclusive educational policies, strengthen social networks, improve knowledge of health risks, and strengthen healthy cultural traditions) (Matlin et al., 2018).

Psychiatric treatment prior to crime and forensic treatment

Independently of migration background status, a considerable proportion of forensic psychiatric patients had already received psychiatric treatment before they were either ordered into a custodial setting or treatment in a forensic psychiatric facility (Weithmann & Traub, 2008; Degl'Innocenti et al., 2014). Routine assessment of risk for violent behaviour and unlawful acts in general psychiatric settings as well as targeted interventions could help prevent serious crime after discharge (e.g., assessing violent thoughts, ownership of weapons, and previous violence at admission to psychiatric treatment or community-based services; Sanders et al., 2000). Including more forensic psychiatric learning contents during psychiatry, psychotherapy, or nursing training may improve the early identification of risks. More specifically, training on culturally sensitive issues and specific needs in the context of ethnic minority treatment is required (Barber Rioja & Rosenfeld, 2018). At the institutional level, strengthening cooperation between forensic services, the local psychiatric and psychosocial networks (Piontek et al., 2013), and community-based services for people with migration backgrounds can help to implement tailored interventions preventing the shift to forensic settings (often referred to as 'forensification') or to criminal justice.

Treatment recommendations for ethnic minorities and patients with a migration background in forensic settings

A recent exploratory study comparing non-European migrants and native European forensic patients diagnosed with schizophrenia in Switzerland found differences in childhood/adolescence variables and therapy-associated factors. Non-Europeans more frequently reported suffering from poverty but less social isolation during childhood and adolescence; they had more language problems during psychotherapy, were more often only engaged in the most basic tasks in ergotherapy, and received a higher antipsychotic dose equivalent to olanzapine at discharge in comparison to native European patients (Huber et al., 2020). These results underline the need for better linguistic and cultural competence in forensic settings. A better understanding of how cultural background may impact an individual's psychopathology and capacity to control behaviour is essential for the current practice of forensic psychiatry, but empirical data on culturally competent practices in forensic settings are scarce (e.g., Kois & Chauhan, 2016).

Several guidelines on cultural competence (APA, 2017) and treatment recommendations for migrants and ethnic minorities have been published (Bhugra et al., 2011; Schouler-Ocak et al., 2015). The DSM-IV Outline for Cultural Formulation (OCF) was developed to help clinicians identify the impact of culture during a clinical evaluation, and the Cultural Formulation Interview (CFI) operationalises the OCF for routine use in the clinical practice (Lewis-Fernández et al., 2017). Healthcare staff may use the information to obtain culturally relevant information during a mental health assessment. The CFI identifies four domains of assessment: cultural definition of the problem; cultural perception of cause, context, and support; cultural factors affecting self-coping and (past) help seeking; and cultural factors of current help seeking. Twelve supplementary modules may help to gain further insights into specific patient groups. There are tailor-made modules for immigrants and refugees, children and adolescents, older adults, and other special populations. In Germany, transcultural aspects of care are still best captured by the 'Sonnenberger Leitlinien' [Sonnenberg Guidelines] (Machleidt, 2002; Machleidt & Callies, 2011) and other recommendations based on these. In recent years, efforts have been made to translate the principles of cultural competence in psychiatry to correctional settings (Kapoor et al., 2013). In forensic psychiatry, the formal guidelines of the OCF have been adapted according to recommendations from the forensic mental health literature (Aggarwal, 2012). The implementation of the CFI on a mixed forensic unit has recently been evaluated in an international field trial (Aggarwal et al., 2020). Although further studies are needed, preliminary results are encouraging with respect to the feasibility, acceptability, and clinical utility of the CFI.

In practice, however, there are many patients with a migration background (especially those of African origin) who may face deportation to their countries of origin. Under these circumstances, it is often difficult to provide medium- or long-term forensic treatment planning for these patients.

Pharmacological treatment

Differences in the responsiveness to medication and in the likelihood of certain adverse drug reactions are known for some ethnic groups (overview in Chaudhry et al., 2008). This must be taken into account when treating ethnic minority individuals diagnosed with schizophrenia. Insights into pharmacokinetics and their clinical application as therapeutic drug monitoring (TDM) now play an important role in the search for effective and well-tolerated psychopharmacological treatments (Hiemke et al., 2018). In addition to interactions between different drugs, pharmacogenetic variants can also lead to significant differences in blood levels. For example, polymorphisms in some isoenzymes of the cytochrome (CYP)-450 families are associated with different catabolism of certain psychotropic drugs in the liver (e.g., Hiemke et al., 2018).

Aftercare

Forensic patients are usually not discharged until a viable concept for adequate aftercare has been established. In addition to mandatory supervision of conduct for as much as five years in Germany, forensic aftercare has a number of options: assisted living, reintegration residential homes, psychiatric residential homes, residential homes for prisoners and individuals with substance use disorders, transfers to other specialised clinics, and admission to a forensic psychiatric outpatient clinic (Bulla et al., 2015). In practice, many providers of aftercare are not yet prepared for dealing with an increasing number of patients with special cultural needs. Treatment and aftercare recommendations for specific ethnic groups need to be translated into practical guidelines in aftercare settings and support patients in finding a balance between their own cultural heritage and the necessary adjustments to the society (Bhugra et al., 2011). To our knowledge, evidence on the effectiveness of specific approaches and interventions for forensic patients with migration backgrounds or ethnic minorities in aftercare settings is still lacking. For non-forensic samples, studies on the differential effects of culturally adapted psychotherapy (Benish et al., 2011) or on community-centred interventions with adult ethnic minority groups reported encouraging results (Baskin et al., 2021).

Notes

1. The HDI (Human Development Index) is a composite statistic of health, education, and per capita income indicators, which are used to rank countries into four main groups of human development. High HDI is associated with longer lifespan, high education level, high gross domestic product (GDP) per capita, low fertility rate, and low inflation rate. Annual reports are published by the United Nations Development Programme (United Nations Development Programme, 2020a).
2. The IHDI (Inequality Adjusted Human Development Index) combines a country's average achievements in health, education, and income with how those achievements are distributed among country's population measured against each dimension's average value according to its level of inequality. Thus, the IHDI is a distribution-sensitive average level of human development. Two countries with different distributions of achievements can have the same average HDI value. Under perfect equality, the IHDI is equal to the HDI but falls below the HDI when inequality rises (United Nations Development Programme, 2020b).
3. The Multidimensional Poverty Index (MPI) identifies multiple deprivations at the household and individual level in health, education, and standard of living. It uses micro data from household surveys. Each person in a given household is classified as poor or non-poor depending on the weighted number of deprivations his or her household, and thus, he or she experiences. These data are then aggregated into the national measure of poverty. The MPI reflects both the incidence of multidimensional deprivation (a headcount of those in multidimensional poverty) and its intensity (the average deprivation score experienced by poor people; United Nations Development Programme, 2020c).
4. In broad terms, there are two types of secure forensic hospitals in Germany: forensic psychiatric hospitals (section 63 of the German Criminal Code) and addiction treatment facilities (section 64 of the German Criminal Code). Only offenders who are found in court to be partially or fully exempt from criminal responsibility can be given a section 63 order which is indeterminate. Section 64 is time limited, reduced, or absent, criminal responsibility is not required, and duration of treatment is time limited. Moreover, individuals suspected to fulfill criteria for one of these sections can be placed in a forensic psychiatric hospital or an addiction treatment facility while awaiting the results of the trial (section 126a of the German Code of Criminal Procedure). Other offenders are usually sentenced to prison or are ordered to pay fines.

   If a person has committed an unlawful act in a state of criminal irresponsibility (section 20 German Criminal Code) or in a state of diminished responsibility (section 21), the court orders that person's placement in a psychiatric hospital under section 63 if the overall evaluation of the offender and of the offence reveals that, due to the offender's condition, he or she represents a danger to the general public on account of it being expected that he or she will in future commit serious unlawful acts which will result in the victims of the offence suffering or being exposed to the considerable danger of severe emotional trauma or physical injury or which will cause serious economic damage. If the unlawful act which has been committed is not an offence as referred to in the previous sentence, the court only makes such an order if special circumstances justify the expectation that, due to the offender's condition, the offender will in future commit such serious offences.

References

Acevedo, A., Miles, J., Panas, L., Ritter, G., Campbell, K., & Garnick, D. (2019). Disparities in criminal justice outcomes after beginning treatment for substance use disorders: The influence of race/ethnicity and place. *Journal of Studies on Alcohol and Drugs, 80*(2), 220–229. doi:10.15288/jsad.2019.80.220

Aggarwal, N. K. (2012). Adapting the cultural formulation for clinical assessments in forensic psychiatry. *Journal of the American Academy of Psychiatry and the Law, 40*(1), 113–118.

Aggarwal, N. K., Lam, P., Diaz, S., Cruz, A. G., & Lewis-Fernández, R. (2020). Clinician perceptions of implementing the cultural formulation interview on a mixed forensic unit. *Journal of the American Academy of Psychiatry and the Law Online*, JAAPL.003914–003920. doi:10.29158/jaapl.003914-20

American Psychiatric Association. (2017). *Multicultural guidelines: An ecological approach to context, identity, and intersectionality*. APA. www.apa.org/about/policy/multicultural-guidelines.pdf

Barber Rioja, V., & Rosenfeld, B. (2018). Addressing linguistic and cultural differences in the forensic interview. *International Journal of Forensic Mental Health, 17*(4), 377–386.

Barnett, T. M., McFarland, A., Miller, J. W., Lowe, V., & Hatcher, S. S. (2019). Physical and mental health experiences among African American college students. *Social Work in Public Health, 34*(2), 145–157.

Baskin, C., Zijlstra, G., McGrath, M., Lee, C., Duncan, F. H., Oliver, E. J., . . . Gnani, S. (2021). Community-centred interventions for improving public mental health among adults from ethnic minority populations in the UK: A scoping review. *BMJ Open, 11*(4), e041102.

Begemann, M., Seidel, J., Poustka, L., & Ehrenreich, H. (2020). Accumulated environmental risk in young refugees—A prospective evaluation. *EClinicalMedicine, 22*, 100345.

Behr, R. (2017). Diskriminierung durch Polizeibehörden. In *Handbuch diskriminierung* (pp. 301–319). Springer VS.

Benish, S. G., Quintana, S., & Wampold, B. E. (2011). Culturally adapted psychotherapy and the legitimacy of myth: A direct-comparison meta-analysis. *Journal of Counseling Psychology, 58*(3), 279.

Bergmann, J., Fontao, M. I., Bulla, J., & Ross, T. (2021). Patienten aus Nord- und Subsahara Afrika im baden-württembergischen Maßregelvollzug. [Patients from North- and Subsahara Africa in Baden-Württemberg forensic psychiatric facilities] *Monatsschrift für Kriminologie und Strafrechtsreform, 104*(1), 2–15.

Bhugra, D., Gupta, S., Bhui, K., Craig, T., Dogra, N., Ingleby, J. D., . . . Tribe, R. (2011). WPA guidance on mental health and mental health care in migrants. *World Psychiatry: Official Journal of the World Psychiatric Association (WPA), 10*(1), 2–10. doi:10.1002/j.2051-5545.2011.tb00002.x

Boon, A., van Dorp, M., & de Boer, S. (2019). Disproportionate minority contact in the Dutch juvenile justice system. *Journal of Ethnicity in Criminal Justice, 17*(1), 42–56. doi:10.1080/15377938.2018.1564717

Boysen, S. (2020). Racial profiling. *JURA – Juristische Ausbildung, 42*(11), 1192–1199. doi:10.1515/jura-2020-2580

Bulla, J., Hoffmann, K., Querengässer, J., & Ross, T. (2017). Socioeconomic disadvantage and schizophrenia in migrants under mental health detention orders. *International Journal of Social Psychiatry, 63*(6), 550–558. doi:10.1177/0020764017716696

Bulla, J., Querengässer, J., Hoffmann, K., & Ross, T. (2015). Forensische Nachsorge von Migranten. *Monatsschrift für Kriminologie und Strafrechtsreform, 98*(5), 415–427.

Bulla, J., Rzodeczko, F., Querengässer, J., Hoffmann, K., & Ross, T. (2018a). Migrants in unlimited detention according to section 63 of the German penal code: Results from the German federal state of Baden-Württemberg. *International Journal of Law and Psychiatry, 57*, 1–8. doi:10.1016/j.ijlp.2017.12.003

Chaudhry, I., Neelam, K., Duddu, V., & Husain, N. (2008). Ethnicity and psychopharmacology. *Journal of Psychopharmacology (Oxf), 22*, 673–680. https://doi.org/10.1177/0269881107082105

Coid, J. W., Ullrich, S., Bebbington, P., Fazel, S., & Keers, R. (2016). Paranoid ideation and violence: Meta-analysis of individual subject data of 7 population surveys. *Schizophrenia Bulletin, 42*(4), 907–915.

Cook, B. L., Hou, S. S.-Y., Lee-Tauler, S. Y., Progovac, A. M., Samson, F., & Sanchez, M. J. (2018). A review of mental health and mental health care disparities research: 2011–2014. *Medical Care Research and Review, 76*(6), 683–710. doi:10.1177/1077558718780592

de Freitas, D. F., Fernandes-Jesus, M., Ferreira, P. D., Coimbra, S., Teixeira, P. M., de Moura, A., . . . Fontaine, A. M. (2018). Psychological correlates of perceived ethnic discrimination in Europe: A meta-analysis. *Psychology of Violence, 8*(6), 712–725. doi:10.1037/vio0000215

Degl'Innocenti, A., Hassing, L. B., Lindqvist, A. S., Andersson, H., Eriksson, L., Hanson, F. H., . . . Anckarsäter, H. (2014). First report from the Swedish national forensic psychiatric register (SNFPR). *International Journal of Law and Psychiatry, 37*(3), 231–237.

Denzel, A. D., van Esch, A. Y., Harte, J. M., & Scherder, E. J. (2016). Ethnic variations in psychotic disorders in the criminal justice system: A systematic review. *Aggression and Violent Behavior, 29*, 20–29.

Gase, L. N., Glenn, B. A., Gomez, L. M., Kuo, T., Inkelas, M., & Ponce, N. A. (2016). Understanding racial and ethnic disparities in arrest: The role of individual, home, school, and community characteristics. *Race and Social Problems*, *8*(4), 296–312.

German Federal Statistical Office [Statistisches Bundesamt]. (2021). *Migrationshintergrund [Migration background]*. Retrieved June 30, 2021, from www.destatis.de/DE/Themen/Gesellschaft-Umwelt/Bevoel kerung/Migration-Integration/Glossar/migrationshintergrund.html

Halvorsrud, K., Nazroo, J., Otis, M., Brown Hajdukova, E., & Bhui, K. (2019). Ethnic inequalities in the incidence of diagnosis of severe mental illness in England: A systematic review and new meta-analyses for non-affective and affective psychoses. *Social Psychiatry and Psychiatric Epidemiology*, *54*(11), 1311–1323. doi:10.1007/s00127-019-01758-y

Harte, E., Herrera, F., Stepanek, M., & Rand, E. (2016). *Education of EU migrant children in EU Member States*. RAND.

Henry, T. L., Jetty, A., Petterson, S., Jaffree, H., Ramsay, A., Heiman, E., & Bazemore, A. (2020). Taking a closer look at mental health treatment differences: Effectiveness of mental health treatment by provider type in racial and ethnic minorities. *Journal of Primary Care & Community Health*, *11*, 2150132720966403.

Hiemke, C., Bergemann, N., Clement, H. W., et al. (2018). Consensus guidelines for therapeutic drug monitoring in neuropsychopharmacology: Update 2017. *Pharmacopsychiatry*, *51*, 9–62.

Huber, D. A., Lau, S., Sonnweber, M., Gunther, M. P., & Kirchebner, J. (2020). Exploring similarities and differences of non-European migrants among forensic patients with schizophrenia. *International Journal of Environmental Research and Public Health*, *17*(21), 15. doi:10.3390/ijerph17217922

Idemudia, E., & Boehnke, K. (2020). Social experiences of migrants. In *Psychosocial experiences of African migrants in six European countries* (Vol. 81, pp. 83–94). Springer.

International Organization for Migration. (2021). *Key migration terms*. Retrieved June 10, 2021, from www. iom.int/key-migration-terms#Migrant

Jocher, P., Bulla, J., Fontao, M. I., & Ross, T. (2021). Patienten mit Migrationshintergrund im Maßregelvollzug gemäß § 63 StGB in Baden-Württemberg. Ein Vergleich von Subgruppen. *Forensische Psychiatrie und Psychotherapie*, *29*(2), 217–234.

Kapoor, R., Dike, C., Burns, C., Carvalho, V., & Griffith, E. E. H. (2013). Cultural competence in correctional mental health. *International Journal of Law and Psychiatry*, *36*(3–4), 273–280. doi:10.1016/j.ijlp.2013.04.016

Kleider-Offutt, H. M., Bond, A. D., & Hegerty, S. E. (2017). Black stereotypical features: When a face type can get you in trouble. *Current Directions in Psychological Science*, *26*(1), 28–33.

Kois, L., & Chauhan, P. (2016). Forensic evaluators' self-reported engagement in culturally competent practices. *The International Journal of Forensic Mental Health*, *15*(4), 312–322. doi:10.1080/14999013.2016.122 8089

Kutateladze, B. L., Andiloro, N. R., Johnson, B. D., & Spohn, C. C. (2014). Cumulative disadvantage: Examining racial and ethnic disparity in prosecution and sentencing. *Criminology*, *52*(3), 514–551.

Lammy, D. (2017). The Lammy review – An independent review into the treatment of, and outcomes for, Black, Asian and minority ethnic individuals in the criminal justice system. https://assets.publishing. service.gov.uk/government/uploads/system/uploads/attachment_data/file/643001/lammy-review-final-report.pdf

Lewis-Fernández, R., Aggarwal, N. K., Lam, P. C., Galfalvy, H., Weiss, M. G., Kirmayer, L. J., . . . Vega-Dienstmaier, J. M. (2017). Feasibility, acceptability and clinical utility of the cultural formulation interview: Mixed-methods results from the DSM-5 international field trial. *British Journal of Psychiatry*, *210*(4), 290–297. doi:10.1192/bjp.bp.116.193862

Machleidt, W. (2002). Die 12 Sonnenberger Leitlinien zur psychiatrisch-psychotherapeutischen Versorgung von MigrantInnen in Deutschland. *Der Nervenarzt*, *73*(12), 1208–1212. doi:10.1007/s00115-002-1460-7

Machleidt, W., & Calliess, I. T. (2011). Transkulturelle Aspekte psychischer Erkrankungen. In *Psychiatrie, psychosomatik, psychotherapie* (pp. 397–427). Springer.

Matlin, S. A., Depoux, A., Schütte, S., Flahault, A., & Saso, L. (2018). Migrants' and refugees' health: Towards an agenda of solutions. *Public Health Reviews*, *39*(1), 1–55.

Mercado-Crespo, M. C., & Mbah, A. K. (2012). Race and ethnicity, substance use, and physical aggression among U.S. High school students. *Journal of Interpersonal Violence*, *28*(7), 1367–1384. doi:10.1177/0886260512468234

Mitjans, M., Seidel, J., Begemann, M., Bockhop, F., Moya-Higueras, J., Bansal, V., . . . Duvar, O. (2019). Violent aggression predicted by multiple pre-adult environmental hits. *Molecular Psychiatry*, *24*(10), 1549–1564.

Morgan, C., Knowles, G., & Hutchinson, G. (2019). Migration, ethnicity and psychoses: Evidence, models and future directions. *World Psychiatry*, *18*(3), 247–258. https://doi.org/10.1002/wps.20655

Oxford Dictionaries. (2021). *Ethnicity: Definition of ethnicity*. Oxford University Press. www.lexico.com/definition/ethnicity

Paradies, Y., Ben, J., Denson, N., Elias, A., Priest, N., Pieterse, A., . . . Gee, G. (2015). Racism as a determinant of health: A systematic review and meta-analysis. *PLoS One*, *10*(9), e0138511. doi:10.1371/journal.pone.0138511

Pearce, J., Rafiq, S., Simpson, J., & Varese, F. (2019). Perceived discrimination and psychosis: A systematic review of the literature. *Social Psychiatry and Psychiatric Epidemiology*, *54*(9), 1023–1044.

Piontek, K., Kutscher, S. U., König, A., & Leygraf, N. (2013). Prädeliktische Behandlungswege schizophrener Patienten der forensischen Psychiatrie. *Der Nervenarzt*, *84*(1), 55–64. doi:10.1007/s00115-011-3409-1

Pyper, D. (2021). *Briefing paper: Race and ethnic disparities*. House of Commons Library. https://commonslibrary.parliament.uk/research-briefings/cbp-8960/

Radua, J., Ramella-Cravaro, V., Ioannidis, J. P. A., Reichenberg, A., Phiphopthatsanee, N., Amir, T., . . . Fusar-Poli, P. (2018). What causes psychosis? An umbrella review of risk and protective factors. *World Psychiatry*, *17*(1), 49–66. doi:10.1002/wps.20490

Ross, T., Fontao, M. I., & Bulla, J. (2020). Rising inpatient numbers in forensic security hospitals of German federal state of Baden-Württemberg: Background and explanatory approaches. *Behavioral Sciences & the Law*, *38*(5), 522–536.

Sanders, J., Milne, S., Brown, P., & Bell, A. J. (2000). Assessment of aggression in psychiatric admissions: Semistructured interview and case note survey. *BMJ*, *320*(7242), 1112. doi:10.1136/bmj.320.7242.1112

Santini, Z. I., Koyanagi, A., Stewart-Brown, S., Perry, B. D., Marmot, M., & Koushede, V. (2021). Cumulative risk of compromised physical, mental and social health in adulthood due to family conflict and financial strain during childhood: A retrospective analysis based on survey data representative of 19 European countries. *BMJ Global Health*, *6*(3), e004144.

Schouler-Ocak, M., Graef-Calliess, I. T., Tarricone, I., Qureshi, A., Kastrup, M. C., & Bhugra, D. (2015). EPA guidance on cultural competence training. *European Psychiatry*, *30*(3), 431–440. doi:10.1016/j.eurpsy.2015.01.012

Schraven, B., Adaawen, S., Rademacher-Schulz, C., & Segadlo, N. (2019). *„Klimamigration"in Subsahara-Afrika: Trends und grundlegende Empfehlungen für die Entwicklungszusammenarbeit*. Deutsches Institut für Entwicklungspolitik (DIE). www.die-gdi.de/uploads/media/AuS_10.2019.pdf

State Statistical Office Baden-Württemberg *[Statistisches Landesamt Baden-Württemberg]*. (2019). *Bevölkerung und Gebiet [Population and territory]*. Retrieved October 16, 2019, from www.statistik-bw.de/BevoelkGebiet/

Tortelli, A., Nakamura, A., Suprani, F., Schürhoff, F., Van der Waerden, J., Szöke, A., . . ., & Pignon, B. (2018). Subclinical psychosis in adult migrants and ethnic minorities: Systematic review and meta-analysis. *British Journal of Psychiatry Open*, *4*(6), 510–518.

United Nations Development Programme. (2020a). *Human development reports: Human development index (HDI)*. Retrieved July 22, 2020, from http://hdr.undp.org/en/content/human-development-index-hdi

United Nations Development Programme. (2020b). *Human development reports: Inequality adjusted human development index (IHDI)*. Retrieved June 07, 2021, from Inequality-adjusted Human Development Index (IHDI) | Human Development Reports (undp.org)

United Nations Development Programme. (2020c). *Human development reports: The 2019 global multidimensional poverty index (MPI)*. Retrieved July 22, 2020, from http://hdr.undp.org/en/2019-MPI

Webb, R. T., Antonsen, S., Mok, P. L. H., Agerbo, E., & Pedersen, C. B. (2015). National cohort study of suicidality and violent criminality among Danish immigrants. *PLoS One*, *10*(6), e0131915. doi:10.1371/journal.pone.0131915

Weithmann, G., & Traub, H.-J. (2008). Die psychiatrische Vorgeschichte schizophrener Maßregelpatienten -Rahmenbedingungen der Deliktprävention durch die Allgemeinpsychiatrie. *Forensische Psychiatrie, Psychologie, Kriminologie*, *2*(2), 38–45. doi:10.1007/s11757-008-0071-y

Whiting, D., Lichtenstein, P., & Fazel, S. (2021). Violence and mental disorders: A structured review of associations by individual diagnoses, risk factors, and risk assessment. *The Lancet Psychiatry*, *8*(2), 150–161. doi:10.1016/S2215-0366(20)30262-5

Witt, K., Van Dorn, R., & Fazel, S. (2013). Risk factors for violence in psychosis: Systematic review and meta-regression analysis of 110 studies. *PloS One, 8*(2), e55942.

Working group process optimization and quality assurance in Baden–Württemberg forensic psychiatric care (Arbeitsgruppe Prozessoptimierung und Qualitätssicherung im MRV-BW, [Arbeitsbericht 2019. Versorgungspolitische Entwicklungen im baden-württembergischen Maßregelvollzug. Kommentierte Auswertungen der Forensischen Basisdokumentation Baden–Württemberg (FoDoBa) 2009 bis 2018 ([FoDoBa Work Report 2019] Unpublished report). Zentrum für Psychiatrie Reichenau, Reichenau.

Chapter 7

Fathers in forensic mental health services

Michelle Wells, Sara Morgan, Leigh Gale, and Christopher Hartwright

Introduction

The purpose of this chapter is to raise awareness of the experiences and needs of fathers in forensic inpatient care and consider its implications for clinical practice. It is recognised that risk assessment is pertinent when working in forensic services, and this has been given elevated focus. In addition, perspectives of healthcare staff and fathers' children have been included to prompt further thinking. The initial focus is on recognising fathers in prison, as parallels to the forensic inpatient context can be drawn from the literature pertaining to incarceration.

Fathers in prison

Qualitative accounts of fathers in prison have been conducted across the globe, including Australia (Dennison et al., 2014), China (Chui, 2016), Norway (Ugelvik, 2014), United Kingdom (Boswell & Wedge, 2002; Akerman et al., 2018; Clarke et al., 2005), and the United States (Arditti et al., 2005). Wells et al. (2020), the authors of this chapter, conducted a systematic review focused on fathers' experiences during their custodial sentences in England and Wales.

The themes developed in the review were reflective of the wider literature, but the importance of recognising the psychological experience of fathers who have no child contact was emphasised. It was concluded that imprisoned fathers experience a complex myriad of emotions associated with identity, loss, hope, and motivation. Further, there seemed to be features of shame and guilt. Imprisonment appeared to be a pertinent time for fathers marked by changes in identity, primarily due to tensions between fatherhood and 'offender' identities. Indeed, it has been identified that the fatherhood role can motivate a future free from offending (Helyar-Cardwell, 2012).

It seemed that some fathers tried to verify their paternal identity by attempting to enact parenting practices and relying on their familial network. Nevertheless, loss was associated with an erosion of fatherhood status, 'missing out' on father–child experiences, and the subsequent adverse impact on their child. Yet, hope and motivation were related to thoughts around crime desistance, to 'keep going' in prison, and improve paternal relationships. It is plausible given the prevalence of MH needs in prison that fathers in the carceral environment may share experiences with those detained in MH services.

Imprisoned fathers, comparably to those in an MH inpatient setting, are detained in an institutional setting and experience separation from their children. The Ministry of Justice (MoJ) in England and Wales identified that a significant proportion of the prison population had MH needs (Bradley, 2009). Many individuals in prison have experienced abusive

DOI: 10.4324/9781003184768-9

parenting in childhood and experience the effects of such trauma into their adult life (Ardino, 2012). Similarly, a study conducted in forensic inpatient care found that over half of the inpatient sample had experienced some form of childhood abuse (Argent et al., 2017).

It is apposite to make reference to the ACEs (Felitti et al., 1998; Public Health Wales, 2015) literature as it is relevant to both fathers in prison and in forensic inpatient settings. The concept of ACEs centres on traumatic events such as physical, sexual, and/or emotional abuse, difficulties in the household environment (e.g., parental imprisonment), or neglect occurring in childhood, which can impact the overall well-being. There are further implications concerning intergenerational patterns of trauma and offending for fathers' children, as parental MH needs and imprisonment are identified as an ACE when experienced in early life.

Parental mental health and inpatient services

In the United Kingdom, it is estimated that one-quarter to one-third of the population in MH inpatient services are parents, some of whom maintain contact and have active child involvement (Chao & Kuti, 2009; Gow et al., 2010). A study conducted in a regional South Wales secure unit recorded higher rates of parental status at 46% (Argent et al., 2017). This study reviewed data over a nine-year period, rather than point prevalence. The MoJ (2018) approximates that 87% of the forensic inpatient population are male. Thus, the majority of parents in such services are likely to be fathers.

Parrott et al. (2015) identified that research focused on parents in forensic inpatient services is sparse, suggesting that when individuals with MH needs who are also parents require hospitalisation, there may be limited understanding on how this may be experienced. This is of concern, as inpatient hospitalisation can be systemically traumatic for the parent, their children, and their wider familial network (Reupert & Maybery, 2007). Trauma may occur on multiple levels for the parent, as they experience heightened MH difficulties, detainment, and separation from loved ones (Akerson, 2003).

Akerson (2003) emphasised that individuals who experience enduring MH difficulties have the same desire to fulfil their parental role as parents who do not have such needs. Further, Akerson (2003) highlighted that during inpatient hospitalisation, there were concerns related to the potential loss of child custody, namely, due to divorce or involvement from child welfare services.

Safeguarding children is of paramount importance, and any decisions made with regard to the parent–child relationship need to ensure they bear the child's best interest in mind. There are, of course, considerations to be made when a parent has MH needs, but it is apt to raise awareness of potential influences on the decision-making process. Reupert and Maybery (2007) identify that inaccurate assumptions may be held around the risk of violence and harm to their child(ren). Argent et al. (2017) reported that men in their secure service sample (regardless of parental status) were unlikely to have ever harmed a child.

Fathers in forensic inpatient services

The current empirical literature base offers a limited understanding of parents' experiences of fatherhood in forensic inpatient settings. The authors are aware of only two relevant qualitative studies: Parrott et al. (2015) and Wells et al. (2021).

Parrott et al. (2015) conducted a qualitative study, recruiting mothers and fathers to investigate their experience of forensic inpatient care. They reported that parenthood remained central to participants' personal identity and the importance of healthcare staff acknowledging parental status was raised. However, due to shame associated with MH difficulties and offending behaviour, some parents chose not to have contact with their children – this was particularly the case for fathers. MH stigma, rather than the shame related to having a criminal record, was the most apparent barrier to child visitation. Fathers appeared to experience difficulties in explaining their MH needs and hospital admission to their child(ren).

Wells et al. (2021) built on the qualitative findings of Parrott et al. (2015). In this project, the core psychological concept of paternal connection was developed via Social Constructivist Grounded Theory (Charmaz, 2014). Paternal connection describes the internal sense of connectivity that men appeared to have to their fatherhood identity. Connection appeared relevant to both fathers who had contact and those who had limited or no contact. The nature and quality of paternal connectivity appeared to be influenced by multiple factors, encompassed under wider themes related to individual psychological processes, interpersonal relationships, and the institutional organisation.

Chao and Kuti (2009) conducted a retrospective study reviewing data from two medium-secure units which found that less than a third of parents had contact with their children. Argent et al. (2017) reported that in their adult forensic inpatient sample of both males and females (*n* = 165), 46% were parents. It was reported that almost half of children under 18 years old had lost all contact with their parents.

In the Parrott et al. (2015) study, fathers were less likely than mothers to maintain child contact. The impact of inpatient admission on the father–child relationship had a detrimental effect on paternal MH. Indeed, the level of distress experienced had led one father to attempt suicide. It was identified that mothers were more likely than fathers to speak about some of the emotional issues related to the child–parent relationship. Parrott et al. (2015) identified that participants experienced loss, shame, and guilt which were related to unmet aspirations they had held as a parent.

It is identified by Evenson et al. (2008) and elsewhere in the literature (Ramachandani & Psychogiou, 2009) that fathers with serious MH needs have been overlooked in research. An exception to this is the study by Evenson et al. (2008), who interviewed fathers who experienced MH difficulties associated with psychosis. Notably, the study was not solely focused on inpatient care, but some fathers described periods of secure care hospitalisation. During inpatient admission, fathers appeared to avoid child contact, namely, due to MH shame and not wanting their child(ren) to witness their MH deterioration. In addition, fathers had concerns regarding visitation which were related to child(ren) being in the presence of other patients and the hospital environment.

The role of fatherhood in forensic mental health risk assessment

Within criminal justice and forensic MH contexts, structured professional judgement (SPJ) tools are used to assess the risk of violence and sexual violence. SPJ tools highlight theoretical and empirically based risk factors, including historical static items and dynamic changeable risk factors in order to identify potential points of intervention.

The HCR-20 version 3 (Douglas et al., 2013) is considered to be the gold standard tool for assessing and formulating the risk of physical violence. Within the HCR-20, a history of problems with relationships is defined as a 'history of serious problems establishing and maintaining stable personal relationships that result in a lack of positive social or emotional support' (p. 72). Assessors are encouraged to consider both intimate and non-intimate relationships, through which the individual's role as a father may be considered. Proposed problems may include conflictual relationships or alienation from family, with indicators presenting as social isolation or emotional distance. Therefore, conflictual or absent relationships with children may be considered relevant within this domain and may be perceived as contributing to an increase in risk.

Furthermore, a gender-sensitive version of HCR-20 has been developed specifically for assessing the risk of violence in females (HCR-20 FAM; de Vogel et al., 2014). In contrast to the original version whereby parenting issues are subsumed within overall 'relationship instability', within the HCR-20 FAM, maternal parenting difficulties are explicitly assessed. This is due to the assumption that parents who abuse their children tend to exhibit difficulties with parenting skills (De Ruiter & De Jong, 2005). Moreover, an exploratory study suggested that women perceive parenting stress as a justification for engaging in violence towards a partner, particularly if they experience low feelings of effectiveness with regard to their parenting role (Simmons et al., 2010). Arguably, risk assessment tools that are generally applied to males are tentative at best in acknowledging the potential impact of fatherhood on risk towards others.

The Good Lives Model of understanding offending behaviour

SPJ tools such as the HCR-20 align primarily with principles of the Risk, Need, and Responsivity model (Andrews & Bonta, 1998). The primary premise of assessment and intervention is to manage risk through the reduction of risk factors, as opposed to enhancing the quality of life (Ward, 2002).

In contrast, the Good Lives Model (GLM) is a strengths-based approach to supporting individuals in desistence from offending (Ward, 2002). The model proposes that offending behaviour occurs in response to individuals seeking out normal human 'goods', for example, excellence in play, agency, and work, creativity, and relatedness. However, individuals may lack the personal skills, capabilities, or environmental means to do this in a prosocial manner. Therefore, criminal behaviour may arise as a maladaptive attempt to meet life values (Ward & Stewart, 2003). Consequently, intervention focuses on supporting the individual to enhance their skills and capabilities to achieve personally meaningful valued outcomes in a prosocial and sustainable way. Thus, in line with the GLM, supporting and empowering fathers to fulfil meaningful relationships with their children may have positive outcomes in terms of desistence from future offending.

The Structured Assessment of Protective Factors for violence risk (SAPROF; de Vogel et al., 2011) aligns with the GLM due to its specific focus on identifying and strengthening protective factors in order to reduce violence. Whilst the SAPROF references social network and intimate relationships as external protective factors, the role of fatherhood and the individual's relationship with their child(ren) is not explicitly assessed.

Assessments of risk and protective factors used commonly within forensic MH potentially overlook the importance of fatherhood in relation to an individual's recovery and future risk of offending. Based upon the principles of the GLM, it could be argued that identifying fatherhood as an unmet 'good' may allow for interventions to be targeted to support the individual to build upon their relationship with their child(ren). In some cases, this would not be deemed appropriate; in line with Child Protection legislation. However, improved relationships with children may also serve to enhance other 'goods' in terms of knowledge, excellence in play, community, and pleasure. Such increases in capability, opportunity, and skills to meet such needs may result in a reduction in offending behaviour.

Care and Treatment Plans (Mental Health [Wales] Measure 2012) in Wales and Care Programme Approach (CPA) documentation in England detail parenting need as part of an overall assessment of the service user. Where parenting needs are identified, the support provided may be practical in nature, for example, checking benefit entitlement or supporting contact if a parent is admitted to the hospital. Support may also extend to emotional support and parenting advice, although specific guidance on the nature of support required for parenting responsibilities is vague.

The Camberwell Assessment of Need (CAN; Phelan et al., 1995) is widely used to understand and address the needs of individuals with serious MH difficulties. The assessment has been adapted for various contexts, including the CAN-M (Howard et al., 2008) for mothers. It appears that no comparable assessment is available for fathers. Consequently, service users and MH professionals undertaking formal care plan documentation lack an assessment tool specifically designed for the robust consideration of the needs of fathers with MH difficulties.

Child perspectives

There is a paucity of research specifically considering the impact on the child of having a father detained in a forensic MH setting. However, it seems likely that the child's exposure to a number of ACEs (including parental mental illness and parental incarceration) increases their vulnerability to developing a myriad of psychological, physical, and MH difficulties that may persist into adulthood. These can include attachment difficulties, complex PTSD, depression, poor school attainment, suicidal behaviour, and externalising behaviours.

Paternal mental illness is understood to both directly and indirectly increase a child's risk of developing emotional and behavioural difficulties, psychiatric disorders, and poor physical health and social outcomes across the lifespan (Manning & Gregoire, 2006; Fisher, 2017). Emerging research also suggests that this vulnerability may be compounded by the intergenerational transmission of paternal ACEs and trauma from father to child. This is of particular relevance because prevalence rates for forensic inpatients experiencing four or more ACEs have been found to be as high as 95.3% for this population (Finch et al., 2020) in comparison to 9.2% of adults in high-income countries in a general population study (Kessler et al., 2010). Furthermore, Finch et al. (2020) found that higher ACEs were significantly related to forensic inpatients reaching diagnostic criteria for complex PTSD, which itself has the potential for intergenerational transmission.

In order to ameliorate the potential impact such experiences will have on the child of fathers in forensic inpatient settings, particularly where there is an ongoing parent–child relationship, it is imperative that the father has access to interventions to address early trauma and abuse and to address attachment issues and to build on their own resilience.

A number of parallels might also be drawn from the literature on the impact on children affected by parental imprisonment. This indicates that children are likely to experience a significant sense of loss, in addition to sigma, social isolation, shame, and fear, and are more likely to become a 'looked after child' and to lose contact with their biological parents (Beresford et al., 2020). Paternal incarceration can lead to financial and residential instability, disrupt caregiving relationships, and is associated with negative child outcomes including mental illness, antisocial, and criminal behaviour (Johnson & Easterling, 2012). In parallel to the children of fathers detained in MH settings, children may also have been 'at risk' prior to incarceration due to, for example, an increased likelihood of parental substance misuse, paternal MH difficulties, and poverty, thus further increasing the child's vulnerability to the negative outcomes discussed.

The impact on the child of paternal hospitalisation in a forensic setting is also likely influenced by the nature and quality of the father–child relationship prior to and during hospitalisation. This includes the father's degree of involvement in parenting and the quality of the parental relationship. For children with a strong father–child relationship or who live with their father prior to hospitalisation, the effects of parental separation on the child should be an important consideration for commissioners and service providers alike. With due consideration given to the father's distance from his child(ren) and whether his children or the father has the necessary support/time/financial means in order to facilitate visits to maintain the relationship.

Encouragingly, emerging research suggests that a number of the mechanisms believed to increase vulnerability to negative outcomes following exposure to ACEs such as paternal mental illness and paternal incarceration/hospitalisation may be ameliorable to intervention. Father involvement has been linked to positive child mental and medical health outcomes from pregnancy to childhood that persist through adulthood (Fisher, 2017). There may therefore be a key role for services in working to mitigate the impact on the child of paternal hospitalisation, particularly when the father has been actively involved in parenting but also where there is potential for them to take a more active and positive parental role whilst detained.

Staff perspectives

The research available on the experiences of staff working with fathers within forensic MH services is very limited. Much of it focuses on specific interventions delivered by staff to patients with the focus being on the outcomes of such interventions, attitudes towards family intervention, or skills needed to deliver them (Absalom et al., 2010; Absalom-Hornby et al., 2012; Gatherer et al., 2020). Despite this, it felt important to highlight staff perspectives in relation to fathers in forensic MH services, as working with fathers within this setting can present with many challenges.

Existing research within adult MH evidences that the staff attitudes can affect the success of a family intervention. Absalom-Hornby (2012) found that staff attitudes towards a family intervention delivered via webcam were positive, though staff did emphasise that there were barriers to its successful application including training and dedicated staff time. Interviews with staff working within adult MH services in Australia revealed that clinicians felt they had two focuses to their work with both the patient–parent needs and the child's needs to consider (Tchernegovski et al., 2018). For some, this 'dual need' was difficult to maintain as their felt sympathy and responsibility aligned with the parent's needs, whilst others had developed ways to manage these feelings enabling a dual focus that held both the needs of the parent and the child in mind. This involved intrapersonal and interpersonal approaches including purposefully keeping both the parent and child perspective in mind, supervision/support/ consultation from objective colleagues, using a strengths-based approach, and enabling parents with choices.

Research that focuses on staff perspectives of parenting in secure services is limited. However, Kalebic et al. (2020) explored social workers' perspectives of parents who were patients within a secure hospital. Themes around the artificial nature of parenting within secure services emerged with resolutions to this being social workers taking an active role in keeping the parent–child relationship in mind and working towards a 'natural' or 'normal' parent–child relationship. Barriers to this, however, included other clinical team members' views of the parent–child relationship, risk to the child, and no access to developing skills in parenting. Enablers included access to facilities such as a family visiting room and family therapy.

Clinical implications

In considering the needs of fathers within the context of a forensic MH service and the wider context of influences on the parental relationship, a number of clinical implications have been identified.

In assessing the father's needs, it is important that this is approached in a systemic way, considering the whole family. This appears relevant to not only the ACEs literature and reducing intergenerational risk but also the father's current risk as their paternal relationship can offer hope and motivation for the future. The need for a thorough assessment is considered imperative regardless of child contact. Thus, the authors recommend enhancing consideration of the emotional, cognitive, and social impact of fatherhood needs as well as the practical needs of fathers on official MH documentation, e.g., CTP/CPA.

In the context of risk assessment, it is important to highlight that risk and protective factors related to fatherhood can be considered within current SPJ tools. Although there are no specific prompts regarding this, it is a potential factor that can influence a patient's risk. Therefore, clinicians undertaking such risk assessments should ensure that they explore the role of fatherhood with patients in order to incorporate relevant information related to fathers' risk/protective factors and support needs.

When considering interventions, supporting a father's role/connection to their child or enhancing their identity as a father even without direct contact with their child could have benefits in terms of enhancing well-being and risk reduction in line with the GLM.

Recommendations for future research

Future research is recommended to focus on fathers who experience under-representation in the empirical literature. Barnett et al. (2019) note ethnic minority groups are disproportionately detained under the MHA (1983, amended 2007). This includes overrepresentation in forensic inpatient care (Coid et al., 2000). The authors recommend that studies actively recruit ethnic minority fathers to ensure consideration of contextual factors, such as variation in cultural expectations of fatherhood.

Research would be welcomed that explores the impact on the father–child relationship and the long-term outcomes for both the father and the child. This could be used to develop interventions that can build upon the strengths of fathers to promote mental well-being whilst also aiming to reduce the risk of harm/offending.

Staff/clinician perceptions and attitudes towards fatherhood within forensic MH services would also be recommended. This would enable the exploration of factors that influence the support/interventions patients receive whilst in secure services. This should include the exploration of potential influences, such as the child's age, offence type, and/or factors within the staff member (e.g., own relationships with fathers/children, values, etc.)

Continuing to conduct research into fathers' experiences of forensic inpatient services and how professionals can support their needs is also recommended. Such research could be expanded to include research with children and other family members to discuss the impact of fathers in forensic inpatient care.

As is available for mothers within MH services, research into an assessment for fathers in forensic inpatient services is also needed. This would formalise the assessment of fathers' needs and consider them within the context of forensic MH services.

Conclusion

Forensic inpatient care offers a valuable opportunity to work with men who may need support to develop a richer relationship with their paternal role. In order to facilitate this, potential unmet needs and the impact of inpatient hospitalisation on fatherhood require recognition, through conducting a thorough assessment and having service support. It is possible that facilitating conversations and systemic interventions focused on the paternal relationship can support MH recovery, motivate desistance from crime, and have beneficial outcomes for fathers' children.

References

Absalom-Hornby, V., Hare, D. J., Gooding, P., & Tarrier, N. (2012). Attitudes of relatives and staff towards family intervention in forensic services using Q methodology. *Journal of Psychiatric and Mental Health Nursing, 19*(2), 162–173.

Absalom-Hornby, V., McGovern, J., Gooding, P. A., & Tarrier, N. (2010). An assessment of patient need for family intervention in forensic services and staff skill in implementing family interventions. *The Journal of Forensic Psychiatry & Psychology, 21*(3), 350–365.

Akerman, G., Arthur, C., & Levi, H. (2018). A qualitative study of imprisoned fathers: Separation and impact on relationships with their children. *Prison Service Journal, 238*, 16–27.

Akerson, B. J. (2003). Coping with the dual demands of severe mental illness and parenting: The parent's perspective. *Families in Society, 84*(1), 109–118.

Andrews, D. A., & Bonta, J. (1998). *The psychology of criminal conduct* (2nd ed.). Anderson.

Ardino, V. (2012). Offending behaviour: The role of trauma and PTSD. *European Journal of Psychotraumatology, 3*(1), 1–4.

Arditti, J. A., Smock, S. A., & Parkman, T. S. (2005). "It's been hard to be a father": A qualitative exploration of incarcerated fatherhood. *Fathering, 3*(3), 267–288.

Argent, S. E., Riddleston, L., Warr, J., Tippetts, H., Meredith, Z., & Taylor, P. J. (2017). A period prevalence study of being a parent in a secure psychiatric hospital and a description of the parents, the children and the impact of admission on parent-child contact. *Criminal Behaviour and Mental Health, 28*(1), 85–99.

Barnett, P., et al. (2019). Ethnic variations in compulsory detention under the mental health act: A systematic review and meta-analysis of international data. *Lancet Psychiatry, 6*(4), 305–317.

Beresford, S., Loucks, N., & Raikes, B. (2020). The health impact on children affected by parental imprisonment. *British Medical Journal Paediatrics Open, 4*, e000275. doi:10.1136/ bmjpo-2018-000275

Boswell, G., & Wedge, P. (2002). *Imprisoned fathers and their children*. Jessica Kingsley Publishers.

Bradley, K. J. C. (2009). *The Bradley report*. Department of Health.

Chao, O., & Kuti, G. (2009). Supporting children of forensic in-patients: Whose role is it? *Psychiatric Bulletin, 33*, 55–57.

Charmaz, K. (2014). *Constructing grounded theory*. SAGE Publications Ltd.

Chui, W. H. (2016). Voices of the incarcerated father: Struggling to live up to fatherhood. *Criminology & Criminal Justice, 16*(1), 60–79.

Clarke, L., O'Brien, M., Day, D., Godwin, H., Connolly, J., Hemmings, J., & Van Leeson, T. (2005). Fathering behind bars in English prisons: Imprisoned fathers' identity and contact with their children. *Fathering, 3*(3), 221–241.

Coid, J., Kahtan, N., Gault, S., & Jarman, B. (2000). Ethnic differences in admissions to secure forensic psychiatry services. *British Journal of Psychiatry, 177*(3), 241–247.

Dennison, S., Smallbone, H., Stewart, A., Freiberg, K., & Teague, R. (2014). 'My life is separated': An examination of the challenges and barriers to parenting for indigenous fathers in prison. *The British Journal of Criminology, 54*(6), 1189–1108.

de Ruiter, C., & de Jong, E. M. (2005). De Ruiter et al., in preparation – parents who abuse have inadequate parent skills.

de Vogel, V., de Vries, M., van Kalmthout, R. W., & Place, C. (2014). *HCR-20 female additional manual, additional guidelines to the HCR-20 v3 for assessing risk for violence in women*. Van der Hoeven Kliniek.

de Vogel, V., de Vries Robbé, M., de Ruiter, C., & Bouman, Y. H. (2011). Assessing protective factors in forensic psychiatric practice: Introducing the SAPROF. *International Journal of Forensic Mental Health, 10*(3), 171–177.

Douglas, K. S., Hart, S. D., Webster, C. D., & Belfrage, H. (2013). *HCR-20V3: Assessing risk of violence – User guide*. Mental Health, Law, and Policy Institute, Simon Fraser University.

Evenson, E., Rhodes, J., Feigenbaum, J., & Solly, A. (2008). The experiences of fathers with psychosis. *Journal of Mental Health, 17*(6), 629–642.

Felitti, V. J., Anda, R. F., Nordenberg, D., Williamson, D. F., Spitz, A. M., Edwards, V., Koss, M. P., & Marks, J. S. (1998). Relationship of childhood abuse and household dysfunction to many of the leading causes of death in adults: The adverse childhood experiences (ACEs) study. *American Journal of Preventative Medicine, 56*(6), 774–786.

Finch, K., Hartwright, C., Lawrence, D., Williams, M., & Thompson, A. (2020). The relationships between adverse childhood experiences, attachment, resilience, psychological distress and trauma among forensic mental health populations [Unpublished Doctoral Thesis]. Cardiff University.

Fisher,. S. D. (2017, May–June). Paternal mental health: Why is it relevant? *American Journal of Lifestyle Medicine*, 200–211.

Gatherer, C., Dickson-Lee, S., & Lowenstein, J. (2020). The forgotten families: A systematic literature review of family interventions within forensic mental health services. *The Journal of Forensic Psychiatry & Psychology*, *31*(6), 1–14.

Gow, R. L., Choo, M., Darjee, M., Gould, S., & Steele, S. (2010). A demographic study of the orchard clinic: Scotland's first medium secure unit. *Journal of Forensic Psychiatry & Psychology*, *21*(1), 139–155.

Helyar-Cardwell, V. (2012). Fathers for good? Exploring the impact of becoming a father on young offenders' desistance from crime. *Safer Communities*, *11*(4), 169–178.

Howard, L. et al. (2008). *Camberwell assessment of need for mothers (Can-M): A needs-based assessment for pregnant women and mothers with severe mental illness*. Royal College of Psychiatrists.

Johnson, E. I., & Easterling, B. (2012, April). Understanding unique effects of parental incarceration on children: Challenges, progress, and recommendations. *Journal of Marriage and Family*, *74*, 342–356.

Kalebic, N., Adams, A., Bezeczky, Z., Argent, S., Bagshaw, R., & Taylor, P. J. (2020). Social workers' perspectives on people parenting while patients in a secure hospital. *The Journal of Forensic Psychiatry & Psychology*, *31*(3), 364–384.

Kessler, R. C., McLaughlin, K. A., Green, J. G., Gruber, M. J., Sampson, N. A., Zaslavsky, A. M., . . . Angermeyer, M. (2010). Childhood adversities and adult psychopathology in the WHO world mental health surveys. *The British Journal of Psychiatry*, *197*(5), 378–385.

Manning, C., & Gregoire, A. (2006). Effects of paternal mental illness on children. *Psychiatry*, *5*(1), 10–12.

Mental Health Act. (MHA, 1983, amended 2007). *Chapter 20*. Retrieved December 29, 2019, from www.legislation.gov.uk/ukpga/1983/20

Ministry of Justice. (2018). *Restricted patients: 2018*. Retrieved February 21, 2020, from www.gov.uk/government/statistics/offender-management-statistics-quarterly-october-to-december-2018

Parrott, F. R., Macinnes, D. L., & Parrott, J. (2015). Mental illness and parenthood: Being a parent in secure psychiatric care. *Criminal Behaviour and Mental Health*, *25*(4), 258–272.

Phelan, M., et al. (1995). The Camberwell assessment of need: The validity and reliability of an instrument to assess the needs of people with severe mental illness. *British Journal of Psychiatry*, *167*(5), 589–595.

Public Health Wales. (2015). *Welsh adverse childhood experiences (ACEs) study. Adverse childhood experiences and their impact on health harming behaviours in the Welsh adult population*. PHW.

Ramachandani, P., & Psychogiou, L. (2009). Paternal psychiatric disorders and children's psychosocial development. *The Lancet*, *374*(9690), 646–653.

Reupert, A., & Maybery, D. (2007, July). Families affected by parental mental illness: A multiperspective account of issues and interventions. *American Journal of Orthopsychiatry*, *77*(3), 362–369. doi: 10.1037/0002-9432.77.3.362. PMID: 17696664.

Simmons, C. A., Lehmann, P., & Dia, D. A. (2010). Parenting and women arrested for intimate partner violence. *Journal of Interpersonal Violence*, *25*, 1429–1448.

Tchernegovski, P., Hine, R., Reupert, A. E., & Maybery, D. J. (2018). Adult mental health clinicians' perspectives of parents with a mental illness and their children: Single and dual focus approaches. *BMC Health Services Research*, *18*(611), 67–76.

Ugelvik, T. (2014). Paternal pains of imprisonment: Incarcerated fathers, ethnic minority masculinity and resistance narratives. *Punishment and Society*, *16*(2), 152–168.

Ward, T. (2002). Good lives and the rehabilitation of sexual offenders: Promises and problems. *Aggression and Violent Behavior*, *7*, 513–528.

Ward, T., & Stewart, C. A. (2003). The treatment of sex offenders: Risk management and good lives. *Professional Psychology: Research and Practice*, *34*, 353–360.

Wells, M., Hartwright, C., Morgan, S., & Gale, L. (2020). *Fatherhood in prison: A narrative synthesis* (Unpublished doctoral thesis). Cardiff University.

Wells, M., Hartwright, C., Morgan, S., & Gale, L. (2021). "My kids will always be around me, if not physically, spiritually they will always be around me": Fatherhood in forensic inpatient services. *Journal of Forensic Psychology Research and Practice*, *27*(3), 404–418. doi:10.1080/24732850.2021.1945840

Part 3

Marginalised and diverse clinical characteristics

Chapter 8

Autism in forensic settings

Emma Longfellow and Julia Skelding

Introduction

Historically, autistic people have been marginalised by virtue of their neurological differences leading to discrimination and barriers to accessing their full human and civil rights (Autism Society, 2017). This already marginalised group is further overlooked due to a lack of representation from experts by experience in clinical review processes, such as mental health review tribunals, and a limited understanding of the links between risk behaviours, offending, and autism. This lack of understanding from professionals concerning autism-related needs leads to care being provided in unsuitable environments that exacerbate several intrinsic difficulties associated with autism (Simpson, 2016). This contributes to extended stays within secure services and, in many cases, high-risk behavioural responses to the environment (CQC, 2020). Further compounding this is the tendency of patients to fall between services where the identification of difficulties is only determined after a significant deterioration in presentation, heightened distress, and when they become a 'management problem'.

This chapter explores current developments within specialist autism services in forensic settings, with specific reference to the United Kingdom's National Learning Disability autism pilot service, and identifies the ongoing areas of development.

Defining autism

Autism spectrum disorder (ASD) is a neurodevelopmental disorder that is characterised by difficulties with social interaction, communication, and the presence of repetitive and fixed behaviour and interests (Beech et al., 2018). ASD is a spectrum disorder, and individuals present with a specific profile of which typical traits would include sensory processing concerns, cognitive strengths and weaknesses, and, frequently, high levels of anxiety (Murphy & Mullens, 2017). The Diagnostic and Statistical Manual fifth edition (DSM-V; American Psychiatric Association, 2013) definition includes two core areas of impairment in ASD: 'persistent deficits in social communication and social interaction' and 'restricted repetitive patterns of behaviour, interests or activities'. These impairments vary in terms of symptoms and levels of severity, hence being described as a *spectrum* disorder. Learning disability and ASD are the most common developmental disorders and 'combined they affect between 3 and 5 percent of the general population' (Srivastava & Schwartz, 2014).

ASD is associated with a high degree of psychiatric morbidity (Beech et al., 2018), the detection of which can be further complicated due to the autistic individual's difficulties in describing their own emotions and experiences. Symptoms of psychiatric or psychological disorders may also present in an atypical way; additionally, there are some disorders such as

DOI: 10.4324/9781003184768-11

social anxiety and obsessive-compulsive disorder that have diagnostic criteria that overlap with ASD (Beech et al., 2018). ASD is often either underdiagnosed as a comorbid difficulty or misdiagnosed as a psychotic disorder, personality disorder, or obsessive-compulsive disorder (Davidson et al., 2014; Dudas et al., 2017).

Throughout this chapter, the terms 'autism' or 'ASD' are used to include all conditions that fall on the autism spectrum, for example, Asperger syndrome, atypical autism, or pervasive developmental disorder. This chapter uses identity-first language, e.g., 'an autistic person' rather than 'a person with autism' (Royal College of Psychiatrists, 2020).

Broader policy trends

There is a growing appetite within general adult services and within the Criminal Justice System (CJS) in the United Kingdom to address the needs of adults with autism. A raft of policy and guidelines exist which emphasise the significance of getting services right for this group.

The introduction of the Autism Act (2009) in the United Kingdom, the only legislation that has been created specifically for a single disability, was hoped to have led to improvements in awareness and understanding by professionals within the public health sector. The statutory guidance accompanying the Act explicitly detailed the actions required by local authorities and the National Health Service (NHS) including training requirements and improved service provision (Archer & Hurley, 2013).

The transforming care agenda set out to improve health and care services with the aim that more people would be able to live in the community with the right support and close to home (NHS England, 2017). This led to the introduction of Care and Treatment Reviews (CTRs) which were designed to support patients and their families to have a voice and support the team around the patient. The main purpose of this review process is to ascertain whether the individual needs to be in hospital and if there are care and treatment needs (NHS England, 2015). The policy and national guidance are clear and consistent in relation to the necessity for patients with learning disabilities and/or autism to be provided treatment within the least restrictive environment (DoH, 2014). The transforming care programme set out guidance to the effect that autistic people with co-morbid learning disabilities need specific care that is tailored to their individual needs and that to provide for this, staff require specialised relevant clinical knowledge to complement their experiences of forensic care.

The 2010 strategy for adults with autism: *Fulfilling and Rewarding Lives* provides a framework for joint working and applies to all public services, including the CJS, with the expectation that reasonable adjustments are made for those encountering agencies (DoH, 2010). It sets out a duty of increasing the awareness and understanding of autism among frontline professionals and a requirement for a clear and consistent pathway for diagnosis.

The new National Autism Strategy included recommendations on improving support within the criminal and youth justice systems and announced a vision to improve the experiences of autistic people (DoH, 2021).

Additionally, the NHS long-term plan (NHS, 2019) signalled an extension to the five-year forward view for Mental Health (The Mental Health Taskforce, 2016) and emphasised a commitment to improving services for those with learning disabilities and autism with a specific focus on reducing long-term inpatient stays and use of restrictive practices.

Reasons why people with ASD may come into contact with the Criminal Justice System

There are many reasons why an autistic person might encounter the CJS, which include being victims of crime, witnesses to crime and incidents, and potential suspects/offenders (Archer &

Hurley, 2013). Although the offending behaviour of an autistic individual may not be related to their difficulties, for some, these difficulties are significant contributory factors (Haskins & Silva, 2006). The offending behaviours that research has linked to autistic people include violence, sexual offending, fire setting, stalking, and cyber-crime (Ledingham & Mills, 2015; Sabet et al., 2015; Allely & Creaby-Attwood, 2016). There is no evidence that suggests autistic people have higher rates of offending behaviour than the general population (King & Murphy, 2014). However, there is a growing body of research that suggests that autistic people who also have co-occurring psychiatric disorders are at higher risk of offending behaviour (Chaplin et al., 2013).

The UK prison system needs to become more autism-informed (Lewis et al., 2015). Autistic people are a challenging group for forensic services due to their specific difficulties, needs, and therapeutic profiles, considerations that these services are not well equipped to meet (Allely, 2018). There is evidence that autistic people experience difficulties in custodial environments due to a mismatch between difficulties associated with ASD and the environmental demands, for example, an autistic individual who is hyper-sensitive to noise may have difficulties in a noisy prison environment with jangling keys, banging doors, and noise from other inmates.

Studies have demonstrated that the average length of stay of autistic patients in forensic mental health hospitals was two to three years longer than the general mental health hospital population (Taylor et al., 1998). Possible explanations for this are the lack of specialist knowledge regarding the rehabilitation needs of this particular patient group and the lack of lower secure services which could provide places for treatment, progression, and discharge (Hare et al., 1999; Haw et al., 2013; Bathgate, 2017).

The process of minimising the potential for offending, which is a central element of the care of patients in psychiatric secure settings (Murphy, 2013), involves the assessment and formulation of risk. Risk assessment involves the consideration of factors such as the specific risk behaviour, its frequency and intensity, as well as other influences such as an individual's specific circumstances, past and current protective and risk factors, and their motivation for offending (Hart, 2001). A risk assessment should base informed decisions on the best available evidence, including knowledge of the individual, social context, and clinical judgement to guide an individual's risk management (Murphy, 2013). A series of guidelines is provided by the UK Department of Health that supports best practice in risk management (DoH, 2007).

The risk assessments that are utilised in the National High Secure Learning Disability (NHSLDS) include the HCR-20 (v3) instrument for violence risk assessment and management. This considers historical, current, clinical, and future risk management factors and is used extensively across forensic settings (Webster et al., 1997). It is recognised that there is a need to examine the application of standard risk assessment tools for autistic patients due to the presence of certain unique needs (Murphy, 2003, 2006). There is a view that risk assessments and formulations for autistic patients in forensic settings should consider associated complications (Staufenberg, 2007), which include cognitive difficulties such as theory of mind (ToM; particularly in relation to empathy and perspective taking), central coherence (the ability to discern meaning from a mass of detail), and dimensions of executive functioning. Social naivety can lead to vulnerability to exploitation, and the pursuit of deviant special interests can also be problematic (Barry-Walsh & Mullen, 2004).

Numerous studies have highlighted psychiatric morbidity as a risk factor for violence in autistic people, yet although this appears to be a significant risk factor, it is likely that the risk of violence is mediated by the cognitive and affective difficulties associated with ASD (Murphy, 2013). For some patients, the possibility is that further cognitive impairment occurs in the presence of psychiatric disorders. Autistic patients in forensic services may have a range of associated vulnerabilities which could increase their risks of violent behaviour in some circumstances; however, the evidence suggests there is no single factor linked to an offence and a combination of difficulties could lead to increased risks (Murphy, 2013).

Features of autism that have been described as factors that, along with environmental conditions, contribute to incidences of offending behaviour include theory of mind deficits and the presence of restricted interests and obsessions (Brewer & Young, 2015). Where autism is relevant to risk formulation, it is important to emphasise that it is a contextual rather than a causal factor. As such, it is the risk factor, not the autism that needs to be addressed. However, the autistic context of the risk factors needs to be considered and support offered in an autism responsive way (Al-Attar, 2019).

A strong case has been made for the development of risk assessment tools that specifically consider the difficulties observed in this patient group. In the absence of this, Al-Attar (2019) developed the Framework for the Assessment of Risk and protection in offenders on the Autistic Spectrum (FARAS) as guidance for risk assessors working with autistic people in the CJS. This framework provides advice on interviewing for risk assessment, autistism-specific risk factors, and how these factors can also be protective. It identifies seven facets associated with autism specifically i) Circumscribed Interests, ii) Visual Fantasy and Impaired Social Imagination, iii) Need for Order, Rules, Routines, and Predictability, iv) Obsessionality, Repetition, and Collecting, v) Social Interaction and Communication Difficulties, vi) Cognitive Styles (Difficulties and Strengths), and vii) Sensory Hyper and Hyposensitivity. These do not map directly onto diagnostic facets but are considered potentially relevant to risk. The FARAS is not a risk assessment tool, and assessors are advised to use it as a supplementary aid to existing risk assessments. However, this provides a guide to address the gap in current risk assessment methodologies. The FARAS guidelines address how to delineate the autistic functions of behaviour and in turn may add depth to risk assessment and inform formulation and rehabilitation pathways (Al-Attar, 2019). Shine and Cooper-Evans (2016) also note the importance of looking at autistic traits within risk formulation and suggest four key areas to consider i) unrelenting and obsessive pursuit of circumscribed interests, ii) deficits in theory of mind leading to impaired social understanding and poor problem solving, iii) seeking sensory stimulation or avoidance of sensory overstimulation, and iv) disruption to idiosyncratic cognitive rules or rigid behavioural routines or difficulties coping with change.

Given the lack of validated instruments for the evaluation of the risk of offending in individuals with ASD, clinicians and forensic practitioners must rely, predominantly, on the research which is based on individuals with no diagnosis of ASD and then extrapolate based on their knowledge of individuals with ASD (Sugrue, 2017).

Prevalence across the Criminal Justice System

Although there is greater consideration of this population in the CJS than in the past, our understanding remains limited and is compounded by difficulties in identifying who and where this population is. There are few studies investigating the prevalence of ASD in forensic settings (Scragg & Shah, 1994; Hare et al., 1999). These studies have shown that although small numbers of autistic patients reside in forensic settings, this is still an overrepresentation in comparison to the general population (Beech et al., 2018). Scragg and Shah (1994) screened the whole male population at Broadmoor high-security hospital in England and found a prevalence rate of 1.5–2.3%; Hare et al. (1999) screened 96% of the high-secure hospital population in England and reported a prevalence rate of 2.4%. To date, studies have not taken place in Scotland or Wales. The prevalence of autistic people in the prison system is unknown (Robinson et al., 2012) although in a study of adult male prisoners, Underwood et al. (2016) found high levels of unrecognised ASD traits with 2% of participants fulfilling the diagnostic criteria.

Considering the difficulties in identifying this population, it is unsurprising that patient experiences are also an under-researched area. This is despite there being a wealth of clinical interest in the field (Esan et al., 2015). What is particularly pronounced is the lack of research on treatment outcomes in forensic services for autistic people and where there has been these are single studies and based primarily on broader frameworks incorporating SPELL (a framework for treating autistic people, 'Sensory, Positive, Environment, Low Arousal, Links'; Esan et al., 2015). More recently, there has been an exploration of relatively innovative interventions such as Radically Open Dialectical Behaviour Therapy (RO:DBT; Lynch, 2015). This has been evaluated with non-forensic autistic populations demonstrating improved outcomes and reduced distress and has been introduced in some forensic settings to work with patients with disorders of overcontrol which would be inclusive of autism. This provision is primarily in specialist hospital services with prison services focused primarily on formulating risk management plans and enabling patients to access existing prison pathways. A study by Murphy and Mullens (2017) identified from patient interviews that in comparison to a prison setting, the high-secure hospital was a less stressful environment with more therapeutic options, but there are practical improvements that would improve outcomes such as specialist trained staff and increased autism awareness amongst staff. Difficulties were described in relation to special interests (e.g., access to items that were not allowed due to security restrictions), sensory aspects, such as noisy environments, and search procedures which were described as particular stressors (Murphy & Mullen, 2017). Some authors have also suggested that autistic individuals benefit from the structured and routine nature of custodial environments (Allen et al., 2008). Worryingly, Hare et al. (1999) noted that autistic people in high secure care were detained significantly longer than those in other treatment settings.

Pilot case study of the service at Rampton Hospital (commenced September 2020)

The National High Secure Learning Disability Service (NHSLDS) based at Rampton High-Security Hospital in England has seen an increase in the number of admissions of patients with a learning disability and/or autism.

It was recognised that the current service delivery and philosophy within the NHSLDS required modernisation in line with best practice. It was proposed that a specialist ward be developed for autistic patients to meet their specialist needs, whether this is support with integration and social skills or to prepare them to move on to a lower security setting. The risks of not implementing the specialist service include this patient group not being provided with reasonable adjustments to access treatment which could potentially lead to an increase in adverse risk behaviours, leading to restrictive practices and an increased length of stay.

The service received funding from specialist commissioners to provide a seven-bed specialist ward for autistic patients with learning disabilities. Additional nursing posts were developed to provide a dedicated nurse specialist and two social communication support workers who are able to assess, plan, and implement autism-informed care for patients and implement the least restrictive practice, provide accessible information to patients, and lead on activities on the ward. Often autistic patients did not engage in the activities offered by the specialist day unit due to anxieties regarding integrating with peers and sensory difficulties relating to noise. The social communication workers were tasked with ensuring that activities were person-centred and tailored to individual needs in recognition of any difficulties experienced and supported patients to access the same opportunities as their peers.

Many autistic individuals have difficulty in processing everyday sensory information, any of the senses may be under- or over-active, or both. These sensory sensitivities can affect behaviour and have a profound impact on a person's life. A sensory-informed environment was established as per National Institute for Health and Care Excellence (NICE) guidance (NIHCE, 2016) using the checklist for autism-friendly environments (Simpson, 2016) whilst maintaining the requirements of a high secure service. For example, building works could not be completed to change doors or windows; however, training was provided to staff to raise awareness of sensory needs and to be mindful when using large key bunches or closing doors. The aim of a sensory-informed environment is to reduce episodes of behaviour that challenge and have a positive impact on patients' mental health.

NICE guidance suggests that care pathways for people with learning disabilities and co-morbid conditions such as autism require that skilled staff care for them and that they are responsive to individual needs (NIHCE, 2016). A specific autism-related training strategy was introduced that utilised the Skills for Health Capabilities Framework for working with autistic people (Health Education England, 2019). Further training was provided to staff which included implementation of the SPELL framework ('Sensory, Positive, Environment, Low Arousal, Links') for working with autistic people (Beadle-Brown & Mills, 2010), and Positive Behaviour Support (PBS; a person-centred approach to supporting people with a learning disability; BILD, 2021), which was led and embedded by staff that had been trained as PBS coaches by the British Institute of Learning Disabilities (BILD), and Sensory Integration Training was completed by an occupational therapist. This ensures a consistent and comprehensive service is delivered and maintained. This training was rolled out across the entirety of the Learning Disability Service (49 beds across four wards) to allow for personalised care to be delivered in line with best practice that is responsive to specific autism spectrum needs.

The multi-disciplinary team across the LD service supports functional analysis, formulation, and development of Positive Behaviour Support Plans which aim to deliver positive outcomes in terms of a reduction in behaviour that challenges and improved quality of life for patients. A trauma-informed approach was also adopted to upskill staff to recognise that many autistic patients have histories involving psychological trauma (Im, 2016). Autistic people could be at an increased risk of experiencing stressful and traumatic life events (Fuld, 2018). The symptoms associated with trauma such as aggression, difficulties in concentrating, social isolation, and relational difficulties can be confused with the symptoms relating to ASD (Bishop-Fitzpatrick et al., 2015; Garcia-Villamisar, D., & Rojahn, J. 2015). It is also important to remember that no two autistic people are the same and that understanding autism is the key to understanding the person (Chaplin et al., 2013).

There is very limited evidence for psychosocial interventions for the management of ASD in adults (Cornwall et al., 2020), and few studies have reviewed the effectiveness of existing interventions with the forensic population (Murphy, 2010; Macdonald et al., 2017). An analysis of therapeutic interventions was considered by the clinical team, and the decision was made to use RO:DBT (Lynch, 2018) to inform treatment. RO-DBT is an evidence-based treatment that targets a range of disorders that are characterised by excessive self-control (otherwise described as 'overcontrol'). It aims to link communicative functions of emotional expression to the formation of social bonds by teaching skills of social signalling and changing neurophysiological arousal (Lynch, 2018). ASDs have been recognised as maladaptive overcontrol conditions, and social signalling (for example, prosocial body language) appears to be a core difficulty in autistic people. Cornwall et al. (2020) evaluated the use of RO-DBT with adults with ASD in a mental health setting and found preliminary evidence for its effectiveness, particularly for adults without intellectual disability. The study suggested that autistic participants were able to learn skills of social signalling; however, evidence was only anecdotal.

The NHSLDS is adapting the treatment program for the needs of patients with both intellectual disability and ASD, and further research is needed to demonstrate the effectiveness with this population.

The dedicated autism and learning disability ward are exclusively for patients who meet the admission criteria within the learning disability pathway, the ward supports patients to receive care that promotes progress in their pathway and prevents delays in moving on in their care pathway via medium-security care, bespoke services, or autism specialised services. The pathway was developed in accordance with NICE guidance and informed by the National Autistic Society (NAS) relating to best practice for autistic patients (see Figure 8.1).

The key benefits and outcomes of having a specialist service are numerous. Patients reside in an environment that meets their needs and are supported by skilled staff. It is hoped that environmental changes will lead to a reduction in incidents and that improving treatment pathways will enable a greater understanding of how to meet patients' needs which should lead to less reliance on more restrictive practices such as seclusion and long-term segregation. The expectation is that this will improve the quality of life for patients and reduce the length of stay. Other proposed benefits are that levels of staff satisfaction will improve, which might lead to reduced sickness absences and improved levels of staff retention. As part of the pilot of the specialist service, a service evaluation project is underway to investigate patient perspectives on their quality of life and how well they perceive their needs are met, patient-reported emotional distress, incidences of behaviour that challenge, and measurement of the use of restrictive interventions such as seclusion and chemical and physical restraints. Staff perceptions will also be explored to understand their level of satisfaction at work, and data on sickness and retention rates will be collected. The pilot was due to be reviewed and evaluated in March 2020 but has been extended to 18 months due to the impact of the global pandemic.

Supporting the development of the specialist ward area is a multi-disciplinary monthly service development meeting. This convenes to review best practices and new legislations and provide support and advice. NICE guidance recommends that strategy groups should be responsible for developing, managing, and evaluating local care pathways; that the aims of the strategy group should be to develop clear policy and protocols; ensure training for staff; and support the integrated delivery of care (NIHCE, 2016). This group is responsible for the audit and review of the performance of the pathway. In addition, the service evaluation meetings feed into a forensic division neurodevelopmental expert group that meets bi-monthly and provides peer support and expert advice.

Future directions

In the future, it is anticipated that the specialist ward team of the NHSLDS will act as a specialist hub for disseminating, consulting, and supporting teams across the hospital and wider forensic division, thus developing a centre of excellence and leadership in an emerging and growing field. Consistent with government legislation, the service is applying for National Autistic Society accreditation which will set out a helpful framework for best practice that can be adopted by other care providers nationally and internationally.

There is a need for further research into the effectiveness of interventions and their impact on outcomes such as length of stay, clinical symptoms and behaviour, experiences of care, and quality of life. Further consideration also needs to be given to the specificity of risk assessment tools and their relevance to autistic patients. What would be particularly helpful would be increased co-production in research to help inform this emerging area.

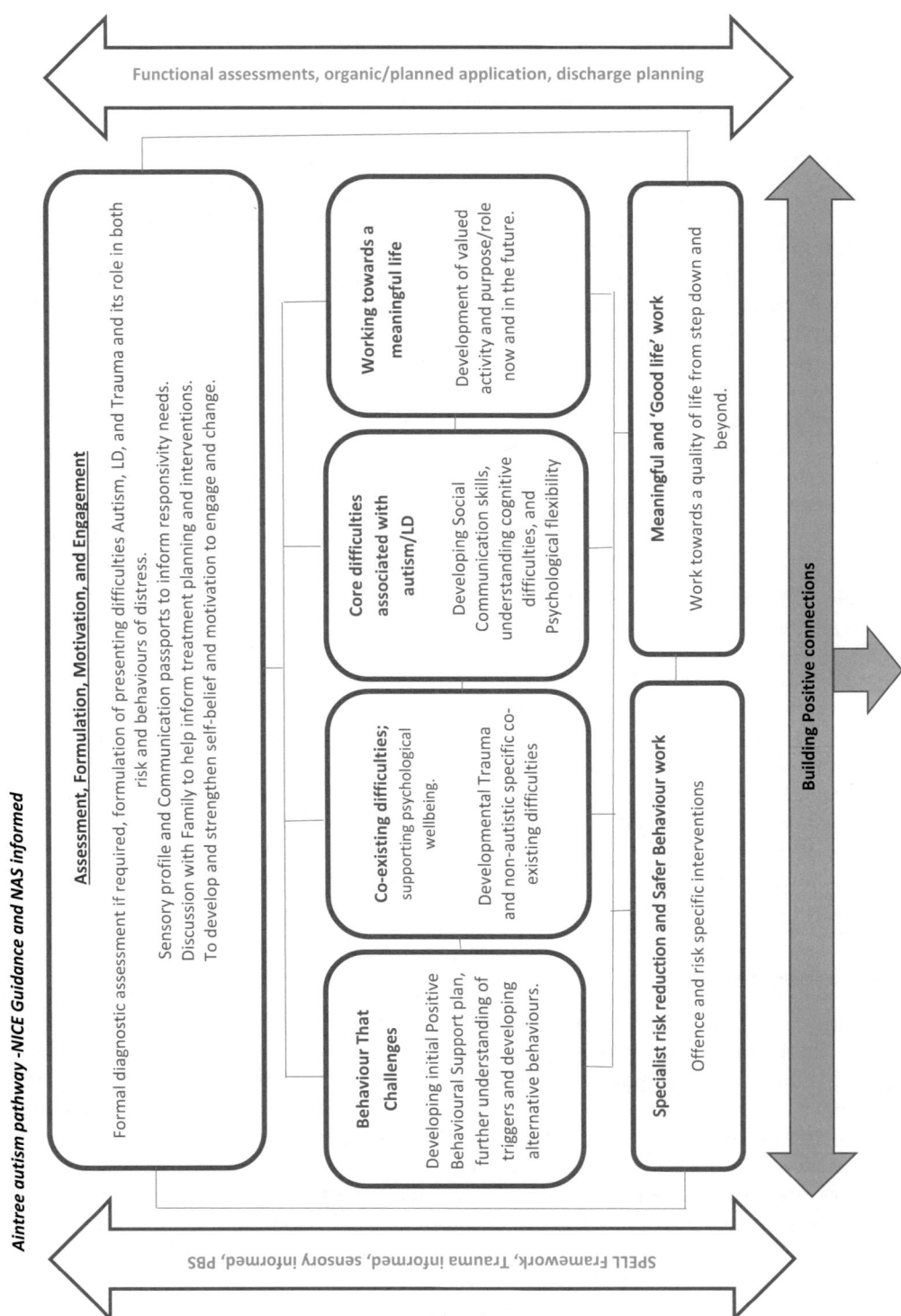

Figure 8.1 Aintree autism pathway – NICE Guidance and NAS informed

Conclusion

People with learning disabilities and autism that encounter the high secure estate have unique needs in comparison to the general high secure population, which can be in relation to both cognitive difficulties and sensory needs as well as the impact of co-morbid conditions. This makes them a highly marginalised group of individuals.

There is a paucity of research in this area, and it is evident that further research needs to be undertaken to understand the specific difficulties that autistic people experience in this environment. There is a lack of validated instruments for both risk assessment and the effectiveness of treatment interventions for this population. In this chapter, we described the only high secure LD/ASD service within the United Kingdom; therefore, comparable services in other countries should be evaluated so that treatment approaches and patient outcomes can be compared and best practices shared.

References

Al-Attar (2019). *Framework for the assessment of risk & protection in offenders on the autistic spectrum.* Retrieved May 5, 2022, from FARAS-Guidelines-Final-1.pdf (nota.co.uk).

Allely, C. S. (2018). A systematic PRISMA review of individuals with autism spectrum disorder in secure psychiatric care: Prevalence, treatment, risk assessment and other clinical considerations. *Journal of Criminal Psychology, 8*(1), 58–79.

Allely, C. S., & Creaby-Attwood, A. (2016). Sexual offending and autism spectrum disorders. *Journal of Intellectual Disabilities and Offending Behaviour, 7*(1), 35–51.

Allen, D., Evans, C., Hidler, A., Hawkins, S., Peckett, H., & Morgan, H. (2008). Offending behaviour in adults with Asperger Syndrome. *Journal of Autism and Developmental Disorders, 38,* 748–758.

American Psychiatric Association. (2013). *Diagnostic and statistical manual of mental disorders* (5th ed.). American Psychiatric Association.

Archer, N., & Hurley, E. A. (2013). A justice system failing the autistic community. *Journal of Intellectual Disabilities and Offending Behaviour, 4*(1/2), 53–59.

Autism Act. (2009). Retrieved February 26, 2021, from www.legislation.gov.uk/ukpga/2009/15/contents

Autism Society. (2017). National Position Statement on Human Rights. *Autism Society.* https://www.autism-society.org/public-policy/national-position-statements/national-position-statement-human-rights/

Barry-Walsh, J. B., & Mullen, P. (2004). Forensic aspects of Asperger's syndrome. *The Journal of Forensic Psychiatry and Psychology, 15*(1), 96–107.

Bathgate, D. (2017). ASD and offending: Reflections of practice in from a New Zealand perspective. *Journal of Intellectual Disabilities and Offending Behaviour, 8*(2), 90–98.

Beadle-Brown, J., & Mills, R. (2010). *Understanding and supporting children and adults on the Autism spectrum (The SPELL framework).* The National Autistic Centre, Tizard, University of Kent and Pavilion Publishing and Media Ltd.

Beech, A. R., Carter, A. J., Mann, R. E., & Rotshtein, P. (Eds.). (2018). *The Wiley Blackwell handbook of forensic neuroscience volume 1.* John Wiley & Sons Ltd, W. Sussex.

Bishop-Fitzpatrick, L., Mazefsky, C. A., Minshew, N. J., & Eack, S. M. (2015). The relationship between stress and social functioning in adults with autism spectrum disorder and without intellectual disability. *Autism Research, 8*(2), 164–173.

Brewer, N., & Young, R. L. (2015). *Crime and Autism spectrum disorder: Myths and mechanisms.* Jessica Kingsley.

British Institute of Learning Disabilities (BILD). (2021). *About PBS.* Retrieved October 02, 2012, from www.bild.org.uk/about-pbs/

Care Quality Commission. (2020). *'Out of sight – who cares? A review of restraint, seclusion and segregation for autistic people, and people with a learning disability and/or mental health condition.* CQC.

Chaplin, E., McCarthy, J., & Underwood, L. (2013). Autism spectrum conditions and offending: An introduction to the special edition. *Journal of Intellectual Disabilities and Offending Behaviour, 4*(1/2), 5–8. https://doi.org/10.1108/JIDOB-05-2013-0012

Cornwall, P. L., Simpson, S., Gibbs, C., & Morfee, V. (2020). Evaluation of radically open dialectical behaviour therapy in an adult community mental health team: Effectiveness in people with autism spectrum disorders. *British Journal of Psychiatry Bulletin*, 1–8.

Davidson, C., Greenwood, N., Stansfield, A., Wright, S. Prevalence of Asperger syndrome among patients of an early intervention in psychosis team. *Early Intervention in Psychiatry*, 8, 138–146.

Department of Health. (2007). *Best practise in managing risk: Principles and Evidence for best practise in the assessment and management of risk to self and others in mental health services*. Document prepared for the National Mental Health Risk Management Programme, Department of Health.

Department of Health. (2010). *Think Autism: Fulfilling and rewarding lives, the strategy for adults with Autism in England*. Department of Health.

Department of Health. (2014). *Positive and proactive care: Reducing the need for restrictive interventions*. Department of Health.

Department of Health. (2021). *The national strategy for autistic children, young people and adults: 2021–2026*. Department of Health.

Dudas, R. B., Lovejoy, C., Cassidy, S., Allison, C., Smith, P., Baron-Cohen, S. (2017). The overlap between autistic spectrum conditions and borderline personality disorder. *PLoS One*, *12*(9), e0184447.

Esan, F., Chester, V., Gunaratna, S. H., & Alexander, R. T. (2015). The clinical, forensic, and treatment outcome factors of patients with autism spectrum disorder treated in a forensic learning disability service. *Journal of Applied Researrch in Intellectual Disabilities*, *28*(3), 193–200.

Fuld, S. (2018). Autism spectrum disorder: The impact of stressful and traumatic life events and implications for clinical practice. *Clinical Social Work Journal*, 1–10.

Garcia-Villamisar, D., & Rojahn, J. (2015). Comorbid psychopathology and stress mediate the relationship between autistic traits and repetitive behaviours in adults with autism. *Journal of Intellectual Disability Research*, *59*(2), 116–124.

Hare, D., Gould, J., Mills, R., & Wing, L. (1999). A preliminary study of individuals with autistic spectrum disorders in three special hospitals in England. *National Autistic Society*, Retrieved March 3, 2013, from www.nas.org.uk/ content/1/c4/38/68/3hospitals.pdf

Hart. (2001). Assessing and managing violence risk. Chapter Two in K. Douglas, C. Webster, S. Hart, D. Eaves, & J. Ogloff (Eds.), *HCR-20 violence risk management companion guide* (pp. 13–26). Mental Health Law and Policy Institute, Simon Fraser University.

Haskins, B., & Silva, A. (2006). Asperger's disorder and criminal behaviour: Forensic psychiatric considerations. *Journal of the American Academy of Psychiatry and Law*, *34*(3), 374–384.

Haw, C., Radley, J., & Cooke, L. (2013). Characteristics of male autistic spectrum patients in low security: Are they different from non-autistic low secure patients? *Journal of Intellectual Disabilities and Offending Behaviour*, *4*(Nos'1/2), 24–32.

Health Education England. (2019). *Core capabilities framework for supporting autistic people*. NHS. Retrieved March 19, 2021, from https://skillsforhealth.org.uk/wp-content/uploads/2020/11/Autism-Capabilities-Framework-Oct-2019.pdf

Im, D. S. (2016). Trauma as a contributor to violence in autism spectrum disorder. *The Journal of the American Academy of Psychiatry and the Law*, *44*(2), 184–192.

King, C., & Murphy, G. (2014). A systematic review of people with autism spectrum disorder and the criminal justice system. *Journal of Autism and Developmental Disorder*, *44*(11), 2717–2733.

Ledingham, R., & Mills, R. (2015). A preliminary study of autism and cybercrime in the context of international law enforcement. *Advances in Autism*, *1*(1), 2–11.

Lewis, A., Pritchett, R., Hughes, C., & Turner, K. (2015). Development and implementation of autism standards for prisons. *Journal of Intellectual Disabilities and Offending Behaviours*, *6*(2), 68–80.

Lynch, T. R. (2018). *Radically open dialectical behaviour therapy. Theory and practice for treating disorders of overcontrol*. New Harbinger Publications.

Lynch, T. R., Hempel, R. J., & Dunkley, C. (2015). Radically open–dialectical behavior therapy for disorders of over-control: Signaling matters. *American Journal of Psychotherapy*, *69*(2), 141–162.

MacDonald, S., Clarbour, J., Whitton, C., & Raynor, K. (2017). The challenges of working with sexual offenders who have autism in secure services. *Journal of Intellectual Disabilities and Offending Behaviour*, *8*(1), 41–54.

The Mental Health Taskforce. (2016). *The five year forward view for mental health*. Retrieved March 19, 2021, from www.england.nhs.uk/wp-content/uploads/2016/02/Mental-Health-Taskforce-FYFV-final.pdf

Murphy, D. (2003). Admission details and cognitive profiles of male patients diagnosed with Asperger's syndrome detained in a special hospital: Comparison with a schizophrenia and a personality disorder sample. *The Journal of Forensic Psychiatry and Psychology*, *14*(3), 506–524.

Murphy, D. (2006). Theory of mind in forensic patients with Asperger's syndrome, schizophrenia and a personality disorder. *Cognitive Neuropsychiatry*, *11*(2), 99–111.

Murphy, D. (2010). Extreme violence in a young man with an autistic spectrum disorder: Assessment and intervention within high security psychiatric care. *Journal of Forensic Psychiatry and Psychology*, *21*(3), 462–477.

Murphy, D. (2013). Risk assessment of offenders with an autism spectrum disorder. *Journal of Learning Disabilities and Offending*. *4*(1/1), 33–41.

Murphy, D., & Mullens, H. (2017). Examining the experiences and quality of life of patients with an autism spectrum disorder detained in high secure psychiatric care. *Advances in Autism*, *3*(1), 3–14.

National Institute for Health and Care Excellence. (2016). *Autism spectrum disorder in adults: Diagnosis and management clinical guideline [CG 142]*. Retrieved March 19, 2021, from www.nice.org.uk/guidance/cg142/resources/autism-spectrum-disorder-in-adults-diagnosis-and-management-pdf-35109567475909

NHS. (2019). *The NHS long term plan*. NHS. Retrieved March 19, 2021, from www.longtermplan.nhs.uk/wp-content/uploads/2019/08/nhs-long-term-plan-version-1.2.pdf

NHS England. (2015). *Transforming care for people with learning disabilities – next steps*. NHS.

NHS England. (2017). *Transforming care. Model service specifications: Supporting implementation of the service model*. NHS England.

Robinson, L., Spencer, M. D., Thomson, L. D., Stanfield, A. C., Owens, D. G., Hall, J., & Johnstone, E. C. (2012). Evaluation of a screening instrument for autism spectrum disorders in prisoners. *PLoS One*, *7*(5), e36078.

Royal College of Psychiatrists. (2020). *The psychiatric management of autism in adults CR228*. RCP. Retrieved March 19, 2021, from www.rcpsych.ac.uk/improving-care/campaigning-for-better-mental-health-policy/college-reports/2020-college-reports/cr228

Sabet, J., Underwood, L., Chaplin, E., Hayward, H., & McCarthy, J. (2015). Autism spectrum disorder, attention-deficit hyperactivity disorder and offending. *Advances in Autism*, *1*(2), 98–107.

Scragg, P., & Shah, A. (1994). Prevalence of Asperger's syndrome in a secure hospital. *The British Journal of Psychiatry*, *165*(5), 679–682.

Shine, J., & Cooper-Evans, S. (2016). Developing and autism specific framework for forensic case formulation. *Journal of Intellectual Disabilities and Offending Behaviour*, *7*(3), 127–139.

Simpson. (2016). *Checklist for Autism-friendly environments*. South West Yorkshire Partnership NHS Foundation Trust: UK

Srivastava, A. K., & Schwartz, C. E. (2014). Intellectual Disability and autism spectrum disorders: Casual genes and molecular mechanisms. *Neuroscience and Biobehavioural Reviews*, *46*(pt 2), 161–174.

Staufenberg, E. (2007). Risk appraisal in developmental forensic neuropsychiatry: An introduction and guide to the existing knowledge and clinical practice basis. *Advances in Mental Health and Learning Disabilities*, *1*(4), 33–43.

Sugrue, D. P. (2017). Forensic assessment of individuals with autism spectrum charged with child pornography violations. In J. D. Lawrence A. Dubin & Emily Horowitz (Eds.), *Caught in the web of the criminal justice system: Autism, developmental disabilities, and sex offenses*. Foreword by J. D. Alan Gershel. Jessica Kingsley Publishers.

Taylor, P. J., Leese, M., Williams, D., Butwell, M., Daly, R., & Larkin, E. (1998). Mental disorder and violence: A special (high security) hospital survey. *British Journal of Psychiatry*, *172*(3), 218–226.

Underwood, L., McCarthy, J., Chaplin, E., Forrester, A., Mills, R., & Murphy, D. (2016). Autism spectrum disorder traits among prisoners. *Advances in Autism*, *2*(3), 106–117.

Webster, C. D., Douglas, K. S., Eaves, D., & Hart, S. D. (1997). *HCR-20 assessing risk for violence – version 2*. Mental Health Law & Policy Institute.

Chapter 9

Learning disability and forensic mental health

Julia Skelding and Emma Longfellow

Introduction

A learning disability (LD) is principally defined by three core criteria: a significantly reduced ability to understand new or complex information in learning new skills, reduced ability to cope independently, and onset in childhood with a lasting effect on development (British Psychological Society, 2015). Individuals with LD are not a homogeneous group, which is evident in varied cognitive, adaptive, social, and emotional functioning (Emerson & Hatton, 2007). To capture the varying degrees of functioning displayed, LD has been further subcategorised into mild, moderate, severe, and profound to support in identifying individual support needs. In the United Kingdom, LD has long been the preferred term for describing these difficulties; however, alternatives exist including the more internationally popular Intellectual Disability (ID) and Intellectual and Developmental Disability. This chapter will refer to difficulties based on the terminology used within the United Kingdom.

This chapter first describes the difficulties of identifying people in forensic settings who have LD. It then discusses what additional challenges are faced by patients with LD in secure settings and the frequent and widespread experiences of trauma they report. Following this, recent developments in UK policy on the treatment and care of people with LD are detailed. Before concluding, the chapter provides a case study of a African-British patient whose reflections should lead readers to contemplate his experiences and patients right to be heard.

Prevalence of learning disability in forensic settings

There are recognised difficulties associated with identifying the proportion of people with LD in forensic settings. These are primarily associated with two key issues: the population is hard to reach, and there are systemic difficulties contributing to underdiagnosis contributing to many difficulties being hidden (Fazel et al., 2008; Hellenbach et al., 2017; Taylor, 2019a; Morris et al., 2019). Prevalence rates of LD in forensic settings vary substantially across studies and are impacted by inconsistently used nomenclature and research methodologies (Murphy et al., 1995; Einat & Einat, 2008; Hayes et al., 2007; Hellenbach et al., 2017; Holland et al., 2002; Jones, 2007). Even within in-patient settings where there has been a significant drive to identify and reduce the LD patient population in response to national Transforming Care and 'Building the right support' initiatives (NHS England, 2015a), there remains inconsistency in figures (Taylor, 2019b).

Although prevalence data remain unclear, Hatton (2016) estimated the number of adults in the general population with LD in the United Kingdom at approximately 2%. From this, the authors calculated the difference between the estimated prevalence and numbers of people

DOI: 10.4324/9781003184768-12

with LD known to healthcare services. He noted a significant discrepancy with only 20% of the estimated prevalence known to services. This has implications for those in forensic settings as there may be a significant group that is not identified. Although there is a lack of clarity on prevalence, the expert consensus is that people with LD are over-represented in forensic settings. UK studies in prisons and police stations have provided a consistent approximation of 7% of people in their services with an identified LD; suggesting that patients with LD are over-represented in forensic settings (Hayes et al., 2007; Søndenaa et al., 2008; Heaton & Murphy, 2013; Dias et al., 2013; Hellenbach et al., 2017). The implication of this in forensic settings is that – despite being overpresented compared to the general population – a significant number of individuals in forensic settings diagnosed with LD have not been identified and are not known to forensic services. This is likely to significantly impact access to available support, reduced recognition for reasonable adjustment, or identification for specialist provision. However, being diagnosed with LD isn't always the 'long straw'. Patients who are identified straddle multiple systems, with differing structures, policy, law, and governance that remain largely disconnected and at times lack fluidity (Stinson & Robins, 2014). This often manifests as a highly fragmented service delivery with frequent movement between agencies and systems in an attempt to address the need (Lunsky et al., 2011; Myers, 2004; Yacoub et al., 2008).

Having learning disability in forensic settings

Individuals with LD often have impacted communication making it harder to understand verbal, written, and receptive communication as well as formulate a response. These difficulties impact obtaining, processing and understanding basic information, providing and giving an accurate account of events, as well as difficulties in understanding and participating in formal proceedings including court and quasi-court settings such as parole boards and tribunals. Forensic patients with LD are often expected to engage in complex cognitive and emotionally intelligent processes dependent on introspection such as reflecting and demonstrating remorse. When this doesn't occur, they can be misinterpreted as wilful and challenging contributing to longer stays in service or ineffective intervention (Marshall–Tate et al., 2020). People diagnosed with LD are protected by the Equality Act (2010). Accordingly, anticipatory and positive steps specific to this population are expected to be taken in forensic settings as they would be in other settings, for example, allowing extra time to improve communication, providing written material in alternative formats, and adapting an environment to make it more conducive to understanding and participation.

People with LD may have more difficulties than others with attention, concentration, memory, and novel intellectual tasks which can put them at a disadvantage in settings reliant on oral communication, multiple instructions, complex constructs, and procedures or sequencing such as forensic hospitals (Marshall–Tate et al., 2020). In 2010, a successful UK-based legal challenge was made after a prisoner with LD evidenced that he was being denied realistic prospects of parole as the interventions being recommended were not accessible or meaningful for him (Straw & Lomri, 2010). Research reports incidents where prisoners with LD were told they were 'not suitable' for interventions, rather than the interventions not being suitable for them, because they could not understand them and they had not been designed for their cognitive functioning difficulties (Straw & Lomri, 2010). This would be accepted within parole boards and categorisation reviews as rationales for why someone had not reduced their risk and warranted continued restriction, despite no alternative being offered. These difficulties are directly associated with being subject to increased restrictions due to a lack of understanding, investment, and provision for people with LD in forensic settings. This is exacerbated further by being unresponsive to needs across settings including a lack of accessible information and instruction on what is required of an individual. For example, some patients have been readmitted to forensic settings from a community or lower security after not adhering to restrictions that they were unable to read or understand.

Ellis (2021) noted that Prison staff and environments did not effectively respond to challenging behaviour displayed by prisoners with LD. He noted there was a lack of understanding of the difficulties being experienced by a prisoner with LD and in particular the impact of difficulties with executive functioning, emotion regulation, and inhibitory control. This, he noted, contributed to unnecessary use of restrictive practice with prisoners with LD and, in many cases, referral to specialist health services as an alternative pathway to prison. Prisoners with LD are five times more likely than other prisoners to experience control and restraint, three times more likely to experience segregation, and three times more likely to have depression or anxiety (Foundation of People with Learning Disability, 2012). This makes difficulties in identifying this population in forensic settings all the more pertinent as it could contribute to retraumatisation of a vulnerable and marginalised population (García-Largo et al., 2020).

Ellis (2021) highlighted the inequity in provision within and between forensic health and prison settings. This includes significant variation in expertise and knowledge of LD and in particular forensic LD, adapted versus bespoke pathways, neuropsychological and allied health specialist availability, and most significantly governance processes. One of the most interesting variations in service provision is the difference in governance for this population across forensic agencies. Transforming Care was a national response to the systemic abuse discovered in Winterborne View, a non-forensic hospital for people with LD (Department of Health, 2012). This policy initiative highlighted the widespread failure to design, commission, and provide services in line with established best practice and a failure to evaluate the quality of care or outcomes. Transforming Care set out an action plan to transform services for people with LD across all agencies, increase community care, and reduce the number of people with LD in inpatient settings. Unfortunately, there have been some difficulties with the implementation of this, and in particular, there is minimal consideration of the specific needs of those in forensic settings. Targets included reduction in physical beds for people with LD which went largely unmet, and in forensic settings, there were protracted lengths of stay and waiting lists increased. In response to limited progress after the implementation of Transforming Care, NHS England introduced Care and Treatment Reviews (NHS England, 2015b). The CTR guidance states that the aim of the review process is to bring a:

> Person-centred and individualised approach to ensuring that the treatment and differing support needs of the person with learning disabilities and their families are met and that barriers to progress are challenged and overcome.
>
> (NHS England, 2015b, p. 5)

CTRs have been rolled out within all health care settings working with LD and have been committed to by NHS England. They identify six core groups of patients and have specific Key Lines Of Enquiry (KLOE) for each, including one specifically for people in secure care. These KLOE's are reviewed by an independent panel including an expert by experience (a person with lived experience of LD). Examples of KLOE's include: 'Is there a clear, safe and proportionate approach to the way risk is assessed or managed?' and 'Is the person receiving the right care and treatment?' (CTR, KLOE workbook, ADULT – Hospital, SECURE). However, these are not used nor particularly known in prison settings, nor has there been a commitment by Her Majesty's Prison and Probation Service (HMPPS) to adhere to these to date. Individuals transferred to the hospital from prison are in fact explicitly precluded from requiring CTR prior to hospital admission (CTR Guidance, 2015). This means there is no governance process to review the appropriateness of transfer to a hospital service until after admission. Although these processes may have varying utility in forensic settings, their absence in some settings suggests further inequality of care and provision. These difficulties affect a complex population with psychiatric, behavioural, trauma, and support needs which are difficult to address in environments with varied and resource-limited specialised care (Stinson & Robins, 2014). Whichever forensic setting individuals are in, ultimately the important issue is the lived reality and experience of these settings and how this impacts treatment outcomes and reduces harmful behaviours.

Trauma and people with learning disability

Current literature suggests that individuals with LD are more likely to experience traumatic and negative life events than those without. More specifically, children with LD are noted to be at increased risk of physical, verbal and sexual violence, emotional abuse, neglect, and disrupted attachment (Miller & Brown, 2014). Adults with LD are at higher risk of exposure to traumas such as systemic abuse and neglect over long periods of time (Ryan, 1994; Hatton & Emerson, 2004; Sobsey & Doe, 1991). Pre-existing trauma symptoms are known to be exacerbated by compulsory detainment in high secure care (Brackenridge & Morrissey, 2010).

Individuals with LD are recognised as a particularly vulnerable group in society, in inpatient settings, and in prison (Gulati et al., 2020). Although there is recognition that individuals with LD are at increased vulnerability to trauma, this is not consistently explored and supported within forensic settings. There are issues with appropriate trauma assessment for people with LD, much of which relies on this having been recognised as trauma by the person with LD, communicated as such, and heard and understood by others. This also impacts understanding of the prevalence and experiences of trauma for people with LD in forensic settings. Additionally, there are limits to appropriate and evidence-based trauma interventions available for people with LD compared with the general population (Wigham et al., 2011; Wigham & Emerson, 2015).

In 2010, Brackenridge and Morrissey (2010) published a service evaluation within the NHSLDS at Rampton Hospital exploring trauma experiences and post-trauma symptoms. These types of abuse were described broadly as physical, psychological, sexual, institutional, discriminatory, financial, and neglect. They assessed this using existing collateral information, self, and observer report. They identified a high prevalence of multiple adverse childhood and lifetime experiences. Specifically, 95% of patients had experienced one or more forms of abuse. This was subsequently broken down into 75% having experienced physical abuse, 50% sexual abuse, and 43% experiencing five or more types of abuse.

Jones (2019) reassessed this population using clinician reporting and existing collateral information. The overall prevalence of trauma wasn't noted; however, 73% were identified as having experienced physical violence, 56% experienced emotional abuse/neglect, 19% experienced physical neglect, and 31% had documented sexual trauma. Despite this review, clinical experience suggested this was an under-representation of trauma prevalence in the population. As such, emphasis was placed on more explicit screening on admission and consideration within annual assessments. This was again evaluated in 2020 (Longfellow & Hicks, 2020) who reviewed available file information and existing assessments that identified trauma presence or absence for each patient. Trauma was defined as any experience of physical or sexual violence, psychological or emotional trauma across lifetime and contexts. From this review, 98% of patients were identified as having experienced some form of trauma. Eighty-six per cent experienced psychological or emotional trauma, 84% experienced physical violence, and 80% experienced sexual violence. Of the 98% who experienced some form of trauma, they were also noted to have all experienced multiple (four or more separate incidences or types) forms of trauma suggesting complex chronic trauma experiences within the population. The variation in prevalence of trauma over the past ten years within one service appears reflective of broader issues in identifying and recording trauma history and symptomology in LD populations (Daveney et al., 2019). This suggests that individuals with LD in forensic settings are exposed to chronic and diverse traumatic events and are at greater risk of re-traumatisation.

Some people with LD have difficulties processing sensory information. They can experience hyper or hyposensitivity to sensations which can cause distress or communication difficulties (Marshall-Tate et al., 2020). This is not easily moderated in forensic settings where it can be busy, loud, bright, and crowded, contributing to sensory overload. Additionally, individuals may engage in sensory-stimulating behaviours such as spinning, rocking, and hand flapping. These behaviours may occur to relieve anxiety, increase sensory stimulation, or because of difficulties processing sensory signals. Unfortunately, these behaviours can at times be misinterpreted as 'challenging' or harmful and restrictions can be put in place to prevent them from potentially adding to distress leading to further traumatising experiences (Marshall-Tate et al., 2020).

Transforming Care

With the introduction of Transforming Care in 2012, the marginalisation and systemic abuse of individuals with LD were brought to the forefront. Subsequent to this, the Building the Right Support national plan published in 2015 laid out an explicit commitment to close hospital beds and develop community services for people with LD. The premise underpinning this was that inpatient settings were being used to manage individuals who could easily be managed in the community with sufficient funding and support. Additionally, it was suggested that the nature of an inpatient setting in many cases contributed to behaviours of distress and an escalation rather than reduction of restrictions (NHS England, 2015a). What is apparent, however, is that this paradigm shift, although welcome in highlighting the difficulties in LD services, inadvertently treats LD as a homogenous group. It supposes the same pathway and community support for mild, moderate, and severe LD and forensic and non-forensic populations. It assumes that families and the community are always better for people with LD and that hospitals do not provide sanctuary, stability, or safety for this group (Taylor et al, 2017). Unfortunately, this commitment, although pertinent for some, is not appropriate for all individuals with LD.

The assumptions made in the Building the Right Support national plan are not appropriate for High Secure ID Services. For many of the people with LD in forensic settings, family and community systems are part of the difficulties. Additionally, communities are noted to be less welcoming of individuals who have been violent, have sexually assaulted, or set fires in their midst (Taylor et al., 2017). More concerning is the added frequency of abuse, aggression, and violence faced by people with disabilities in the community (Taylor et al., 2017). The pursuit of least restrictive practices – a central tenet of mental health services in the United Kingdom – is also applicable in secure services, including to individuals who are at high risk of violence and self-harm, some of whom have been in care for extended periods of ten or more years. The increasing pressure to discharge individuals with LD quickly to meet national plans can contribute to some individuals being progressed before they are ready or community services can appropriately support them. Conversely, patients might not progress to conditions of lower security or the community when ready as recommended bespoke outpatient environments have yet to be developed (in some cases built) or because medium and low secure beds have been occupied or settings closed before a community alternative has been provided. This in many cases leads to prolonged stays in restrictive settings beyond that necessary to manage risk safely.

The right to be heard: a case study

Awareness and understanding of the experiences of individuals with LD are firmly on the agenda with a range of government initiatives being launched including the 'Right to be heard' and understood prompting large-scale LD awareness training initiatives co-produced with service users (Department of Health and Social Care, 2019). This corresponds with one of the most pertinent issues in forensic LD and what cements this population as marginalised: their lack of voice. In some cases, this can be due to inherent difficulties in understanding, self-awareness, and communication. More often, it is because of 'othering' and microaggressions including environmental invalidation and assumptions on abilities that result in forensic LD populations being viewed as lesser, incapable, and ultimately not being asked their perspective. For this chapter, we wanted to provide an insight into the experience of a current patient with LD residing within a secure forensic setting. For the purpose of this, he chose the pseudonym 'Devonte'.[1] This section includes exerts from our conversation with Devonte and explores a difficult childhood, family dynamic, harmful behaviours, and experiences in academic and secure settings. Devonte also highlights examples of othering and microaggressions that can be commonplace.

Devonte is a 24-year-old African–British male, who was diagnosed with LD and attention deficit and hyperactivity disorder at the age of 7 years. Devonte's developmental history involves multiple adverse life events including parental neglect, physical abuse from siblings and carers, witness to intimate partner violence, exposure to substances, disrupted carer attachment, and an internalised sense of being unwanted.

Devonte describes being bullied in school and engaging in behaviour including violence towards peers and siblings and setting fires in school. He came to the attention of his local authority when he was approximately 11 years old following a referral from the Child and Adolescent Mental Health Services team (CAMHS). There were suggestions of involvement in sexual contact with siblings, and after becoming subject to a child protection plan, Devonte was placed in foster care aged 13. He would regularly run away from his foster home and the placement ultimately broke down due to his aggressive behaviour. He was placed into a children's home and subsequently a residential unit for adolescents with emotional and behavioural disorders. Devonte describes experiencing bullying within this unit, and he subsequently committed his index offence aged 15 years which was a sexual assault on a member of staff, resulting in his transfer to a CAMHS unit and receiving a hospital order under s. 37/41 of the Mental Health Act, 1983 (as amended). Within hospital placements, Devonte has engaged in frequent physical violence towards staff members and peers resulting in him being placed under increased restriction culminating in him being managed in high secure conditions.

Devonte described his experience of being in forensic settings with an LD diagnosis. He recalled receiving his diagnosis in school and described this as being in response to him not being able to 'keep up' as the work was too difficult. He discussed the positives and negatives of receiving a diagnosis. He felt things were broken down more for him and that he received more explanations from those involved in his care. Conversely, he described feeling judged by others and felt he was not capable of things other people were. Devonte also discussed feeling 'mocked by others' particularly those without an LD diagnosis, believing people 'underestimate me, think they are cleverer than I am'. Devonte also noted that relating to others was difficult at times, with carers and peers struggling to understand 'how I feel or where I am coming from'. He also found it difficult to 'get my point across, feel misunderstood'. This is something that he attributed to becoming frustrated and at times getting 'into trouble', usually involving verbal or physical aggression. Despite this, Devonte described experiencing a supportive environment, particularly in relation to having his needs met and being supported with basic needs such as writing, reading, and maintaining contact with people in the community. He felt that he was able to have some sense of agency, albeit limited within the environment.

Devonte discussed his views on prison versus hospital environments for someone with LD. He described not knowing when he would be able to leave the hospital and this being difficult. At times, he felt that you stay longer and probably 'longer than you need to when you have stopped misbehaving'. He felt that with prison you 'knew better when you will get out but here you don't know'. However, he felt that hospital services provided him with a host of treatment and therapies as they 'have everything you need'. Devonte also felt like he had some say and involvement in services in the hospital although he did not always fully understand the processes involved including patient-centred forums such as monthly 'ward rounds', tribunals, bi-annual pathway meetings, or Care and Treatment Reviews (CTRs). Devonte also thought that formal reports were inaccessible at times and that these should be easier to read.

Devonte discussed that as an 'African-British' male his culture was something that was difficult to fully acknowledge within the hospital. There are only a small number of Black and Asian Minority Ethnic (BAME) patients within the service and this contributed to him struggling to fully celebrate his culture and background including his culinary heritage. Additionally, Devonte described experiencing racist abuse within the service from peers and finding this incredibly difficult to manage. He discussed that at times he felt that his voice was not heard by services in particular when reporting incidents to the police. He described feeling powerless in institutions in relation to this issue or being subject to punishment if he reacted negatively to chronic racial abuse. He commented that it 'feels like when I report things that have happened to me I don't get the outcome I want'. Similarly, Devonte noted that he would regularly experience 'staff speaking with attitude towards me and then when I have one back I get done'. This experience of inequity is one that he described experiencing throughout his time in services from reporting bullying, racism, and engaging in 'banter'. He described a regular pattern of othering whereby his comments and behaviours would be recorded, sanctioned, and reprimanded whereas others, including staff, would not.

Overall, Devonte described his experiences as 'mixed', influenced not only by being diagnosed with LD but also by being an African-British male in services. He identified some of the common themes associated with diagnostic labels, including increasing access to services and support but corresponding negative labels from others, assumption of inability, and feeling like he is in a lesser 'out' group. Devonte also described not feeling he could communicate effectively at times and that this contributed to him getting into trouble or expressing himself with behaviours of distress that challenge staff. He also felt at times that he could engage in comparable behaviour to staff; for example making jokes but would 'get done' for this. Devonte recognised himself as having a mild form of LD and felt that others in services struggled more profoundly with the complexity of the system they were in. Devonte ended the discussion with: 'My hopes for the future are to be eventually back in the community, live a better life, get a job, and maybe have a family of my own'.

This is just one example of what it is like to be in forensic services with LD. It is Devonte's story; however, it is reflective of some of the experiences of marginalised patients discussed in the literature.

Conclusion

This chapter has discussed a range of ways in which people with LD in forensic settings are marginalised. This is exacerbated by systematic and interpersonal features of forensic mental health settings and because there is a lack of understanding and adjustments for this patient group. There are a number of initiatives for improving the lives of individuals with LD with the Transforming Care agenda being an important catalyst. Unfortunately, in the ten years since an infamous inquiry into abuses committed at Winterbourne View hospital, there remain significant systemic, procedural, and interpersonal improvements that still need to be made. There also remains inconsistency in service provision and a failure to recognise heterogeneity in the population, particularly in forensic settings when developing national policies, agendas, and ultimately care and treatment. There is also an emerging recognition of microaggressions that impact people with LD in forensic settings, suggesting there is a need for systemic and cultural review. Some positive steps have been taken in the form of heavily commissioned national training initiatives to help understand this population.

Most problematic is a clear lack of emphasis on agency in this population despite a range of capabilities, and this contributes to this group having little or no voice in what happens to them. There is a clear recognition in the pertinently titled policies in recent years including 'Out of sight' (Mencap, 2012), 'Out of sight- who cares' (Care and Quality Commission, 2020), and 'The right to be heard' (Department of Health and Social Care, 2019) that marks what the critical issue in this population is. This has culminated in an increasing focus on co-production in forensic LD populations across all levels. Unfortunately, operationalising this like many other initiatives in this population remains to be seen. However, it remains essential that individuals with LD in forensic settings are given the opportunity to help shape current provision, identify what some of the critical issues in treatment are, and describe what the unique difficulties are for those with vulnerabilities and neurodevelopmental difficulties. This should include ensuring that services are neurodevelopmentally informed and that service users contribute to this. Much remains to be done to achieve the cultural and systemic change that is needed to best care for this patient group. There is a long road ahead.

Note

1. 'The person going by the pseudonym Devonte gave his full consent to have these excerpts included in this chapter'.

References

Brackenridge, I., & Morrissey, C. (2010). Trauma and post-traumatic stress disorder (PTSD) in a high secure forensic learning disability population: Future directions for practice. *Advances in Mental Health and Intellectual Disabilities, 4*(3), 49–56. https://doi.org/10.5042/amhid.2010.0544

British Psychological Society. (2015). *Guidance of neuropsychological testing with individuals who have intellectual disabilities*. British Psychological Society.

Care Quality Commission. (2020). *Out of sight-who cares? Restraint, seclusion and segregation*. https://www.cqc.org.uk/sites/default/files/20201218_rssreview_report.pdf

Daveney, J., Hassiotis, A., Katona, C., Matcham, F., & Sen, P. (2019). Ascertainment and prevalence of post-traumatic stress disorder (PTSD) in people with intellectual disabilities. *Journal of Mental Health Research in Intellectual Disabilities, 12*(3–4), 211–233. https://doi.org/10.1080/19315864.2019.1637979

Department of Health. (2012). *Transforming Care: A National Response to Winterbourne View Hospital*. NHS England. https://assets.publishing.service.gov.uk/government/uploads/system/uploads/attachment_data/file/213215/final-report.pdf

Department of Health and Social Care. (2019). *'Right to be heard': The Government's response to the consultation on learning disability and autism training for health and care staff*. https://assets.publishing.service.gov.uk/government/uploads/system/uploads/attachment_data/file/844356/autism-and-learning-disability-training-for-staff-consultation-response.pdf

Dias, S., Ware, R. S., Kinner, S. A., & Lennox, N. G. (2013). Co-occurring mental disorder and intellectual disability in a large sample of Australian prisoners. *Australian & New Zealand Journal of Psychiatry, 47*(10), 938–944. https://doi.org/10.1177/0004867413492220

Ellis, S. (2021). *How suitable is prison for people with Learning Disabilities or autism?* Paper presentation, what good looks like – Supporting Neurodiversity in prisons, conference 2021.

Emerson, E., & Hatton, C. (2007). Mental health of children and adolescents with intellectual disabilities in Britain. *British Journal of Psychiatry, 191*, 493–499. doi:10.1192/bjp.bp.107.038729

Einat, T., & Einat, A. (2008). Learning disabilities and delinquency: A study of Israeli prison inmates. *International Journal of Offender Therapy and Comparative Criminology, 52*(4), 416–434. doi:10.1177/0306624X07307352

Fazel, S., Xenitidis, K., & Powell, J. (2008, August–September). The prevalence of intellectual disabilities among 12,000 prisoners – a systematic review. *International Journal of Law and Psychiatry, 31*(4), 369–373. doi:10.1016/j.ijlp.2008.06.001. Epub July 21, 2008. PMID: 18644624.

García-Largo, L. M., Martí-Agustí, G., Martin-Fumadó, C., & Gómez-Durán, E. L. (2020). Intellectual disability rates among male prison inmates. *International Journal of Law and Psychiatry, 70*, 101566. https://doi.org/10.1016/j.ijlp.2020.101566

Gulati, G., Cusack, A., Kilcommins, S., & Dunne, C. P. (2020). Intellectual disabilities in Irish prisons: Could Article 13 of the UNCRPD hold the key? *International Journal of Law and Psychiatry, 68*, 101540. https://doi.org/10.1016/j.ijlp.2019.101540

Hatton, C. (2016). Specialist inpatient services for people with learning disabilities across the four countries of the UK. *Tizard Learning Disability Review, 21*(4), 220–225. https://doi.org/10.1108/TLDR-08-2016-0023

Hatton, C., & Emerson, E. (2004). The relationship between life events and psychopathology amongst children with intellectual disabilities. *Journal of Applied Research in Intellectual Disabilities, 17*(2), 109–117.

Hayes, S., Shackell, P., Mottram, P., & Lancaster, R. (2007). The prevalence of intellectual disability in a major UK prison. *British Journal of Learning Disabilities, 35*, 162–167. https://doi.org/10.1111/j.1468-3156.2007.00461.x

Heaton, K. M., & Murphy, G. H. (2013). Men with intellectual disabilities who have attended sex offender treatment groups: A follow-up. *Journal of Applied Research in Intellectual Disabilities, 26*, 489–500. https://doi.org/10.1111/jar.12038

Hellenbach, M., Karatzias, T., & Brown, M. (2017). Intellectual disabilities among prisoners: Prevalence and mental and physical health comorbidities. *Journal of Applied Research in Intellectual Disabilities, 30*(2), 230–241. doi:10.1111/jar.12234

Holland, T., & Clare, I., & Mukhopadhyay, T. (2002). Prevalence of 'criminal offending' by men and women with intellectual disability and the characteristics of 'offenders': Implications for research and service development. *Journal of Intellectual Disability Research: JIDR, 46* (Suppl 1), 6–20. doi:10.1046/j.1365-2788.2002.00001.x

Jones, J. (2007). Persons with intellectual disabilities in the criminal justice system: Review of issues. *International Journal of Offender Therapy and Comparative Criminology, 51*(6), 723–733. https://doi.org/10.1177/0306624X07299343

Jones, L. (2019). New developments in interventions for working with offending behavior. In D. L. L. Polaschek, A. Day, & C. R. Hollin (Eds.), *The Wiley international handbook of correctional psychology* (pp. 669–685). Wiley Blackwell. https://doi.org/10.1002/9781119139980.ch42

Legislation.gov.uk. (2021). *Equality act 2010.* Retrieved June 1, 2021, from www.legislation.gov.uk/ukpga/2010/15/contents

Longfellow, E., & Hicks, R. (2000). *Developmental trauma and learning disability.* Paper presentation, Trauma informed care in forensic settings, 2020, Nottingham.

Lunsky, Y., Gracey, C., Koegl, C., Bradley, E., Durbin, J., & Raina, P. (2011). The clinical profile and service needs of psychiatric inpatients with intellectual disabilities and forensic involvement. *Psychology, Crime & Law, 17*(1), 9–23. doi:10.1080/10683160903392277

Marshall-Tate, K., Chaplin, E., McCarthy, J., & Grealish, A. (2020). A literature review about the prevalence and identification of people with an intellectual disability within court Liaison and Diversion services. *Journal of Intellectual Disabilities and Offending Behaviour.* https://doi.org/10.1108/JIDOB-10-2019-0023

Mencap. (2012). *Out of Sight: Stopping the neglect and abuse of people with a learning disability.* https://www.mencap.org.uk/sites/default/files/2016-08/Out-of-Sight-Report.pdf

Miller, D., & Brown, J. (2014). *'We have the right to be safe': Protecting disabled children from abuse.* www.nspcc.org.uk/preventing-abuse/research-and-resources/ right-to-be-safe/

Morris, D. J., Shergill, S., & Beber, E. (2019). Developmental trauma in a forensic intellectual disability population. *Journal of Intellectual Disabilities and Offending Behaviour, 11*(1), 35–48. https://doi.org/10.1108/JIDOB-06-2019-0011

Murphy, G. H., Harnett, H., Holland, A. J. (1995). A survey of intellectual disabilities amongst men on remand in prison. *Mental Handicap Research, 8*(2), 81–98. ISSN 0952–9608. doi:10.1111/j.1468-3148.1995.tb00147.x

Myers, F. (2004). *On the borderline? People with learning disabilities and/or autistic spectrum disorders in secure forensic and other specialist settings.* Scottish Development Centre for Mental Health.

NHS England (2015a). Building the Right Support. NHS England. www.england.nhs.uk/wp-content/uploads/2015/10/ld-nat-imp-plan-oct15.pdf [Google Scholar].

NHS England (2015b). Care and Treatment Review: Policy and Guidelines. NHS England [Google Scholar].

Ryan, M. (1994). Caring for People with Learning Difficulties in Scotland: Comparative Costs. *British Journal of Learning Disabilities, 22*(2), 57–61. https://doi.org/10.1111/j.1468-3156.1994.tb00116.x

Sobsey, D., & Doe, T. (1991). Patterns of sexual abuse and assault. *Sexuality and Disability, 9*(3), 243–259.

Søndenaa, E., Rasmussen, K., Palmstierna, T., & Nøttestad, J. (2008). The prevalence and nature of intellectual disability in Norwegian prisons. *Journal of Intellectual Disability Research, 52*(12), 1129–1137. https://doi.org/10.1111/j.1365-2788.2008.01072.x

Stinson, J. D., & Robbins, S. B. (2014). Characteristics of people with intellectual disabilities in a secure US forensic hospital. *Journal of Mental Health Research in Intellectual Disabilities, 7*(4), 337–358. https://doi.org/10.1080/19315864.2014.930549

Straw, A., & Lomri, S. (2010). Public law update: Failing prisoners with learning disabilities. *Criminal Law and Justice Weekly, 174*, 292–293.

Taylor, J. (2019a). Exploring the experiences and perceptions of people with learning disabilities. *Lancaster University.* https://doi.org/10.17635/lancaster/thesis/796

Taylor, J. (2019b). Delivering the transforming care programme: A case of smoke and mirrors? *BJPsych Bulletin, 43*(5), 201–203. doi:10.1192/bjb.2019.3

Taylor, J. L., McKinnon, I., Thorpe, I., & Gillmer, B. T. (2017). The impact of transforming care on the care and safety of patients with intellectual disabilities and forensic needs. *BJPsych Bulletin, 41*(4), 205–208. doi:10.1192/pb.bp.116.055095. PMID: 28811914; PMCID: PMC5537574.

Valuing People. (2001). A new strategy for learning disability for the 21st century. Department of Health.

Wigham, S., & Emerson, E. (2015). Trauma and life events in adults with intellectual disability. *Current Developmental Disorders Reports, 2*(2), 93–99. https://doi.org/10.1007/s40474-015-0041-y

Wigham, S., Hatton, C., & Taylor, J. L. (2011). The effects of traumatizing life events on people with intellectual disabilities: A systematic review. *Journal of Mental Health Research in Intellectual Disabilities, 4*(1), 19–39. https://doi.org/10.1080/19315864.2010.534576

Yacoub, E., Hall, I., & Bernal, J. (2008). Secure in-patient services for people with learning disability: Is the market serving the user well? *Psychiatric Bulletin, 32*(6), 205–207. doi:10.1192/pb.bp.107.018523

Chapter 10

The problematic nature of transitions amongst adolescents with multiple and complex needs in secure care

An overview of institutional transitions

Maria Livanou and Vivek Furtado

Introduction

The following chapter will focus on young people moving from adolescent secure services to adult care, including inpatient hospitals and community settings. Transitions of care have turned into a priority across services due to infrastructural barriers and the great divide between adolescent and adult services. The period of adolescence is marked by developmental, emotional, psychological, and social changes that elevate the risk for poor transition outcomes. The transition process for young people discharged from adolescent secure hospitals has been described as being fragmented, abrupt, and unsupportive. This distinct group of young people presents with complex needs, multiple vulnerabilities, and high risk to self and/or others. Previous research has indicated several risk factors in periods of transition, such as limited pre-admission familiarisation with the adult placement, shortage of beds in adult services, lack of emotional readiness, and lack of specialised pathways for those with neurodevelopmental needs. Services follow a *one-size-fits-all* approach that disregards individual needs and neurodiversity. There is a need to design age-appropriate services and targeted transition programmes aiming to improve life opportunities and reduce mental health symptoms post-transition and length of stay (LoS) during secure care.

The term that best describes young people's journey across and between services is known as 'transition'. This refers to an ongoing, goal-oriented, and purposeful process and should not be used interchangeably with 'transfer', which describes a single and discrete event linked to disrupted clinical and institutional practice (Singh & Tuomainen, 2015). A successful transition integrates good preparation and management including parallel and joint working with adult services, handover planning, transition meetings and visits, and family involvement. Continuity of care is a concept commonly discussed in the extant literature, as an optimal outcome following transitional care (Paul et al., 2015). However, continuity of care is meaningful only if designed in the best interest of the young person. Services and healthcare professionals should aim for after-care tailored around individualised needs and the presenting complexities of each case.

Transitions from child and adolescent mental health services (CAMHS) to adult-oriented settings have received increasing attention over the past two decades globally (Hovish et al., 2012). The period of moving from CAMHS to adult care is known in the literature as 'transitional care'. However, this term does not encompass a standard transitional package across and/or approach across CAMHS. Transition makes up a complex phenomenon in young people's care because of the overlapping nature of institutional transitions with developmental and diagnostic transitions (Pontoni et al., 2021). Young people experience significant psychosocial changes as part of entering adulthood, such as independence, employment,

DOI: 10.4324/9781003184768-13

and housing. Biological, psychosocial, cognitive, and emotional changes emerge simultaneously during early and mid-adolescence, which can be overwhelming and intimidating for the young person. Young people with pre-existing and ongoing mental health problems and other chronic medical conditions are called to manage developmental, healthcare, and institutional transitions regardless of readiness, maturity, and life context (Dunn, 2017). The intersectionality of multiple synchronous forms of transition can be traumatic for the young person's overall well-being.

There is substantial evidence that transitions from child and adolescent services to adult care are linked to exacerbation of medical and mental health symptoms and poor life opportunities (Campbell et al., 2016). Young people moving from CAMHS to adult care are more likely to experience poorly planned transitions because of inconsistent care and lack of emotional and developmental readiness (Lepkowska, 2017). The current divide between CAMHS and adult services perpetuates the problematic nature of transitions because these are disconnected services (Signorini et al., 2018). Fundamental differences in treatment approaches and care priorities have forged a substantial gap between child and adult services. Young people newly admitted to adult services from CAMHS are expected to self-manage presenting psychosocial needs (e.g., managing finances, self-care, and social interactions) without parallel transitional preparation and support (O'Connell & Petty, 2019). Those with neurodevelopmental disorders such as autism spectrum disorder (ASD) and learning disabilities are further disadvantaged given that services for this group are underdeveloped (Devapriam & Alexander, 2012). There are only a few specialist services providing inpatient care for adults with neurodevelopmental problems in the United Kingdom, where local geographic access is limited (Xenitidis et al., 2004). Health-associated costs for adults with learning disabilities in secure care are estimated at over 300 million annually (Hackett et al., 2027). Poorly managed transitions can lead to enduring use and dependency on mental health services associated with long-term financial burden, limited employment opportunities, and social functioning (Levy et al., 2020).

Literature on mental health transitions describes the process as particularly complex and problematic (Singh et al., 2008). Service provision for young people in mental health services during transition periods cannot meet precipitating and ongoing needs, and this especially applies to those with neurodevelopmental problems, emerging personality disorders, and comorbid mental health difficulties. Previous research has identified barriers to successful transitions from mainstream CAMHS to adult mental health services (AMHS) including waiting time, rigid referral criteria, inconsistent continuity of care, age cut-off, lack of communication between services, limited understanding of developmental needs, abrupt transitions, and limited staff training (Singh et al., 2010). Historically, there has been a great divide between the two services because of different treatment approaches and care priorities. This gap in culture and philosophy pertains to AMHS adopting a more independent care model and CAMHS using a multimodal line, which integrates biological, psychological, and developmental factors towards treatment and rehabilitation (Paul et al., 2015).

What has been done so far at a national level to improve transitions from CAMHS to adult services?

The Department of Health (DoH) has prioritised the overall well-being of young people experiencing transitions in education and healthcare given the developmental challenges inherent in the process. Most research has focused on transitions from child and adolescent mental healthcare to adult services for young people with chronic medical conditions such as diabetes, heart disease, cancer, cerebral palsy, and haemophilia (Singh & Tuomainen, 2015). Specific transition intervention models have been designed for service users, carers, and healthcare professionals. Randomised control trials (RCTs) have been conducted in test-ing out interventions for those leaving paediatric services with physical health conditions such as transition preparation training and educational interventions (Campbell et al., 2016). However, the outcomes and effectiveness of such programmes are not conclusive. The largest European Trial, MILESTONE, focusing on transitions from CAMHS to AMHS included services across eight European countries to assess outcome measures and improve service delivery. Preliminary findings show that detached, non-specific care and low levels of family involvement in the transition process comprise key barriers to smooth transitions of care in mental health services (Signorini et al., 2018).

During transition periods, service input declines and therefore widens the gap between child and adult services. Research findings echo the need to improve transition outcomes for young people accessing AMHS and to design age-appropriate care with the implementation of specialised transition programmes. There is limited evidence on how transitional inter-ventions may improve the care pathway of vulnerable populations such as young offenders (Campbell et al., 2016).

Secure inpatient services for adolescents in the United Kingdom

Adolescents with mental health problems detained in secure settings are doubly stigmatised and neglected in research despite their complex and multitude needs (e.g., 'looked after chil-dren', trauma history, comorbidity, and high risk to self and/or others). Young people may be admitted to adolescent secure services and be treated under the jurisdiction of the Mental Health Act, 1983 (as amended in 2007) due to committing an offence and presenting a high risk to self or others. Eighty per cent of young people in medium-secure units (MSUs) have at least two mental disorders (Hales et al., 2018). The implications of poor transition outcomes extend to poor mental health and high re-offending rates upon returning to the community (Hales et al., 2019). However, very little has been done to address these issues considering how few people are adequately trained in adolescent forensic psychiatry (Hindley et al., 2017).

Looked After Children (LAC) – children in contact with social services, in foster care, or in residential homes when parents are unable to take care of them – and young people in contact with the youth justice system with mental health problems encounter additional chal-lenges engaging with services due to multiple vulnerabilities such as their legal status, mental health and risk presentation, and lack of family support (Singh & Tuomainen, 2015). There are very few studies on transitional care among young offenders, and these include small sam-ples because of challenges in recruitment and engagement of this group in research studies. In England and Wales, young people committing an offence can be transferred to a young offender institution (YOI), a secure children's home (SCH), or a secure training centre (STC). In case they present with persistent mental health problems which cannot be managed in the secure estate (UK youth custody for young people below 18 years which consists of three secure establishments: YOIs, SCHs, and STCs), they can be transferred to adolescent low- or medium-secure mental health units (forensic hospitals which provide treatment and care for young people with severe mental health problems and high risk) depending on the severity of the symptoms and presentation of risk in order to receive treatment. However, there are no longitudinal outcomes about this group's transitional experiences once they reach 18 years and have to move to adult services and settings.

The UK DoH has recently developed practice guidelines on transitions of care for young people moving from adolescent secure services to adult secure hospitals (NHS, 2020). These guidelines illustrate the importance of graded and flexible transitions aiming for a needs-based care model rather than an age-based model. Effective and supportive transitions foster independence in young people and facilitate confidence in their treatment. National Institute for Health and Care Excellence (NICE, 2016) – evidence-based quality standards about clinical practice drafted by independent groups of professionals and members of the public in the United Kingdom) – guidelines explicitly state that self-efficacy (managing one's own health) is a key priority for service commissioners and policymakers and recommend evidence-based research in self-management training to improve transition preparation for special groups.

NHS England (2014) identifies the transition process from child mental health services to adult services as a significant risk factor to the mental health of young people. In the same service specification document, NHS England reports that young people experiencing poor transitions are more likely to have poor education outcomes. For instance, many of the young people admitted to forensic inpatient services have either dropped out from school or their neurodevelopmental level lags behind their chronological age. There is empirical evidence that integrated youth mental health services for children and young people aged 12–25 years can implement a holistic approach that addresses psychosocial and developmental needs (Fusar-Poli, 2019). Research also suggests that services need to adopt developmentally appropriate and youth-friendly services to overcome existing barriers during the developmental period aiming to prevent the course and progression of mental health disorders.

Barriers and challenges to transitions from adolescent secure services

A broad range of factors – biological, developmental, emotional, and social – mark adolescence as a vulnerable period for the emergence of mental disorders. Little is known about young people discharged from adolescent secure hospitals (inpatient care) such as MSUs and low-secure units (LSUs), psychiatric intensive care units, and high dependency units. According to a national scoping exercise, as of 2016, there were 1,283 young people in secure hospitals across England (Hales et al., 2018). About 43% of young people in secure care did not have a placement address when transitioning to the community. This can have further implications on young people including re-offending, relapse, and lifelong institutional dependency.

Young people in contact with the youth justice system are more likely to experience multiple transitions across a range of services including secure establishments to forensic inpatient hospitals (McAra & McVie, 2010). Six per cent of young people in secure care have been in ten or more placements before (Hales et al., 2018). Each setting follows different principles in its care approach and delivers different treatment models to the young people they accommodate. These constant changes in principles and care are harmful and especially challenging for young people with learning disabilities, autism, and other neurodevelopmental disorders (Gomot & Wicker, 2012). A five-year applied health research programme revealed that young people with autism need a 'developmentally appropriate healthcare' approach that clearly addresses psychosocial needs and autonomy (King et al., 2019). Parental involvement during transition times though remains a significant protective factor for young people with autism (Levy et al., 2020).

Transitional care has become a national priority in the United Kingdom in order to minimise the risk of poor transition preparation and increase positive outcomes such as better employability prospects, desistance, housing, and managing an independent lifestyle. The National Health Service (NHS) outlined within its five-year forward view (NHS, 2014) that mental health services should strive to work within the capacity of 'personalised care' and co-production, whereby individuals are empowered using a strength-based approach.

Most available interventions are in line with adult models of care and possibly fail to identify developmental perspectives (Hales et al., 2019). Currently, there are no interventions targeting transitional care in secure settings and there is limited clinical and policy guidance on the development of transitional care for young people in secure services. There is a lack of clear planning and knowledge about the feasibility of specific models of transitional care which may reduce the public health burden of emerging adults at risk. Implementing systematic interventions during institutional and healthcare transitions is highly likely to be cost-effective considering the costs associated with enduring mental health issues and secure hospital admission.

Care pathways for young people with autism and learning difficulties

National findings including a representative sample from all six adolescent medium-secure hospitals in England discharged to adult services within a designated period (January 2016 to December 2017) have shown that transition outcomes are poor for the majority of these young people (Livanou, 2018). Thirty-four young people were initially identified to participate in this study; the annual number of young people eligible to transition from adolescent secure services is quite low estimated at around six to eight adolescents. This study followed up 18 young people and parents/carers in adult placements and used qualitative interviews to reflect on their transitional experiences (Livanou, 2018). Thirty-four mental health professionals across 15 adolescent and adult services were interviewed to further understanding of transition management and preparation and address barriers and facilitators to the process (Livanou et al., 2021). This was the first prospective study that recruited this cohort across England to identify transition outcomes nationally.

Common subthemes that emerged from interviews with mental health professionals included transitional delays, transition preparation and management, inflexible age boundaries disregarding emotional and developmental readiness, specific pathways for young female offenders presenting with emerging borderline personality disorder (BPD) and self-harming, risk presentation and developmental readiness, reluctance of community services to take on high-risk patients, difficulties in multi-agency collaboration, an inadequate number of community placements for young people with learning disabilities and ASDs, and lack of readiness to move onto adult services. Females with emerging BPD who recently moved to adult services relapsed and those with neurodiversity were often bullied by older peers in adult wards. The majority of young people reported they did not know the transition date and had not received sufficient preparation which intensified feelings of anxiety. Another challenge was in the environment of an adult placement considering a significant change in status and being surrounded by much older service users in either secure hospitals or community support accommodation. It is unsurprising that families and carers described transitions to adult services as anxiety-provoking events.

The findings show that young people transitioning from forensic child and adolescent mental health services experience several difficulties throughout the transition period. Poor transition planning increases levels of uncertainty and leads to the deterioration of their mental health symptoms. Young people with neurodevelopmental problems comprise the most vulnerable group with increasing complex needs; this problem is amplified by a lack of local specialist services which leads to inappropriate placements. Neurodiversity and emerging BPD symptoms should be considered carefully when preparing these cohorts for future transitions to adult services. These groups are more likely to encounter additional difficulties due to their high vulnerability, pertinent to risk, self-harming, and ward victimisation (Livanou et al., 2021). Age flexibility would enable smoother transitions by identifying more suitable placements for young people tailored to their individual needs. Young people's voices should be taken into consideration to inform policy and clinical practice decision-making.

The Care Quality Commission (CQC, 2019) released a report about young people with neurodiversity recently admitted to adult inpatient services and indicated that they were more likely to spend time in long-term segregation due to a lack of familiarity with adult placements' staff and culture. These findings reflect the abrupt nature of transitions to AMHS and the difficulty for vulnerable young people with neurodevelopmental needs to adjust to adult wards. Young people with autism and/or learning disabilities experience greater distress in unfamiliar environments, which can explain higher risk presentation during transition periods (Hollins, 2019).

Young people's needs change over time and services should adjust care models accordingly. Designing and tailoring services around individualised needs by adopting person-centred approaches makes up the primary long-term aim for improving current service delivery which acknowledges diversity. However, to enhance existing care models and facilitate transitional care, we need to first develop and test out early integrative intervention models to assess whether they have the potential to improve quality of life outcomes by reducing risk and increasing social functioning and minimise the prospect of re-institutionalisation.

Culture change and differences between adolescent and adult services

Adult services reinforce a more isolated model for the young person compared to the supportive and contained environment provided by adolescent secure services. The shift in age status affects the well-being of young people moving to adult services, and they are less likely to experience secure relationships with adult healthcare professionals and/or peers (Livanou, 2018). Lower staffing and lack of trained staff for young people who need specialised services may account for these relational changes. Family members such as parents and/or carers often experience the difference in culture reflected in policy and care approach. Young people with ASD and LDs are more likely to be marginalised and stigmatised in adult wards because of their vulnerability to changes (Livanou et al., 2021).

Multi-agency/service collaboration challenges are heightened by the gap between child and adolescent mental services and AMHS (Davis, 2003). Young people transitioning back to their communities present with the poorest outcomes and are more likely to receive inadequate care (Wright & Liddle, 2014). We know that about 68% of children discharged from the secure estate to the community will re-offend within one year (Beyond Youth Custody, 2016). Chitsabesan and colleagues (2006) found that young people released from custody encounter major challenges including housing, unemployment and limited life opportunities, and mental health relapse in the community. Service provision declines once young people enter adulthood, 18–20 years, and often lose benefits and associated support they were eligible for as children (Davis, 2003). Adolescent and adult key workers must liaise to ease the process through parallel care provision which includes dynamically young people and their families.

Young people in secure services present with a greater difficulty of 'letting go' and, therapeutic endings may be more traumatic considering that majority have experiences of trauma and loss early in their childhoods (Broad et al., 2017). However, they are more likely to build secure bonding with key workers from adolescent secure services. As Lindgren et al. (2014) pointed out, young people feel ambivalent about their prospective transitions because of the uncertainty of moving to a new service where they have to start all over again in forming relationships with staff. Young people discharged from forensic services are less likely to establish trusting relationships with authorities, as they have received inconsistent care from parents and services in the past.

Females in adolescent secure services

Females in forensic services are likely to present with emerging personality disorders (Hill et al., 2014). Despite the relatively high prevalence rates of emerging personality disorders in this group, they do not meet the criteria to be detained under the Mental Health Act if this is the only presenting mental health problem. Once they enter adulthood, they can be transferred to an adult MSU. Hill et al. (2014) report that female young offenders mostly present with severe features of emerging BPD such as recurrent self-harming episodes and unstable mood. This group is considered to develop BPD in adulthood and, therefore, a review of adult services' current service provision needs to be undertaken in order to address ongoing and emerging needs with the aim of tailored individual-basis interventions.

Gendered clinical pathways would significantly facilitate adjustment to adult services. This group of female offenders presents with a set of very special needs that require clinical attention. Severe self-harming increases during periods of transition and this is an area that needs to be considered from different perspectives. Some young females may not feel ready to move to AMHS, and by engaging in self-harming, they can delay their transition and/or change their transition pathway. However, at the moment there is no clinical consensus on how best to address emerging personality disorder needs.

Young people moving to the community

Young people transitioning from adolescent secure services to community placements are perceived as a highly unwanted group considering the stigma and index offence they have committed (Livanou et al., 2021). They may present with very challenging behaviours not easily managed in community placements due to lack of training and associated anxiety to work with high-risk young people with comorbid mental health problems. Risk is a concerning factor along with past forensic history which may act as a barrier for community mental health professionals to engage in treatment provision. The number of previous offences though varies. Community services are likely to turn down young people with severe risk of offending and complex mental health presentation. However, it has been reported that young people may not be able to manage a more independent lifestyle in community support accommodations and they return to adolescent secure services. Adult services are less likely to adopt trauma-informed care and employ a developmental understanding of young people's adverse experiences; therefore, they are more likely to exclude and/or reject them (Wright & Liddle, 2014). Currently, there is a wider consensus amongst professionals about the value and effectiveness of trauma-informed care, especially in young people with highly complex needs. NHS England has recently implemented this framework in the secure estate aiming for a developmentally informed approach that addresses complex difficulties.

Unsuccessful transitions, as discussed earlier, can bring additional confusion to the young people and the clinicians who have to identify a new placement for the young person. Some young people are 'returned' to forensic services due to their difficulty in becoming truly independent. These transition outcomes have a regressive character which may re-traumatise the young person and their families and can extend to poor mental health and increased risk presentation. This process could be seen as a 'double punishment' considering social and institutional pressures (Wright & Liddle, 2014).

Young people in adult placements

Research studies report that many young people are placed in adult psychiatric hospitals before moving to secure adolescent services due to bed shortages in appropriate services.

Young people have described this experience as 'shocking' (Livanou et al., 2021). The existing literature along with NICE guidelines recommends that young people should not be placed in adult mental health hospitals when they are below 18 years. Placing adolescents in adult settings intensifies existing vulnerabilities such as being subjected to bullying by much older peers. It needs to be emphasised that young people are leaving adolescent secure units where they are the oldest amongst their peers and are transferring to adult hospitals, where they are the youngest amongst much older peers in their late 50s and 60s. This shift in social status and hierarchy in the institution they are placed can turn into a very complex issue for the young person. Concurrently, the young person has to adjust to a new environment and also accept a new assigned status that is inferior to the one they had previously in the institution where they felt safer. Transition to adult placements can become a particularly terrifying experience for young people wherein they lose relationships with key figures and peers, and their social and personal identity is shaken.

The impact of transitional delays on young people

Waiting time to be discharged to adult secure inpatient services may account for the deterioration of mental health problems, violent incidents on the ward, disengagement from therapeutic relationships and education, isolation, bullying, and safeguarding issues. Young people's response to untimely transitions is often reflected in violent acts and/or social withdrawal, such as aggression against staff and/or peers (Livanou, 2018). Young people experiencing isolation might be disengaged from any ward activities and spend the day in their rooms. Transitional delays mostly result from organisational and infrastructural weakness of current services. Both child and adult healthcare professionals need to overcome presenting challenges and facilitate transitions to services. However, delays can impact negatively healthcare professionals, families, and young people but they were all affected to different extents. The level of a young person's risk can change as a result of delayed transitions and healthcare professionals must identify new placements considering that community settings will not take over young people with recent violent incidents who are not ready to deal with the challenges in the community.

The protective role of parental involvement

Parental involvement constitutes a protective factor for young people's transitions. However, recent research in adolescent secure services shows that only in a few cases, the parent is involved throughout the different stages of transition (Livanou et al., 2021). Geographical distribution of current national services does not facilitate travelling for parents living far away from these secure units. Unequal geographical distribution of services has further implications on young people and their families and can be linked to poor transition outcomes. Some families cannot visit their children in hospital units frequently due to geographical distance and associated expenses and cannot liaise with adolescent healthcare professionals about the upcoming transition to adult services.

Parents can facilitate transitions, and their involvement in this process is critical for young peoples' resocialisation and reintegration into the community. However, parents can be a destabilising factor in young people's lives during periods of transition, in case they cannot provide adequate care or if they have their own mental health difficulties. Many of these parents have mental health disorders and can reinforce antisocial lifestyles, which have been adopted by their children and have played a role in their care and criminal trajectories. The findings from a case note review study (Livanou et al., 2020) revealed that several young people transitioning to adult services and in contact with the youth justice system from an early age had parents with psychopathology and/or criminal histories.

Transition preparation

Lack of or limited transition preparation can emerge from poor liaison with AMHS, poor multi-agency collaboration, uncertainty about transition destination, and the young person's resistance to accept that they have to leave child services. Transition preparation is not a single event and requires ongoing support from the multidisciplinary team of each service. It needs to be a collaborative effort between child and adult services with parallel care from both services (NHS, 2020). However, transition preparation needs tend to vary and must not follow a one-size fits-all model and should take into account neurodiversity, complex trauma, and comorbidities. Attending CPA meetings can facilitate parallel and joint working between adolescent and adult services in the best interest of the young person. These meetings have an interdisciplinary character and aim to provide an agreed structured treatment plan and close monitoring of the transition process.

Risk presentation can have a strong impact on transition preparation and management. Young people presenting with high risk are often not informed about their transition date due to safeguarding issues and to prevent any adverse events during the transition. Although a young person may have shown significant improvement mental health-wise, they might still present with high risk to others and therefore more focus is given to presenting risk and transition care pathway reflects risk needs rather than developmental needs. However, risk focus during the transition period may be appropriate in a number of cases, whereas young people with serious concerns of risk or with severe index offence history need to be transferred to adult secure hospitals of medium or high security – if there has not been a suitable reduction in risk previously. In such cases, a transition key worker such as a nurse should visit the receiving adult placement to build relationships with adult staff and prepare the team for the young person's admission (NHS, 2020).

Continuity of care

The concept of continuity of care can be understood differently for young people moving to the community than those transferring to adult secure inpatient services. Those returning to the community need a distinctive care approach compared to young people remaining in the forensic system. The dynamics of transition depend heavily on the new placement. Presumably, transition for young people moving between secure hospitals is smoother based on national findings (Livanou, 2018). For example, one study following up young people in adult hospitals found that young males transferring to adult secure hospitals were more likely to report positive outcomes short term (three to six months) (Livanou et al., 2021). However, there are no longitudinal reports about the mental health and risk presentation of young people moving to the community. Young people placed in community settings need the involvement of multiple services to ensure community integration reinforcing self-efficacy and institutional independence which currently is limited. A more graded approach to community transitions should be planned to include short leaves, multiple visits, and self-management interventions (NHS, 2020). However, for young individuals moving to adult medium- or high-secure hospitals issues surrounding hope need to be examined considering their detention in such services might be indefinite.

References

Beyond Youth Custody. (2016). *Trauma and young offenders: A review of the research and practice literature*. http://www.beyondyouthcustody.net/wp-content/uploads/BYC-Trauma-Young-Offenders-FINAL.pdf

Broad, K. L., Sandhu, V. K., Sunderji, N., & Charach, A. (2017). Youth experiences of transition from child mental health services to adult mental health services: A qualitative thematic synthesis. *BMC psychiatry*, *17*(1), 380.

Campbell, F., Biggs, K., Aldiss, S. K., O'Neill, P. M., Clowes, M., McDonagh, J., . . . Gibson, F. (2016). Transition of care for adolescents from paediatric services to adult health services. *Cochrane Database of Systematic Reviews* (4).

Care Quality Commission. (2019). *Segregation in mental health wards for children and young people and in wards for people with a learning disability or autism.* Retrieved October 1, 2020, from www.cqc.org.uk/sites/default/files/20190626_rssinterimreport_full.pdf

Chitsabesan, P., Kroll, L., Bailey, S. U. E., Kenning, C., Sneider, S., MacDonald, W., & Theodosiou, L. (2006). Mental health needs of young offenders in custody and in the community. *The British Journal of Psychiatry, 188*(6), 534–540.

Davis, M. (2003). Addressing the needs of youth in transition to adulthood. *Administration and Policy in Mental Health and Mental Health Services Research, 30*(6), 495–509.

Devapriam, J., & Alexander, R. T. (2012). Tiered model of learning disability forensic service provision. *Journal of Learning Disabilities and Offending Behaviour*, (3), 175–185.

Dunn, V. (2017). Young people, mental health practitioners and researchers co-produce a transition preparation programme to improve outcomes and experience for young people leaving child and adolescent mental health services (CAMHS). *BMC Health Services Research, 17*(1), 1–12.

England, NHS. (2020). *Transitions from adolescent secure to adult secure inpatient services: Practice guidance for all secure services.* NHS England. www.england.nhs.uk/wp-content/uploads/2020/03/camhs-adult-secure-transition-practice-guidance.pdf

Fusar-Poli, P. (2019). Integrated mental health services for the developmental period (0 to 25 years): A critical review of the evidence. *Frontiers in Psychiatry, 10*, 355.

Gomot, M., & Wicker, B. (2012). A challenging, unpredictable world for people with autism spectrum disorder. *International Journal of Psychophysiology, 83*(2), 240–247.

Hackett, S. S., Taylor, J. L., Freeston, M., Jahoda, A., McColl, E., Pennington, L., & Kaner, E. (2017). Interpersonal art psychotherapy for the treatment of aggression in people with learning disabilities in secure care: A protocol for a randomised controlled feasibility study. *Pilot and Feasibility Studies, 3*(1), 1–8.

Hales, H., Holt, C., Delmage, E., & Lengua, C. (2019). What next for adolescent forensic mental health research? *Criminal Behaviour and Mental Health, 29*(4), 196–206. https://doi.org/10.1002/cbm.2124.

Hales, H., Warner, L., Smith, J., & Bartlett, A. (2018). *Census of young people in secure settings on 14 September 2016: Characteristics, needs and pathways of care.* NHS Central and Northwest London, St George's University of London.

Hill, S. A., Brodrick, P., Doherty, A., Lolley, J., Wallington, F., & White, O. (2014). Characteristics of female patients admitted to an adolescent secure forensic psychiatric hospital. *The Journal of Forensic Psychiatry & Psychology, 25*(5), 503–519.

Hindley, N., Lengua, C., & White, O. (2017). Forensic mental health services for children and adolescents: Rationale and development. *BJPsych Advances, 23*(1), 36–43.

Hollins, L. (2019). Review of restraint, prolonged seclusion and segregation for people with a mental health problem, a learning disability or autism. *International Journal of Positive Behavioural Support, 9*(1), 50–51.

Hovish, K., Weaver, T., Islam, Z., Paul, M., & Singh, S. P. (2012). Transition experiences of mental health service users, parents, and professionals in the United Kingdom: A qualitative study. *Psychiatric Rehabilitation Journal, 35*(3), 251.

King, J., O'Neill, B., Ramsay, P., Linden, M. A., Medniuk, A. D., Outtrim, J., & Blackwood, B. (2019). Identifying patients' support needs following critical illness: A scoping review of the qualitative literature. *Critical Care, 23*(1), 1–12.

Lepkowska, D. (2017). Preparing transition to adult services: New guidance. *British Journal of School Nursing, 12*(6), 279–282.

Levy, B. B., Song, J. Z., Luong, D., Perrier, L., Bayley, M. T., Andrew, G., . . . Munce, S. E. (2020). Transitional care interventions for youth with disabilities: A systematic review. *Pediatrics, 146*(5).

Lindgren, E., Söderberg, S., & Skär, L. (2014). Managing transition with support: Experiences of transition from child and adolescent psychiatry to general adult psychiatry narrated by young adults and relatives. *Psychiatry Journal.* https://doi.org/10.1155/2014/457160

Livanou, M. I. (2018). Transition of care among young offenders with ongoing mental health problems in England: Young offenders in transition (Doctoral dissertation). University of Warwick.

Livanou, M. I., D'Souza, S., Lane, R., La Plante, B., & Singh, S. P. (2021). Challenges and facilitators during transitions from adolescent medium secure units to adult services in England: Interviews with mental healthcare professionals. *Administration and Policy in Mental Health and Mental Health Services Research*, 1–16.

Livanou, M. I., Lane, R., D'Souza, S., & Singh, S. P. (2020). A retrospective case note review of young people in transition from adolescent medium secure units to adult services. *The Journal of Forensic Practice, 22*(3), 161–172.

McAra, L., & McVie, S. (2010). Youth crime and justice: Key messages from the Edinburgh study of youth transitions and crime. *Criminology & Criminal Justice, 10*(2), 179–209.

National Health Service. (2014). *Five year forward view.* www.england.nhs.uk/wp-content/uploads/2014/10/5yfv-web.pdf

National Institute for Health and Care Excellence. (2016). *Transition from children's to adults' services for young people using health or social care services.* Clinical Guideline: NG43.

O'Connell, A., & Petty, J. (2019). Preparing young people with complex needs and their families for transition to adult services. *Nursing Children and Young People, 31*(1).

Paul, M., Street, C., Wheeler, N., & Singh, S. P. (2015). Transition to adult services for young people with mental health needs: A systematic review. *Clinical Child Psychology and Psychiatry, 20*(3), 436–457.

Pontoni, G., Di Pietro, E., Neri, T., Mattei, G., Longo, F., Neviani, V., . . . Galeazzi, G. M. (2021). Factors associated with the transition of adolescent inpatients from an intensive residential ward to adult mental health services. *European Child & Adolescent Psychiatry*, 1–14.

Signorini, G., Singh, S. P., Marsanic, V. B., Dieleman, G., Dodig-Ćurković, K., Franic, T., . . . O'Hara, L. (2018). The interface between child/adolescent and adult mental health services: Results from a European 28-country survey. *European Child & Adolescent Psychiatry, 27*(4), 501–511.

Singh, S. P., Paul, M., Ford, T., Kramer, T., & Weaver, T. (2008). Transitions of care from child and adolescent mental health services to adult mental health services (TRACK study): A study of protocols in Greater London. *BMC Health Services Research, 8*(1), 135. https://doi.org/10.1186/1472-6963-8-135

Singh, S. P., Paul, M., Ford, T., Kramer, T., Weaver, T., McLaren, S., . . . White, S. (2010). Process, outcome and experience of transition from child to adult mental healthcare: Multiperspective study. *The British Journal of Psychiatry, 197*(4), 305–312.

Singh, S. P., & Tuomainen, H. (2015). Transition from child to adult mental health services: Needs, barriers, experiences and new models of care. *World Psychiatry, 14*(3), 358.

Wright, S., & Liddle, M. (2014). *Young offenders and trauma: Experience and impact.* A Practitioner's Guide, Beyond Youth Custody.

Xenitidis, K., Gratsa, A., Bouras, N., Hammond, R., Ditchfield, H., Holt, G., . . . Brooks, D. (2004). Psychiatric inpatient care for adults with intellectual disabilities: Generic or specialist units? *Journal of Intellectual Disability Research, 48*(1), 11–18.

Chapter 11

'Long-Stay' in forensic mental health

Prof Birgit Völlm

Introduction

Forensic psychiatry deals with patients who have a mental disorder as well as having committed an (often serious) offence. Depending on the country, there are different requirements for admission to a forensic mental health setting. Often diminished or totally absent criminal responsibility and a clear link between the disorder and the offence are needed. There are also countries, however, where admission to forensic mental health care is possible on the basis of a high risk to self or others even if no offence has (yet) been committed or at least not one that has resulted in a criminal conviction. Unlike in other specialties of psychiatry, the issue of risk is central to the treatment and management of mentally disordered offenders (MDOs) and might even be more focal than the disorder itself. Modern concepts of treatment of MDOs, e.g., the Risk Needs Responsivity principle (Bonta & Andrews, 2017), also emphasise that treatment 'dose' should be tailored towards risk level (as opposed to, e.g., the severity of illness or individual suffering). For doctors working in the field of forensic psychiatry this dual role, treating individuals as well as having responsibility for the protection of the public often entails uncomfortable dilemmas and role conflicts.

Patients in forensic mental health settings present with multiple challenges: early deprivation; disrupted upbringings; emotional, physical, and sexual abuse; neglect; poor educational and vocational opportunities; drug and alcohol abuse; victimisation; prior offending; institutionalisation including in psychiatric care and imprisonment; and physical ill-health comorbidity with poor treatment response are all more common in patients in forensic mental health care compared to other patient cohorts (Taylor & Farrington, 2014). Patients have often experienced poor care, including in institutions, and can be very suspicious particularly at the beginning of their stay. For all these reasons, treatment is complex, even without considering the additional requirement to target and reduce risk factors. It is therefore hardly surprising that LoS is considerably higher in forensic mental health care compared to other mental health facilities. But: How long is (too) long? What is the prevalence of 'long-stay' and which factors are associated with lengthy stays? How do patients experience long-stay? What kinds of services are appropriate for long-stay patients? These are the topics this chapter will elaborate on. Understanding these issues is not only important from a clinical point of view. Long stay also poses significant ethical questions given the highly restrictive and resource-intensive nature of forensic mental health care. Long-stay patients represent some of the most socially excluded groups in society.

DOI: 10.4324/9781003184768-14

How long is (too) long?

There is no generally, or even locally, accepted standard for LoS in forensic mental health care. A review by Huband et al. (2018), including 69 studies from 14 different countries covering different aspects of long stay in forensic mental health care, identified 20 papers that had reported a prospectively chosen LoS threshold. Studies from Germany, Israel, and Malaysia used an LoS of ten years as a cut-off, studies from Ireland and some from the United Kingdom used a considerably shorter LoS of two years to indicate long stay. A survey of 18 European countries by Edworthy et al. (2016) showed that thresholds of five to ten years were used to define long-stay. The Netherlands as the only country providing a formal designated service for long-stay patients (see later) uses a cut-off of six years as a criterion to be considered for this service.

Countries that operate a system with clearly demarcated security levels, like, e.g., the United Kingdom, might use different thresholds for different levels of security. When medium-secure services were introduced in the United Kingdom in the 1970s (before then there had only been high secure care), it was recommended that LoS should be limited to two years (e.g., Butler, 1975); however, in practice, LoS often turned out often be much longer than that (Shah et al., 2011). To complicate matters further some patients stay in high- and medium-secure care consecutively; therefore to calculate a patient's total LoS in forensic mental health care, the two time periods, as well as any time spent in low secure settings, have to be added. In a multi-centre study in the United Kingdom looking at patients in medium and high secure settings, Völlm et al. (2017) suggested the following definition of long stay: having been in a high secure setting for more than 10 years, in a medium-secure setting for more than five, or in a combination of both for more than 15 years. The authors explain

> this decision was guided by the consideration that the population included should be large enough in size to provide meaningful conclusions for service developments (i.e. not so small that only a very limited number of patients would be included and not so large that a substantial proportion of patients would be captured).
>
> (p. 12)

While we have so far considered different concrete time periods to define long stay, an alternative approach might be to link the long-stay definition to the average LoS in that country, security level, or even specific patient group. For example, one might consider a patient to be a long-stay patient if their LoS falls outside two standard deviations from the mean of a sufficiently similar patient group. Such an approach would have the advantage of being much more tailored to the circumstances in specific countries, types of services, and so on. However, it would be impractical to use and would make the identification of long-stay patients rather cumbersome.

Finally, one might consider defining long stay without reference to a specific time period. Someone could have stayed for 'too long' if they should have progressed according to their characteristics and needs – even if they had not stayed for a long time period. The definition of long stay from the COST action IS1302[1] used this approach when suggesting: 'Forensic psychiatric inpatients with needs for security and care who are not able to safely progress to a level of lower security due to internal and/or external factors' (Bulten, personal communication). Also important to note in this definition is the recognition that factors hindering progress could lay within or outside the individual patient.

Methodological issues

There are a number of ways to measure LoS (Huband et al., 2018). Which approach is the best to use depends on the individual question to be answered. The three main methods are:

1. Admission samples (considers all patients admitted on a particular date or during a particular time period with LoS calculated from admission to discharge)
2. Discharge samples (considers all patients discharged on a particular date or during a particular time period with LoS calculated from admission to discharge)
3. Cross-sectional samples (sampling all patients resident in the particular unit on a particular date or during a particular time period with LoS calculated from the date of admission to this time point).

Admission samples have the advantage that the political and service provision context is very similar for all patients in the sample at the point of admission, they are also well suited to identify factors that predict LoS. Discharge samples, similarly, capture context at the time of discharge. Neither of these two methods, however, consider patients who have not (yet) been discharged, thereby underestimating LoS. Cross-sectional samples capture these patients but cannot make any observations about LoS up to discharge. However, the advantage of cross-sectional samples is that they include patients who may never be discharged which is a group of particular interest in long-stay research. The necessity to not only consider current care spells but add periods of stay in different units during the same treatment episode (that is following the same index offence/conviction) has already been pointed out earlier.

Length of stay in forensic mental health settings

Not surprisingly, LoS in forensic mental health settings is far higher than in general psychiatric services, e.g., 1367 compared to 79 days in a one-night census of a catchment area of 1.2 million people in North London (Sharma et al., 2015). LoS in high secure care has been identified as eight years in the United Kingdom (Dell, 1987). For UK medium-secure care, Völlm et al. (2017) found five studies reporting mean LoS in their review, ranging from 30 weeks to 26 months based on admission and discharge samples. Given the methodology of these studies, LoS is likely to be considerably underestimated which is confirmed by findings in the same review concluding that up to 50% of patients' LoS was over two years and about 10% of over five years. A recent study (Tomlin et al., 2021) reporting on LoS in Europe with data based on a survey of experts from 17 different countries reported broad differences in the average LoS, ranging from under three years in Italy, Latvia, Lithuania, Macedonia, Poland, and Slovenia to eight years in Germany and Scotland and ten years in the Netherlands.

From a patient as well as service provision point of view those who 'get stuck' in highly restrictive settings are of particular concern. In the United Kingdom, e.g., in the 1990s, studies using needs assessments identified that between one-third and two-thirds of patients resident in a high secure hospital did not have to be managed at that high level of security (e.g., Thomas et al., 2004) and that issues around inadequate care provision at lower levels of security as well as delays in the transfer of patients were to blame. These findings led to the 'accelerated discharge programme' (Department of Health, 2000), which aimed to reduce the number of patients in high secure care. This was successful in that high secure bed numbers reduced from 1700 at the beginning of the 1990s to about 800 twenty years later (Craissati & Taylor, 2014), while at the same time, medium-secure beds increased from about 600–3,200 (NHS England, 2015). Despite this significant shift, a more recent study (Völlm et al., 2017) again found a prevalence of long stay of 23.5% for high secure patients and 18.1% for medium-secure patients based on the criteria described earlier. While percentages in the three high secure hospitals showed little variation (22–26%), the proportion of long-stay patients in medium-secure care ranged from 0% to 50% indicating probably significant differences in the type of patients different units accept as well as their approaches to treatment and discharge.

Some studies have reported an increase in LoS over time though others have found opposite trends. Ricketts et al. (2001), in a UK medium-secure sample, found that the percentage of patients staying for more than two years increased from 7% in 1983–7 to 16.2% in 1991–5 before falling again to 12.3% in 1995–9. More recently, Earnshaw et al. (2019) showed a significant increase in LoS in one MSU in the United Kingdom over a 30-year period. In addition, they observed an increase of discharges to other psychiatric settings and a decrease of those discharged to independent living. This could not be explained by differences in the diagnostic composition of the samples. Despite these findings, as will be reported later, there is some evidence to suggest that active management of LoS with clear targets to reduce it can be successful.

Factors associated with long stay

A number of studies have aimed to identify factors associated with LoS. Possible factors include patient characteristics (e.g., age, gender, diagnoses, offences, behaviour in the unit), service and wider care provision factors (e.g., legal sections, availability of care in lower or non-secure settings), as well as societal issues (e.g., risk adversity). By far the largest number of studies have investigated patient factors, probably not least as they are much easier to measure than the other two types of factors.

Huband et al. (2018) reviewed the international literature regarding long stay. In the 40 studies describing characteristics of long-stay patients, 90 variables of potential relevance were examined, 48 of those were mentioned in more than one study. The most common association with long stay was severity of index offence. Those with violent index offences, in particular murder or homicide, were significantly more likely to be in the long-stay group (or had a longer LoS depending on whether a group comparison or correlational analysis was used). Other offending characteristics related to long stay included parallel prison sentence, longer prior prison sentence(s), and younger age at offence. By contrast, the number of previous convictions was not found to be associated with LoS in most studies that examined this variable. Diagnosis was also frequently studied, here most, though not all, studies showed a positive association between schizophrenia or other psychotic disorders and LoS, some, however, found a negative or no relationship. Other factors related to mental health commonly identified included: longer history of prior psychiatric treatment, prior substance abuse, more severe symptoms as well as organic/cognitive deficits. Maybe somewhat surprising, personality disorder, including psychopathy, did not emerge as a factor consistently associated with LoS. Gender was also not associated with LoS showing equal numbers of positive and negative associations while most studies did not report a relationship between gender and LoS. Findings relating to ethnicity were also conflicting. Younger age at admission was associated with longer LoS and so was older age at discharge or no discharge address, poor education, and the absence of a close relationship. Behaviour during the current stay was also relevant to non-compliance with treatment, aggressive or violent behaviour, as well as seclusion or restraint during the current stay all associated with longer LoS, while attendance at psychological treatment sessions was related to shorter LoS. Other factors associated with shorter LoS were prior employment, ongoing contact with family, and being a parent.

This review was therefore able to identify patient characteristics associated with LoS but contributes little to relevant factors outside patient characteristics. Some UK studies looked at the legal basis of detention and found that criminal (as opposed to civil) sections as well as having a 'restriction order'[2] were associated with longer LoS. Lack of step-down facilities was suggested in some studies though this was offered more as a possible explanation of LoS than an actual scientific finding. The same is true for suggestions that a more risk-adverse society contributes to increases in LoS over time. Tomlin et al. (2021) contribute important information regarding LoS and wider societal factors. They report significant positive correlations between LoS and gross domestic product (GDP) per capita as well as GDP spending on healthcare and democracy index scores.

Another approach was used in Völlm et al. (2017); they asked consultants in charge of the treatment of long-stay patients in high and medium-secure care (data relate to 169 patients in total) in the United Kingdom to give their opinion as to the possible obstacles for discharge for their individual patients. The main factor impeding a move to lower secure care in their view was psychopathology, followed by risk to others, personality traits, institutionalisation, patient anxiety, and lack of suitable facilities to move to. High media attention towards specific patients was rated the lowest. Therefore, in the view of those in charge of the treatment of long-stay patients, patient characteristics also play a more significant role compared to external factors.

Patient experience of long stay

Only few studies have thus far considered patients' experiences of residing in a forensic setting for a long period of time. In a qualitative study as part of a multi-centre study, interviews with 40 patients resident in high- and medium-secure settings fulfilling the long-stay criteria described earlier were conducted (Völlm et al., 2017). The main topics of the interviews were patients' views on reasons for long stay, how they experience their current situation, and what they expect for themselves in the future. The study found a wide range of different views and experiences. Regarding attribution of long stay, patients could be divided into those who saw the reasons for their long stay mainly within themselves (e.g., their illness or behaviour) and those who attributed their situation to external factors, examples being a change in clinical team, unfair emphasis on their past compared to the current presentation, lack of facilities to move to, and so on. Those who saw the severity of their index offence as an important reason for their LoS, mainly felt that it was justified that they were detained for a long period of time. With regard to their current situation, some patients felt positive about their current treatment and felt and expected that it would help them to get better and eventually move on. They generally were active in the unit and engaged in a range of daily routines and therapies, including medication. Others felt that therapies were not effective, often repetitive, and did not help them move on. As a consequence of that view, these patients often did not fully engage in the treatment programme. With regard to moving on, most patients expected to eventually move on and also wanted to physically move to a less secure setting which was an important goal for them. A smaller group of patients, on the other hand, appeared to have given up on the idea of moving on, did not expect this to happen, and often also said this was not something they were striving towards. Sometimes this might be due to having lost hope for the future; some patients, however, also described that they felt comfortable in their current setting and did not want to have to get used to a new place and start all over again.

Based on the emerging themes – attribution, outlook, approach, and readiness for change – the authors identified four groups: The 'dynamic acceptance' group comprised patients who attributed their long stay to themselves; they felt positive about therapy overall but felt they were ready to move on. Patients in the 'static acceptance' group attributed the reason for long stay internally and externally, were somewhat less positive about therapies, and did not believe they were ready to move on. The groups 'dynamic resistance' attributed their long stay to external factors, felt negative about their current situation but still believed they would eventually move on. A smaller group 'static resistance' shared the first two attributes with the former group but had largely given up on the prospect of moving on despite their belief that they did not need to be in secure care.

Recognising these different patient perspectives is important in both working with individual long-stay patients and when thinking about service models for long-stay patients.

Service provision

Currently, patients who experience long stay are in most countries resident on wards with patients with a mix of LoS; they therefore experience others around them moving on, while they don't. Whether this is positive in terms of motivation or rather frustrating will depend on the specific patient; service providers and those who care for long-stay patients also have different views about how care should be provided for long-stay patients, e.g., whether there should be a separate ward/service tailored to their needs or not.

A useful starting point when thinking about service provision is to consider the needs of long-stay patients. The review by Huband et al. (2018) identified several needs which were reported in more than one study. Most commonly noted were needs around the treatment of a severe mental illness, specifically psychosis, as well as substance abuse treatment. Psychological distress, risk to self, and physical health were also often identified. Also commonly reported were needs related to treatment programmes for violent and/or sexual offending and/or arson. The remaining needs found in more than one study were: daytime activities, social skills, understanding sexual experiences, and placement needs. The group of long-stay patients thus has a range of needs in different domains pointing towards the necessity of a multi-professional approach with a high level of resources.

Völlm et al. (2017) describe a small survey of 36 senior professionals (e.g., clinical managers with nursing background) in the United Kingdom on the need for and possible specifications of a long-stay service. The majority of professionals agreed that there is a need for a separate secure long-stay service, 70% of respondents agreed that the main aim of this service should be to provide optimum quality of life with care rather than cure as the main philosophy, providing a stable and secure living environment. They felt that the service was likely to be considered 'home' for the patient and that staff working there needed to understand this. Maybe somewhat contradictory, respondents largely still considered risk reduction work an important treatment focus. There was no agreement on possible admission criteria, but respondents seemed to favour a mix of the actual LoS and other characteristics as entry criteria. They thought that admission should also be possible on a compulsory basis. With regard to the specific characteristics of the service, few statements reached more than 70% agreement (agree or strongly agree). Those statements reaching such high level of concordance regarded the need to emphasise the importance of physical healthcare and the need to have a high level of occupational therapy input. Participants were split on the question of whether there was more or less medical and psychological input needed compared to other types of services. Agreement could also not be reached on the (relative) importance of physical and relational security and on the flexibility of policies and routine reporting. A range of challenges on all levels (government, commissioners, staff, and patients) was foreseen in setting up a long-stay service though none was supported by more than 50% of respondents. Interestingly, participants themselves felt uncomfortable with the name 'long-stay' and suggested a range of other names for such a service: enhanced recovery, extended care, continuing care, forensic recovery service, ongoing treatment, and slower-stream rehabilitation.

Individual interviews and focus groups with managers, doctors, and other professionals were also conducted as part of the study by Völlm et al. (2017). They revealed a strong attachment to a model of cure (as opposed to long-term care), particularly in the medical professionals. Participants felt uncomfortable with the idea of a long-stay service associating this with 'warehousing' and giving up on patients. The same group of professionals (i.e., those caring for long-stay patients in high- and medium-secure settings in the United Kingdom), however, identified the placement needs of their high-secure patients in five years' time as 'high secure' in over 40% of cases and 'medium secure' in over 50% of cases, suggesting a very low expectation of patients moving to lower levels of security even after a relatively long period of time.

The only country to my knowledge currently providing an actual long-stay model with clear entry criteria and service specifications is the Dutch long-stay service. The Dutch forensic service, TBS (Terbeschikkingstelling), has developed the following criteria for 'long-stay': Treatment of at least six years in at least two different TBS-clinics but nevertheless very little treatment success, meaning no relevant risk reduction. If a patient fulfils these criteria, their team can ask for long-stay status for the patient which is decided by a panel outside the treatment team. If agreed, the person is moved to one of two long-stay services in the country. There the focus is on quality of life rather than on risk reduction. Patients do, however, still have reviews regarding the ongoing need for detention – they could still be discharged or move back to the mainstream TBS service if their circumstances change and treatment is expected to be more successful. This service is understandably much debated. While opponents fear warehousing and neglect, those in favour point to the better quality of life, reduced stress levels (e.g., due to not being forced to participate in certain treatment groups), and the fact that patients often speak positively about the service.

Other countries provide long-stay services (wards) on a more local and 'ad hoc' basis, borne out of the need to provide for this patient group, but without a legal or even policy framework to support it. Vaughan (2000) described some characteristics he thought important for services catering to patients with lengthy LoS including the importance of an individualised approach and a structured timetable with sport, social, and leisure groups. These activities as well as physical health care are generally thought to be more important than psychological care in this patient group.

Initiatives to reduce LoS

What helps to reduce LoS is a matter of much debate and no clear answers can thus far be identified. Huband et al. (2018) found only two papers describing such initiatives. The first paper from the Netherlands (Nagtegaal et al., 2011) described an approach trying to focus on improving aftercare services by increasing the length of compulsory aftercare as well as improving the quality of such services. However, the evaluation of this approach is not reported. What is reported though is the success of financial penalties for services providers which exceed certain LoS levels in the TBS system. Glorney (2010) in the United Kingdom described a model effectively trying to improve the efficiency of inpatient services, thereby enabling patients to move through the treatment programs quicker. Again, the outcomes of this model are not reported.

Conclusions

Research has identified a group of patients in forensic mental health services who stay there for extended periods of time, potentially lifelong, and thus represent a highly excluded social group. Sociodemographic, clinical, and offending parameters have been described for this group while information on the experience of these long-stay patients themselves remains limited. Nevertheless, it is clear that the long-stay patient group is a heterogeneous group likely to consist of patients who might yet make progress albeit slow, those who are stuck currently but who might make progress again later, and those who are very likely to spend the rest of their life in a secure environment. Obviously, what is needed in terms of service provision will be very different for these groups. Those who are still on a trajectory of progress and risk reduction might be suitably catered for in mainstream services. Those who are currently 'stuck' might need approaches such as motivational interviewing to identify possible next steps in care delivery. Those for whom moving on and out of the secure system is not possible need first of all to be recognised as a group for whom society has a particular responsibility given they are, after all, mainly detained for the protection of *others* based on imperfect risk assessments with the possibility of false-positive assessments. They are also often detained for longer than they would have been had they not been diagnosed with a mental disorder, an issue some would argue goes against the principles of the United Nations Convention on the Rights of People with Disabilities. This is also why some countries, including Croatia, Italy, and Portugal, now have legal provisions such that detention in a hospital can no longer exceed the length of a prison sentence the individual would have been given had they been convicted as a non-MDO.

Notes

1. COST stands for 'Cooperation in Science and Technology', an EU funding stream. The COST action IS1302: Towards an EU research framework on forensic psychiatric care focused on long-stay in forensic psychiatric care.
2. In UK mental health law a 'restriction order' stipulates that decisions regarding leave, transfer, and discharge cannot be made by the clinical teams without agreement of the Ministry of Justice or a tribunal decision.

References

Bonta, J., & Andrews, D. A. (2017). *The psychology of criminal conduct* (6th ed.). Routledge.
Boyd-Caine, T. (2012). *Protecting the public? Detention and release of mentally disordered offenders*. Routledge.
Butler. (1975). *Report of the committee on mentally abnormal offenders* (chairman Lord Butler). Cmnd 6244. HMSO.
Craissati, J., & Taylor, P. (2014). Forensic mental health services in the United Kingdom and Ireland. In J. Gunn, C. Johnson, & P. Taylor (Eds.), *Forensic psychiatry: Clinical, legal and ethical issues* (pp. 589–619). Taylor and Francis.
Dell, S., Robertson, G., & Parker, E. (1987). Detention in Broadmoor. Factors in length of stay. *Journal of Psychiatry, 150*, 824–827.
Department of Health. (2000). *Report of the review of security at the high security hospitals*. HMSO.
Earnshaw, C. H., Shaw, L., Thomas, D., & Haeney, O. (2019). A retrospective study comparing the length of admission of medium secure unit patients admitted in the three decades since 1985. *The British Journal of Psychiatry, 43*, 154–157.
Edworthy, R., Sampson, S., & Völlm, B. A. (2016). Inpatient forensic-psychiatric care: Legal frameworks and service provision in three European countries. *International Journal of Law and Psychiatry, 29*, 18–27.
Glorney, E., Perkins, D., Adshead, G., McGauley, G., Murray, K., Noak, J., & Sichau, G. (2010). Domains of need in a high secure hospital setting: A model for streamlining care and reducing length of stay. *International Journal of Forensic Mental Health, 9*, 138–148.
Huband, N., Furtado, V., Schel, S., Eckert, M., CheuNg, N., BultEn, E., & Völlm, B. (2018). Characteristics and needs of long-stay forensic psychiatric inpatients: A rapid review of the literature. *International Journal of Forensic Mental Health, 17*, 45–60.
Nagtegaal, M. H., Horst, R. P. V. D., & Schönberger, H. J. M. (2011). Inzicht in de verblijfsduur van tbs-gestelden: cijfers en mogelijke verklaringen [Understanding the duration of forensic psychiatric patients: Numbers and possible explanations]. WODC, Ministerie van Veiligheid en Justitie.
NHS England. (2015). *NHS standard contract for high secure mental health services (ADULTS). C02/S/a 2014/15.* www.england.nhs.uk/wp-content/uploads/2013/06/c02-high-sec-mh.pdf

Ricketts, D., Carnell, H., Davies, S., Kaul, A., & Duggan, C. (2001). First admissions to a regional secure unit over a 16-year period: Changes in demographic and service characteristics. *The Journal of Forensic Psychiatry, 12*, 78–89.

Shah, A., Waldron, G., Boast, N., Coid, J. W., & Ullrich, S. (2011). Factors associated with length of admission at a medium secure forensic psychiatric unit. *The Journal of Forensic Psychiatry & Psychology*, 496–512.

Sharma, A., Dunn, W., O'Toole, C., & Kennedy, H. G. (2015). The virtual institution: Cross-sectional length of stay in general adult and forensic psychiatry beds. *International Journal of Mental Health Systems, 30*(9), 25.

Taylor, P. J., & Farrington, D. P. (2014). The psychosocial milieu of the offender. In J. Gunn & P. J. Taylor (Eds.), *Forensic psychiatry: Clinical, legal and ethical issues* (2nd ed., pp. 170–185). CRC Press.

Thomas, S., Leese, M., Dolan, M., Harty, M., Shaw, J., Middleton, H., et al. (2004). The individual needs of patients in high secure psychiatric hospitals in England. *The Journal of Forensic Psychiatry & Psychology, 15*, 222–243.

Tomlin, J., Lega, I., Braun, P., Kennedy, H. G., Tort Herrando, V., Barroso, R., Castelletti, L., Mirabella, F., Scarpa, F., Völlm, B., & the experts of COST Action IS1302 (2021). Forensic mental health in Europe: Some key figures. *Social Psychiatry and Psychiatric Epidemiology, 56*, 109–117.

Vaughan, P. (2000). Developing service specifications for secure provision. *The British Journal of Forensic Practice, 2*, 13–18.

Völlm, B., Edworthy, R., Holley, J., Talbot, E., Majid, S., Duggan, C., Weaver, T., & McDonald, R. (2017). A mixed-methods study exploring the characteristics and needs of long-stay patients in high and medium secure settings in England: Implications for service organisation. *Health Services and Delivery Research, 5*, 11.

Part 4

Developing responsive interventions and models of care

A tripartite model of cultural, clinical, and operational governance in the planning and delivery of culturally informed care for Indigenous Māori forensic mental health service users

James Cavney

Introduction

When one considers the delivery of care to marginalised and minority groups within forensic mental health care settings, it is difficult to overlook the plight of indigenous peoples. Numerous international epidemiological studies, particularly from Australasia and Canada, have demonstrated that indigenous populations are grossly overrepresented in both prison and mental health populations when compared to non-indigenous groups within the same jurisdictions.

In New Zealand, the focus of this chapter, Māori are the indigenous population group. They experienced 7.5 times the risk of imprisonment compared to non-Māori, with a rate of 704 per 100,000 population (Skipworth, 2019). Repeated large-scale prison epidemiological studies have also identified Māori as having significantly disproportionate rates of serious mental illness (Brinded et al., 2001) with significantly higher rates of psychotic illnesses than any other ethnic groups (Indig et al., 2016).

Similarly, in Australia, indigenous people (Aboriginal and Torres Strait Islanders) experience a relative risk of imprisonment 15.2 times that of the non-indigenous population. Although they constitute 3% of the population, they represent 27% of the prison population, with an imprisonment rate of 2,434 per 100,000 population compared to 160 per 100,000 population for non-Aboriginal (Skipworth, 2019) with a 12-month prevalence of mental disorder to be 73% amongst men and 86% amongst female (Heffernan et al., 2012).

Likewise, in Canada, indigenous people (First Nations, Inuit, and Métis) represent 4.3% of the general population but constitute approximately 21% of the total federal prison population (Gutierrez et al., 2017). They too have high rates of serious mental illness including psychotic and mood disorders (Simpson et al., 2013). However, understanding the root cause of these adverse health and social justice outcomes for indigenous people requires more than a point prevalence analyses.

Colonisation: Outcomes Versus Process

It is widely accepted that the poor mental health and social justice outcomes among indigenous people have worsened over time due to the intergenerational transmission of the adverse impacts of Western colonisation. The development of social institutions and policy by colonial governors promoted and consolidated inequalities in power and resources through the erosion of indigenous cultural identity in favour of assimilation and compliance (Shepherd et al., 2018).

DOI: 10.4324/9781003184768-16

The deleterious impact of colonisation upon indigenous populations is numerous and well described (see Cavney & Hatters Friedman, 2018). These include racial discrimination, unemployment, poverty, substance abuse, poor education, and the disruption and breakdown of family systems, all recognised risk factors for mental illness and incarceration within indigenous groups. However, it is the process of 'political colonisation' that is the root cause of their intergenerational transmission. Specifically, the cultural disenfranchisement, divestment of political capital, and erosion of autonomy in decision making in relation to their own interests (Anderson et al., 2016).

A full analysis of the historical colonisation process over multiple jurisdictions is well beyond the scope of this chapter. However, understanding how social justice and health policy development has often served to maintain structural racism against indigenous people within forensic mental health settings is helpful (Came et al., 2021) and discussed in this chapter in relation to New Zealand's experiences.

This is not to suggest there are easy or universal solutions to these complex issues. Indeed, the cultural diversity of indigenous peoples internationally in itself complicates identifying any specific cross-cultural strategy to redress these disparities. Rather, it is proposed that a process to engage indigenous peoples in the development of policy and service design is the critical mechanism to better meet their diverse needs and could be more readily applied across international forensic settings.

International governance and legislation

Recognition of the negative impact of colonisation upon indigenous peoples has been recognised at the highest levels of international governance bodies and reconceptualised the most fundamental of definitions. In classic anthropological terms, indigenous people are defined as members of an ethnic group descended from the original inhabitants of a particular geographical region. They collectively identify with and retain at least some aspects of the traditions, knowledge, and values of their ancestral culture (Sanders, 1999).

However, the term 'indigenous peoples' has more recently evolved to implicitly recognise the subjugation, disenfranchisement, and marginalisation of these groups from economic and socio-political influence within their traditional lands (United Nations, 2009). The United Nations has thus decreed the importance of protecting the rights of indigenous peoples and elevating their interests in decision-making processes.

The Declaration on the Rights of Indigenous Peoples (United Nations, 2007) established requirements for engaging indigenous peoples in constitution making to enhance their autonomy. A number of auditing branches such as the Committee on the Elimination of Racial Discrimination (CERD) have also provided mechanisms to monitor the compliance of member states in meeting their human rights commitments to indigenous peoples (see later).

National governance: a New Zealand perspective

At a national level, New Zealand's obligations to the United Nations decrees are further reinforced by a somewhat unique colonial history that, on 6 February 1840, led to the signing of a treaty between Māori tribes (iwi) and the British Crown. The so-called Treaty of Waitangi (Te Tiriti o Waitangi) is now recognised as the legitimate foundation for constitutional government in New Zealand (Came, 2021).

However, aspects of the original Treaty were critically mistranslated from the English version to the Māori version and resulted in a profound misunderstanding that has resonated over subsequent generations (Orange, 1987). A central and recurrent tension has pivoted around issues of governance. In the English version of the Treaty, Māori ceded sovereignty to the Crown in exchange for the protection of Māori culture and equal standing as Crown subjects. Māori in contrast believed they had entered into an equal partnership and retained absolute sovereignty and self-determination (*Tino rangatiratanga*) over their land and cultural assets.

As the reality of colonial governance began to exert its authority over Māori, a series of armed conflicts arose between 1845 and 1872 that led to a cascade of legislation that divested Māori from their traditional resources and cultural identity. Over a period of less than 50 years, the combination of war, land confiscation, disease, forced assimilation, poverty, alcoholism, and demoralisation caused a rapid decline in the health of Māori. Durie (1999) identified that process as the forerunner of Māori offending, imprisonment, and poor mental health outcomes.

In 1975, the Waitangi Tribunal was established as a permanent commission of inquiry tasked with researching breaches of the Treaty by the Crown and suggesting means of redress. Whereas claims initially related to land confiscations, this broadened to include the concepts of *taonga* (cultural treasures) and matters of social justice and health. The Treaty of Waitangi Amendment Act in 1985 provided a more contemporaneous interpretation of the Treaty's principles providing Māori additional legislative rights to revisit many previously neglected grievances (Orange, 1987).

These principles, the so-called three 'P's', became mandated obligations for all New Zealand governmental policy and practice development to ensure equity between Māori and non-Māori. *Partnership* reflected a commitment to collaborative processes between Māori and the Crown. *Participation* ensured Māori could engage in policy development. *Protection* recognised the duty of Crown to respect and preserve Māori cultural beliefs, values, and practise within those processes (Crocker, 1989).

And yet, despite international obligations and national imperatives, New Zealand has continued to struggle to achieve equity in health and social justice outcomes for Māori. In 2013, the CERD (CERD, 2013) urged New Zealand to 'intensify its efforts' to address the overrepresentation of Māori within the criminal justice system which they found little progress on in a 2017 review (CERD, 2017). In 2015, the United Nations Working Group on Arbitrary Detention similarly urged New Zealand to identify the root causes of the systemic bias that contributed to that overrepresentation (Waitangi Tribunal, 2017).

In 2017, the Waitangi Tribunal reviewed a claim concerning the Crown's failure to make a long-term commitment to reducing the high rates of Māori incarceration and reoffending (ibid). The Tribunal heard arguments that institutional racism 'pervaded' the criminal justice system and concluded that the Crown had breached the principles of equity and protection by having not prioritised the needs of Māori offenders.

As Came et al. (2021) summarised, the health disparities for Māori within New Zealand also resulted in the lodging of similar claims of systematic discrimination and racism within the health system. Following an umbrella claim, the Waitangi Tribunal concluded there had been an overall failure of the legislative and policy framework of the New Zealand's primary health system to improve Māori health outcomes (Waitangi Tribunal, 2019). The Tribunal again argued that existing entrenched health policies were 'non-compliant' in relation to the Crown's treaty responsibilities.

Whilst mental health services, and more specifically forensic mental health, have not yet been subject to a Waitangi Tribunal claims process, a recent national enquiry into mental health services (He Ara Oranga, 2018) noted that mental health services had also failed to meet the needs of Māori. Māori participants in that enquiry identified that current services, strategies, and policies did not reflect a genuine partnership between the Crown and Māori. Rather, approaches to mental distress and illness reflected a colonising worldview that often contrasted with Māori understanding of well-being.

In sum, the New Zealand experience would suggest that operationalising aspirational commitments to protect the rights and well-being of indigenous people in relation to health and social justice is difficult, particularly as there are no clear guidelines on how to translate policy into tangible interventions creating a daunting challenge for those working within these systems, particularly forensic mental health settings.

Whilst legislative imperatives, whether at a national or international level, are strategically important, it is clear that a 'top-down' approach is insufficient in addressing the complexity of the problem. It also requires a commitment at an organisational level to generate mechanisms to include indigenous people in the development of policy and service delivery to ensure more equitable outcomes for indigenous people within forensic mental health settings. The central argument of this chapter is that the critical mechanism to that end is robust clinical governance.

Clinical governance: a tripartite model

Clinical governance is an internationally recognised model for health delivery that arose after a number of failings of Britain's National Health Service (NHS) in the late 1990s. A key finding was an imbalance between the fiscal priorities of managers and the clinical priorities of clinicians. Clinical governance was thus defined as 'a framework through which NHS organisations are accountable for continuously improving the quality of their services and safe-guarding high standards of care by creating an environment in which excellence in clinical care will flourish' (Scally & Donaldson, 1998).

Clinical governance has since been adopted by a number of jurisdictions although has come to be defined in different ways. Variations in those definitions have reflected the different activities and relationships within different health organisations and the organisational structures that link governance, management, clinicians, and stakeholders (Health Quality & Safety Commission, 2017). Despite these variations, there are common elements that relate to seven primary 'pillars': clinical effectiveness, risk management, patient experience and involvement, communication, resource effectiveness, strategic effectiveness, and learning effectiveness.

New Zealand has yet to formalise its own definition of clinical governance but utilises variations of the Australian Council on Healthcare Standards' (2004) definition that places service users at the centre. Clinical governance in New Zealand is thus a system by which the 'governing body, managers, clinicians and staff share responsibility and accountability for the quality of care, continuously improving, minimising risks, and fostering an environment of excellence in care for [service users]' (ibid.).

The New Zealand Health Safety and Quality Commission also recommended developing clinical leadership at all levels of health organisations as a way of effecting change and enhancing quality (Gauld, 2014). It further recommended that clinical governance aligns to strategic quality goals defined by Ministry of Health (2003) to include people-centredness; access and equity; safety; effectiveness; and efficiency that rested on the Treaty of Waitangi principles: partnership, participation, and protection.

Notwithstanding the tacit acknowledgement of the Treaty of Waitangi's principles in relation to the delivery of health care to Māori, there was still no clear process identified to ensure the engagement of Māori in developing policy and process at an organisational level. Whilst clinical and managerial partnerships were prioritised, exactly how these governance dyads were to engage with Māori at the different levels of the health system remained unclear.

Although the Treaty of Waitangi does not impose an absolute duty on the Crown to consult with Māori, it does bestow an obligation on the Crown and its organisations to inform itself of Māori interests when making decisions that affect Māori. However, the 2540 Waitangi Tribunal Report (2017) argued this was not enough. Instead, it recommended that good governance required mechanisms to ensure co-design by engaging Māori as stakeholders including service users, their families (whanau), and tribal groups (iwi).

The New Zealand Department of Corrections and Ministry of Health have since established Māori advisory boards. However, one commentator contributing to the 2017 report noted that Māori are treaty partners, not treaty advisors and such entities cannot simply be token gestures. There must be frameworks that provide accountability to those stakeholders and enable them to offer solutions or recommendations (ibid).

Nor is it not enough to simply add Māori concepts to mainstream programmes. Services need to be funded and co-designed in consultation and engagement with Māori. In summary, the central premise of this chapter is that the development of effective Kaupapa Māori services (designed by Māori for Māori) requires a commitment to a 'tripartite model' of clinical governance that includes cultural, clinical, and operational partnerships at all levels of an organisation.

The Mason Report

The foundations for a tripartite model of clinical governance within a forensic mental health setting in New Zealand were first laid out in The Mason Report (Mason, 1988). Commissioned in 1987 by the New Zealand Ministry of Health, it was the culmination of some 16 inquiries, working parties, and other investigations that had examined the plight of mentally disordered offenders in New Zealand institutions. It followed a high number of prison suicides between 1983 and 1987 and a number of high-profile homicides in 1985–86 committed by people known to community mental health services.

From the outset, the committee charged with undertaking the enquiry consulted with prominent Māori and Pacific Island community organisations and representatives. It appointed a Kaumatua (Māori tribal leader) to join the committee and consulted widely with all other stakeholders including mental health and correctional staff, unions, service users, prison inmates, academics, police, the judiciary, and reviewed international forensic mental health services.

The enquiry committee also reviewed the poor outcomes of Māori and Pacific Island mental health service users both in the community and in prison. It concluded that 'there was a tremendous lack of Māori input' to the prisons including cultural, spiritual, and educational and that mainstream mental health facilities were also deficient in meeting the needs of Māori. Throughout their investigations, the psychiatrists on the committee were struck by the response from Māori inmates to the Māori team members and concluded that their participation had added a 'cultural enrichment' to the social and psychological assessments of the inmates they interviewed.

The Māori committee members in turn noted that it was important to 'marry up' the psychiatric and Māori perspectives 'to get an even balance'. This observation was particularly poignant when the committee reviewed an early example of a Kaupapa Māori unit (Whare Paea) that had some success in managing patients deemed too dangerous for other services in low-level security settings.

However, the committee was critical of that facility noting that it seemed to act independently of the main hospital management and that cultural imperatives prevailed whilst evidence-based medicine was side-lined. It had no criteria for admission, no stated function, no stated role, and no stated method of practice. There was no cultural leadership and little understanding of either the Māori language or Māori cultural practices.

The Mason Report concluded that Whare Paea's self-imposed isolation from external scrutiny risked aberrant practice. These concerns ultimately led to the closure of the unit and a recommendation in the Mason Report that culturally based forensic services should not be developed in isolation. Nevertheless, the report did strongly recommend the establishment of specialist forensic mental health services that had a bicultural focus that aspired to both cultural and clinical excellence.

It recommended the establishment of forensic mental health services staffed by multidisciplinary teams who had skills and understanding of Māori culture in addition to specialist cultural advisors. In addition to a Clinical Director, it also recommended the establishment of a Director of Cultural Services. Following the Mason Report, Auckland Regional Forensic Psychiatric Services (ARFPS) (the Mason Clinic) was established and has upheld a high degree of fidelity to its founding document and its commitment to the principles of the Treaty of Waitangi and working in partnership with Māori has been a process that has continued to evolve.

Auckland regional forensic psychiatric services: the Mason Clinic

The Mason Clinic is the largest provider of forensic mental health services in New Zealand with a catchment region of approximately 1.5 million people. The service has approximately 130 inpatients and 50 outpatients at any given time, including people with serious mental illnesses and/or intellectual disabilities. Of those, approximately half are Māori and 20% Pacific Islanders. It also provides services to the courts and prisons as well as forensic community liaison to four District Health Boards.

The Mason Clinic's executive team is led by a triumvirate of a Clinical Director, an Operational Manager, and a Kaumatua with reporting lines to the Waitemata District Health Board. Its funding to date has been a priority area within the Ministry of Health expenditure that has over time seen significant financial investment in buildings, funding for leadership positions, and the appointments of both clinical and cultural staffing positions.

There are Clinical Governance meetings once per month that are attended by the executive, clinical subspeciality leaders, leads from each sub-service, service user representatives, family and whanau representatives, programme governance leadership, and cultural representation. Cultural representation is additionally enhanced with a parallel monthly meeting of the 'Taumata', a Māori focused forum where service issues of importance to Māori are robustly debated to provide direct feedback to the clinical governance forum.

There are numerous sub-committee forums that consider programme governance, security, restrictive practices, documents and forms, key performance indicators, and research, each of which has a requirement for cultural representation. In recent years, an admissions panel and a discharge panel have also been established to provide independent oversight of those key steps, again with cultural representation in those processes. There is a culture of audit and research that has contributed to the establishment of clear models of care for the prisons (Pillai et al., 2016), rehabilitation stream, community settings, and intellectually disabled offenders.

Cultural advisors (Taura whiri) are embedded within all parts of the service to provide cultural engagement with service users and their families (whanau), to undertake cultural assessments, and to provide cultural guidance and supervision for other staff. The workforce in general, but leadership in particular, are expected to have some knowledge and appreciation of Māori culture (Sweetman, 2016).

In addition, staff are expected to have an awareness to recognise and act on the inequities experienced by Māori in relation to the colonisation process. This requires recognition of one's own ethnocentric biases to understand the importance of engaging with and empowering Māori staff and service users. A critical consciousness is referred to as cultural safety (Curtis et al., 2019).

As a model for the application of a tripartite system of clinical governance that gives voice to indigenous people within a forensic mental health setting, the Mason Clinic could thus reasonably claim to be an exemplar service if not an international centre of excellence in that regard. However, the strategic goal of reducing inequitable health and social justice outcomes for Māori as an indigenous people remains an aspirational journey and not a final destination.

Indeed, despite the Mason Clinic's many positive steps forward on that journey, there have also been mis-steps although the service has yet to grapple with metrics to fully articulate the costs and benefits of those. The remainder of this chapter thus presents a 'case study' of sorts as an anecdotal account of tripartite clinical governance in action from the perspective of the author, the inaugural Lead Clinician for the Kaupapa Māori and Pasifika Service. It gives examples of what has worked well and what has not and what work is yet to be done.

Outcomes of tripartite clinical governance: the good, the bad, and the ugly

In 2006, the Mason Clinic opened Te Papakainga o Tane Whakapiripiri, a ten-bed Kaupapa Māori forensic unit based on the functions of a traditional Māori village (papakainga). It developed a model of care that provided a therapeutic milieu of programme delivery that merged clinical and cultural knowledge based on contemporary rehabilitation models as well as Durie's (1985) Whare Tapa Wha model of Māori health.

This model overtly recognised Te Ao Māori (the Māori worldview), through seven core values: wairuatanga (spiritual health), tikanga/kawa (boundaries/rules), whanaungatanga (family health), tinana (physical health), hinengaro (mental health), tūmanako (hope for the future), and whakapaitia (excellence in service delivery). The key point of difference from general rehabilitation units was a focus on wairuatanga (spiritual health) that included an emphasis on karakia (Māori prayer), kapahaka (traditional song and dance), and communal living, for example, where staff shared meals with service users (Sweetman, 2016).

However, there was no independent governance of that unit and any decisions in relation to admissions or discharges were brokered externally to the operation of the unit itself. This led to a heterogeneous configuration of service user security classifications and specific rehabilitation needs that created inefficiencies in delivering targeted programming. This resulted in lost opportunities for most Māori to be admitted to the unit due to long waiting lists and delays in discharge.

This significantly changed in 2012 when the service sought to reconfigure its operations and improve its efficiency and effectiveness. There was an extensive process of consultation with stakeholders, including cultural advisors, based on the corporate 'lean thinking' model (Womack et al., 1990) designed to improve performance and eliminate waste. As a result of that collaboration, the rehabilitation units were restructured to develop paired units with stepped medium/minimum security ratings into three rehabilitation streams, a mixed-gender general stream, a male-only general stream, and a mixed-gender Kaupapa Māori stream.

Each stream was assigned a lead clinician and subservice manager with cultural advisors embedded into the MDTs. Admissions decisions continued to be independently vetted by an admissions panel but enhanced with representation from a combination of cultural and clinical expertise. A new 15-bed medium-secure Kaupapa Māori was commissioned that had extensive cultural input in design that included art and carving with images and motifs depicting Te Ao Māori and the whare tapa wha that signalled the entry to a cultural space (McKenna and Cavney, unpublished).

However, two key events were to have profound implications for the implementation of the new Kaupapa Māori stream. The first was related to a critical failure in the structural integrity of an older unit with an urgent need to move those service users to another decanting unit. The second was related to the implementation of the DUNDRUM quartet (Kennedy et al., 2016) as a mechanism to objectively quantify service user's security classification and to better target programme delivery across seven pillars of recovery (including physical health, mental health, alcohol and drugs, problem behaviours, and social and occupational functioning).

An executive decision was thus made for the new Kaupapa Māori unit to be used as a decanting unit on its completion, thus delaying its cultural operation by several years. Similarly, implementation of the DUNDRUM quartet resulted in a drive to standardise programme delivery across the service and to redevelop clinical forms and assessment processes that effectively usurped the Whare Tapa Wha model and overlooked the significance of culturally based programming.

These decisions resulted in the demoralisation of staff committed to developing a bicultural way of working who, in numerous personal discussions with the author, characterised these decisions as a re-capitulation of the colonisation process that had divested Māori of land and eroded its cultural heritage. Although these events were arguably the nadir in the Mason Clinic's development of a culturally informed and responsive setting, they also provided some critical lessons and opportunities.

For example, the decisions of the executive were made in good faith but at a time when the service had no Kaumatua and thus occurred without any rigorous consultation, advice, or input from Māori. However, the ramifications of those decisions were later passionately aired within the Taumata and, in turn, the Clinical Governance meetings.

There was eventually a reprioritisation of the Kaupapa Māori stream taking possession of the second unit which subsequently occurred some two years ahead of the decanting schedule. It also resulted in an invigoration of service research strategies with new 'action research' methodologies to validate cultural initiatives and innovation to supplement the use of more mainstream tools such as the DUNDRUM quartet (Wharewera-Mika et al., 2020).

Concluding Remarks

For the author, the aforementioned events represented a genuine 'stress test' of the Mason Clinic's commitment to listening to the voice of Māori in the planning and delivery of forensic mental health services. It demonstrated how robust and culturally safe governance processes can provide a mechanism for transparency and accountability to achieve that strategic goal. It was as a participant observer in those processes and experiences that the author's concept of a tripartite model of clinical governance took form.

Challenges for the Mason Clinic moving forward include the development of sound metrics, key performance indicators, and auditable outcomes to evaluate whether these systems are in fact meeting the strategic goals of improving the outcomes of Māori, the indigenous people of New Zealand. However, there would seem an unlimited potential to develop new innovations in care and programme delivery by harnessing the expertise of Māori as masters of their own destiny in a genuine partnership with a mainstream forensic service.

Although the operationalisation of a culturally informed tripartite clinical governance model has at times been challenging, it has provided a transparent, dynamic, and innovative approach to service planning and delivery for Māori within the Mason Clinic. It is recommended here as a critical mechanism by which forensic mental health services in other international jurisdictions might consider engaging with their own indigenous populations to assist in developing culturally informed practice. It will hopefully enable an enhanced approach to service planning and delivery specific to their own local needs to better comply with the international conventions that compel them to do so.

References

Anderson, I., Robson, B., Connolly, M., et al. (2016). Indigenous and tribal peoples' health (The lancet – Lowitja institute global collaboration): A population study. *The Lancet*, *338*(10040), 131–157.

Australian Council on Healthcare Standards. (2004). Clinical governance defined. *ACHS News*, *12*, 1–4. www.achs.org.au/media/15289/achsnews_issue12_spring2004

Brinded, P. M., Simpson, A. I. F., Laidlaw, T. M., Fairley, N., & Malcom, F. (2001). Prevalence of psychiatric disorders in New Zealand Prisons: A national study. *Australian and New Zealand Journal of Psychiatry*, *35*, 166–173.

Came, H., Baker, M., & McCreanor, T. (2021). Addressing structural racism through constitutional transformation and decolonization: Insights for the New Zealand health sector. *Journal of Bioethical Inquiry*, *18*(1), 59–70.

Cavney, J., & Hatters Friedman, S. (2018). Culture, mental illness and prison: A New Zealand Perspective. In A. Mills & K. Kendall (Eds.), *Mental health in prisons: Critical perspectives on treatment and confinement* (pp. 211–234). Palgrave Studies in Prisons and Penology.

CERD. (2013). *Concluding observations on the eighteenth to twentieth periodic reports of New Zealand (CERD/C/NZL/CO/18–20)* (pp. 3–4). CERD.

CERD. (2017). *Concluding observations of the CERD on the New Zealand government (CERD/C/NZL/CO/21–22)*. United Nations.

Crocker, T. (1989). *Principles for crown action on the treaty of Waitangi*. Treaty of Waitangi Research Unit, Stout Research Centre for New Zealand Studies, Victoria University, Wellington.

Curtis, E., Jones, R., Tipene-Leach, D., Walker, C., Loring, B., Paine, S., & Reid, P. (2019). Why cultural safety rather than cultural competency is required to achieve health equity: A literature review and recommended definition. *International Journal for Equity in Health*, *18*, 174.

Durie, M. H. (1985). Māori perspective of health. *Social Science and Medicine*, *20*(5), 483–486.

Durie, M. H. (1999). *Imprisonment, trapped lifestyles, and strategies for freedom*. Paper presented at the Indigenous People and Justice Conference. www.firstfound.org/vol.%201/masont.htm

Gauld, R. (2014). Clinical governance development: Learning from the New Zealand experience. *Postgraduate Medical Journal*, *90*, 43–47.

Gutierrez, L., Helmus, L. M., & Hanson, R. K. (2017). *What we know and don't know about risk assessment with offenders of indigenous heritage*. Public Safety Canada. www.publicsafety.gc.ca/cnt/rsrcs/pblctns/2017-r009/index-en.aspx

He Ara Oranga. (2018). *Report of the government inquiry into mental health and addiction*. www.mentalhealth.inquiry.govt.nz/

Health Quality & Safety Commission New Zealand. (2017). *Clinical governance: Guidance for health and disability providers*. www.hqsc.govt.nz/assets/Capability-Leadership/PR/HQS-ClinicalGovernance.pdf.

Heffernan, E., Anderson, K., Dev, A., & Kinner, S. (2012). Prevalence of mental illness among aboriginal and torres strait islander people in Queensland prisons. *Medical Journal of Australia*, *197*(1), 37–41.

Indig, D., Gear, C., & Wilhelm, K. (2016). *Comorbid substance use disorders and mental health disorders among New Zealand prisoners*. Wellington, Department of Corrections.

Kennedy, H. G., O'Neill, C., Flynn, G., Gill, P., & Davoren, M. (2016). *The Dundrum toolkit. Dangerousness, understanding, recovery and urgency manual* (The DUNDRUM Quartet) V1.0.26 (01/08/13). Trinity College Dublin.

Mason, K., Bennett, H., & Ryan, E. (1988). *Report of the Committee of Inquiry into procedures used in psychiatric hospitals in relation to admission discharge or release on leave of certain classes of patient* ("The Mason Report"). Department of Health.

McKenna, B., & Cavney, J. (unpublished). Cultural service delivery in forensic mental health.

Ministry of Health. (2003). *Improving quality (IQ): A systems approach for the New Zealand health and disability sector*. Ministry of Health.

Orange, C. (1987). *The treaty of Waitangi*. Allen and Unwin New Zealand Ltd.

Pillai, K., Rouse, P., McKenna, B., Skipworth, J., Cavney, J., Tapsell, R., & Madell, D. (2016). From positive screen to engagement in treatment: A preliminary study of the impact of a new model of care for prisoners with serious mental illness. *BMC Psychiatry*, *16*(9).

Sanders, D. (1999). Indigenous peoples: Issues of definition. *International Journal of Cultural Property*, *8*, 4–13.

Scally, G., & Donaldson, L. J. (1998). Looking forward: Clinical governance and the drive for quality improvement in the new NHS in England. *British Medical Journal*, *317*, 61–65.

Shepherd, S., Delgado, R., & Paradies, Y. (2018). Inter-relationships, cultural identity, discrimination, distress, agency, and safety among indigenous people in custody. *International Journal of for Mental Health*, *17*, 111–121.

Simpson, A., McMaster, J., & Cohen, S. (2013). Challenges for Canada in meeting the needs of persons with serious mental illness in prison. *Journal of the American Academy of Psychiatry and the Law*, *41*, 501–509.

Skipworth, J. (2019). The Australian and New Zealand prison crisis: Cultural and clinical issues. *Australian and New Zealand Journal of Psychiatry*, *53*(5), 472–473.

Sweetman, L. (2016). Ngā Waiata O Tāne Whakapiripiri (the music of Tāne Whakapiripiri): Cultural expression, transformation, and healing in a Māori forensic psychiatric unit (Unpublished PhD dissertation). New York University.

United Nations. (2007, October 2). *Declaration on the rights of Indigenous peoples*. Adopted by the General Assembly. www.un.org/development/desa/indigenouspeoples/declaration-onthe-rights-of-indigenous-peoples.html.

United Nations. (2009). *State of the world's indigenous peoples, secretariat of permanent forum on Indigenous issues*. www.un.org/development/desa/indigenouspeoples/publications/state-of-the-worlds-indigenous-peoples.html

Waitangi Tribunal Report. (2017). *Tū mai te rangi – Report on the Crown and disproportionate reoffending rates: Wai 2540 Waitangi tribunal report*. https://waitangitribunal.govt.nz/publications-and-resources/waitangitribunalreports

Waitangi Tribunal Report. (2019). *Hauora – Report on stage one of the health services and outcomes Kaupapa inquiry: Wai 2575 Waitangi tribunal report*. https://waitangitribunal.govt.nz/publications-and-resources/waitangitribunalreports

Wharewera-Mika, J., Cooper, E., Wiki, N., Prentice, K., Field, T., Cavney, J., Kaire, D., & McKenna, B. (2020). The appropriateness of DUNDRUM-3 and DUNDRUM-4 for Māori in forensic mental health services in New Zealand: Participatory action research. *BMC Psych*. 20, 61, 1–9.

Womack, J. P., Jones, D. T., & Roos, D. (1990). *The machine that changed the world*. Rawson Associates.

Chapter 13

The Elders Project

Bringing Black African-Caribbean collectivism in from the outside

Beresford Dawkins, Dawn M. Sutherland, Kimberly Sham Ku, Patrick Bennett, and Abdullah Mia

Introduction

This chapter discusses the challenges of establishing a project that aims to connect male forensic inpatients with African-Caribbean members of the community. Specifically, it describes the security, organisational, and ethical conundrums and issues that arose from the conception of the project in 2017, through the recruitment of community Elders and patients, the provision of training, until the first meetings between community Elders and patients. It begins by offering some context to the African-Caribbean experience in the United Kingdom including experiences of exclusion and racism. It then describes in detail the steps undertaken to recruit and arrange training for community members, patients, and staff involved in the Elders Project. Finally, we ask where we go from here and share lessons learnt.

Background and context

The African-Caribbean community has been present in the United Kingdom since the mid-18th century. A significant number of the community migrated in the 1950s and 60s as part of the United Kingdom's attempt to address the severe labour shortages following World War II. These migrants were known colloquially as the 'Windrush generation'. The challenges of settling into UK life are documented well (see Olusoga (2016) and Fryer (2018)), and within the community itself, stories were shared as a way of providing validation and support. Thus, the community has been solving and resolving issues within for decades; these issues rarely come to the attention of statutory services.

Due to the threat of racial violence and to ensure the community spirit and ethos continued to be valued, the African-Caribbean community had to be self-reliant in many ways. There was a strong sense of community where it was felt everyone knew everyone else; it was known that people would look out for you. As the community developed a lot of thought was given to where people lived, the bus routes to take, and the sharing of knowledge of what was safe and what was not, this largely remains the case today. There were well-known go-to spaces, family, clergy, or community members who provided solutions and resolve. The community provided security, through discussion with elders who had experienced life in the United Kingdom. Of experiences outside the safety of the community, stories were spoken, shared, and heard about the racism and violence from White communities, which spoke to the experience of the African-Caribbean community. The trauma of racism was held within bodies and minds and within stories that are told from generation to generation, in order to ensure the continued safety of Black bodies and minds.

DOI: 10.4324/9781003184768-17

Whilst sharing stories of racial trauma, the African-Caribbean community also built strength in their connectivity, wholeness, and citizenship, this generally centred within the Christian faith community. Having experienced animosity and being asked to leave Anglican churches due to the perceived impact on the congregation, many African-Caribbean community members set up their own churches, to provide a space for their religious practice and a focus for the burgeoning community. Community and family were, and continue to be, important in that they became a source of protection from racist attacks and poor access to state-funded services. The strength of this *collectivism* (see Laugani (2007) for further information) was seen as families ate together, said grace, looked after children in the streets with play and community discipline, and also shared a religion, meetings, and connectedness.

The elders of the community were deferred to with regard to decision-making for the benefit of individuals and the community. The community may meet, often in church, to make decisions in order that ensure you were looked after and cared for and compassion was provided where statutory services were not providing this. Should someone become mentally unwell, because of the overt anti-Black narrative within healthcare, the responsibility to support and look after the individual would be taken by the community through prayer and scripture amongst other means. Self-reliance on the community was learned by the community, and central to this was the role of the elder.

Racism is constant and racial weathering erodes and breaks the spirit, drive, motivation, and identity of many in the African-Caribbean community. The role of the elders in the community provides a space of strength, resolve, and reminder of who we are. As Beresford Dawkins (Elders Project Lead) notes:

> Spending time with family, nothing has to be said, we have food and drink and there is this thing that happens, where we all know and feel there is safety and care for you. These words are not spoken, it's in the behaviours, the simple hand holding, arm around, the value of your life as a Black man. It helps me connect as an individual, as a being and where my Caribbean heritage fits, being rooted, grounded in safety and growth.

As the community developed, and people got older, the community recognised what the elders have tolerated and lived through. There has also been an intergenerational disconnect, young people's racial trauma is now seen through the eyes and experience of first and second generations; how this was managed, and with the knowledge that it is not to be tolerated. The modern experience of racism and the impact of 'everyday' microaggressions have been at the forefront of people's minds with a resurgent interest in race relations, following the murder of George Floyd in America. The disproportionate impact on Black and minority ethnic communities of COVID-19 has also led to an exploration of the impact of structural racism (see Majors, 2020). Of note here, is the distinction between structural (or systemic), institutional, and interpersonal racism (see Nazroo et al., 2019 for definitions). Whilst overt interpersonal racism is not routinely encountered or observed within UK healthcare, there are numerous reports outlining the impact of institutional racism within mental healthcare (see Fernando, 2017; Runnymede, 2021 for further exploration).

It is known that people of colour are more likely to be detained under the English Mental Health Act 1983 (MHA), more likely to die in custody, and more likely to be diagnosed and admitted to a mental health facility for treatment (Bhui et al., 2018). Therefore, one element of the institutional practices that need to be considered is the appropriateness and applicability of psychological and psychiatric practices to diverse communities. When considering the applicability of mental health practices across cultures, this includes the epistemological position held, as science is not conducted in a cultural and political vacuum (Kuhn, 1970). The Elders Project aims to address conflicts that the African-Caribbean community may experience in receiving ethnomonocultural interventions by incorporating the breadth of cultural, social, and political experiences.

The Elders Project

The project uses the following definitions for the following terms:

- 'The Elders Project': a psychosocial intervention supporting the transition of African-Caribbean men from admission to an inpatient secure unit to discharge into the community, with the support of community Elders. Elders provide support through a range of methods, including individual support, group social events, and through community integration and involvement efforts.
- 'Elders': Community volunteers from the African-Caribbean community who have strong community ties and family relationships within the local area of Birmingham, United Kingdom. They bring these life experiences into the forensic setting.
- 'Facilitators': Staff members who are part of the core group leading the Elders Project. They provide support to the Elders and patients.
- 'Patients': This term is used here for clarity and to avoid confusion. In the actual delivery of the project, patients were referred to as 'the men' involved to emphasise their identities beyond being inpatients.

Developing the Elders Project

The Elders project began from a hope for change within the NHS, utilising the African-Caribbean communities' strong faith connections to stimulate progressive and liberative social change (Shannahan, 2013). The project recognised the need for community engagement within forensic services and the need to appreciate grass-root approaches within institutional care. Project Lead Beresford's desire to understand and make sense of the world alongside the community and statutory, charity sector, and faith organisations initiated this work. This desire was shared by the other facilitators, identifying the conflicts of working within structures and organisations whose practices can be oppressive and discriminatory towards the Black community.

The transformation sought was for volunteers, workers, institutions (NHS and Church), and the community at large. The Elders Project developed on the UK Government's guidance that 'local areas should consider how community-centred approaches that build on individual and community assets can become an essential part of local mental health plans and strategies' (Public Health England, 2018). In developing the Elders work, facilitators connected their shared experiences across several domains: occupational, social, religious, educational, and personal. The personal connection to this work was important to all facilitators, as it ensured motivation was maintained from its inception in 2017 to the start of delivery post-pandemic in 2021.

The Elders Project was given financial support via the NHS Trust's[1] internal funding process, as it hoped to improve discharge processes. There was a mixture of excitement and trepidation; we recognised 'it was not something that the service at the Tamarind Centre, or even across Secure Care were used to' (Facilitator), and with this came anxiety from individuals and the organisation as to what it meant to invite the community in, bringing with them psychospiritual ways to enhance mental health and well-being.

It may be interpreted that following the initial interest, the challenges in delivery were also impacted by how the organisation broadly and locally managed the anxiety of difference in the delivery of mental health care; Menzies-Lyth ([1959] 1988) and Hinshelwood and

Skogstad (2000) give further exploration of how organisational anxiety is managed within healthcare systems via a process of 'anxiety-*culture*-defence'. The Elders Project may have activated organisational defences at an unconscious level with regard to the conflict between knowing the organisation is there to care, but also part of a system that has been indicated as perpetuating practices that disadvantage ethnic minorities. At a conscious level, the organisation and its employees may also be balancing depleted energy levels, increased workloads, and the fear that their personal practices may be experienced and shown to be discriminating against ethnic minorities. The fear of this can lead to a number of social defences being enacted and/or embodied, disrupting the work and task.

Delivering the Elders project

Recruitment

The project facilitators recruited Elders through networks already known to the NHS Trust and to the community engagement team. Adverts were distributed through community meetings, presentations at churches, community events, and community halls. A key part of recruitment was Beresford utilising his relationships with the community and also his knowledge of Biblical texts to put a 'call to action' to support those with mental health difficulties.

Ninety-six people from the community responded to the recruitment drive, they were invited to the medium-secure service (MSU), which was the first step in breaking down some of the metaphorical 'walls' and inviting the community in. This was a meaningful experience for the NHS Trust and MSU; it indicated the level of interest within the community to contribute to care and to learn about mental health services. This event had to hold in mind the logistics of safely and securely supporting people to move across the site, whilst ensuring minimal disruption to the delivery of care for service users.

Following the event, 22 people volunteered for the project, from a range of backgrounds including faith, music, and sports communities. These skills were sought as it would be something that interested the service users. Thirteen people were interviewed and accepted onto the project following the successful completion of standard NHS employment checks. This process involved emails and phone calls, which breaks from normal human resources (HR) practice, whilst there was initial HR communication, HR support throughout was minimal as the HR department conveyed there were 'other priorities' that needed to be met; therefore, meetings between HR and facilitators were cancelled. This was mirrored in panel interviews having to be cancelled due to appropriate documentation not being sent to applicants by HR. During facilitator meetings, this was reflected upon as to what impact this interaction had on community members. Specifically, this may reinforce negative experiences of the NHS, building upon experiences shared socially and historically.

Patients were recruited utilising a similar process. An information event shared details about the project, purpose, and hopes. In order to bring the community ethos to the MSU, there were performances by Black community members combined with food. Recruitment was also enhanced by discussing with mental health teams as to who was likely to engage and benefit from the project. Thirty patients attended the event, with 15 patients identifying as being of African-Caribbean heritage agreeing to take part.

Training of the Elders prior to meeting patients

Content of training

We implemented a training programme to address the unfamiliarity of the MSU and create connections between project facilitators and the Elders. Training balanced sharing an awareness of the risk posed by service users, along with a strong focus on compassion. This was chosen following conversations with the Elders on the seriousness of the risks associated with some of the men.

The training covered the following topics:

- Background to the project and an introduction to secure services
- Introduction to, and expectations of, the role
- Integrating clinical, risk, and operational procedures, including administrative aspects of the visits such as incident reporting, de-briefing, supervision, and reflective practice
- The importance of boundaries (role and therapeutic)
- Mental health awareness, including diagnoses, MHA sections, and restrictions.

It was hoped the Elders would feel more confident and comfortable to work with us and extend this experience to community members, encouraging them to also work within secure services. By honestly sharing the experiences, the Facilitators aimed to ensure that barriers and misunderstandings of the MSU, use of medication, and delivery of therapy would be demystified.

A central element of the training was that this was not delivered in a traditional model of didactic teaching but incorporated the values of collectivist cultures. Acknowledging the respect afforded to Elders within the community, it was important to emphasise a dialogic process of learning.

Context

Facilitators spoke about their anxiety, and that of the service, in training a group of people who had no experience in mental health service delivery, particularly within forensic environments. Whilst the Elders were aware that patients may be dangerous, the context and reach of danger were not fully understood. In devising and delivering the training, Facilitators also had to consider what basic skills were important for the Elders and what was important to address some of the staff and service needs and anxieties.

The training allowed time for a relationship to be developed between Elders and Facilitators, sharing knowledge, learning, and involving them as peers in the process. The training also helped increased awareness of process and procedure whilst also involving the meaning of recovery and how the community could contribute. Importantly, it addressed the risk of blurring boundaries and how this could result in adverse experiences.

Joining with the community

The training was an inclusive experience, for example, Facilitators asked Elders about their faith but not from an evangelical position. Opening these conversations is unusual for mental health services within the United Kingdom, incorporating faith and spiritual beliefs in an informal way alongside food and drink. The purpose of this was to bring in the community values of the Elders and Facilitators, ensuring training was informal and professional, valuing the Elders' needs, and balancing this with the organisational needs.

Facilitators were considerate of age in terms of respect and value within the community. As some Facilitators belonged to the same or similar communities as the Elders, their understanding of the cultural context from which the Elders came was important and came through in the delivery of the training. Through reflective conversations, Facilitators became mindful of using a different language to describe their everyday clinical experiences. The connections and relationship building with the community went beyond using cultural terms and literal translations. Whilst these were helpful, it was the quality of the relationships that ensured connections were meaningful rather than just a shared vocabulary. Facilitators behaved less as clinicians, and instead as 'themselves', this was unusual in comparison to the usual 'clinical' approach to working with the service users and families. The project is built on the relationships the facilitators have with the community and Elders, and this involves knowing the Elders personally and sharing parts of themselves as Facilitators.

> I was able to be myself, still professional, but be natural. With other professionals there, I have to think about what I say, here we can be ourselves, and this was transmitted to the Elders.
>
> – Facilitator

> Being myself made sense to me, I used my own knowledge, experience and background. It involved drawing on my experiences of where Elders may be coming from, and talking about cultural understanding of mental health.
>
> – Facilitator

> I can talk in a way that brings my whole self, in a way that shows I am connected to them [Elders] which I can trust in, and they can trust me.
>
> – Facilitator

There was an awareness of how 'trust' is established, the warmth involved in being authentic, and relating a sense of belonging and togetherness. This involved explicitly discussing the history of bad experiences shared as community members, yet also challenging Facilitators to integrate community views into the delivery of mental health services. The training encouraged curiosity, about the patients within the MSU, and about the types of offences people committed. Whilst the training was intended for the Elders, it provided an opportunity for humility to be shown and for learning for Facilitators. In particular, the recognition that being invited was not the same as being welcomed, with the Elders and African-Caribbean community experiences of health services in the United Kingdom often being that there was an invitation, but not a welcoming.

> The training wasn't straight faced and boring, it was about value and the Elders' worth, details were remembered, for example, they remembered what music we liked, it let us know that they valued and respected us.
>
> – Elder

Maintaining the relationship was equally as important as developing the relationship; therefore, the Facilitators scheduled in regular 'catch-up' meetings with the Elders, ensuring that the relationship deepened. Through these meetings, often virtually due to the COVID-19 pandemic, conversations developed and helped shape the content of the training and delivery of the project.

Setting up the training

It was important that the project and training were flexible right from the start. The training day was chosen to be a Saturday, which fell outside of the normal working hours for the Facilitators. Facilitators recognised the importance of making adjustments to routine practices, acknowledging that Elders being invited in also came with their own lives, and volunteers were also to be respected and valued.

The Facilitators recognised that being flexible with boundaries to deliver the training, it would also show the value and importance placed on the project itself. Facilitators were aware that projects like this had historically been driven by top-down agendas to meet targets, asking a lot of the community with little return. Therefore, there was an explicit desire to redress this balance in practice.

As discussed previously, food is important as a focal point within African-Caribbean communities, and providing food during the training events contributed to the difference between the experience of being invited and being welcomed. Operationally, this was challenging as the catering department worked on a skeletal rota during the weekend; therefore, changes to additional departments needed to be considered.

Whilst simultaneously developing and building relationships with the community, the Facilitators invested time in supporting the security team and senior staff within the MSU to manage anxieties as this would bring about sustained change to established practices. This included developing local policies and practice papers to be passed through governance meetings ensuring anxiety was managed by documents and relational risk management was known.

In order to maintain security standards and manage the dynamics of training, Elders were split into two groups, with each group attending a full day of training. The first day of training was completed face to face, and due to COVID-19, the second day of training was delivered virtually.

Connecting the Elders with patients

In order to match the Elders with the Patients who volunteered, both parties were asked to complete information sheets including their interests, skills and abilities, strengths, and why they were interested in the project.

Knowing both groups of people, Facilitators met and matched Elders with Patients according to the information they shared and their past experiences. Once the matching process was completed, an event was arranged where both groups met, engaged with some icebreakers, shared food, and had a space to get to know each other through conversation.

Following the meeting event, each pair arranged to meet on a weekly basis for one hour. The visits would remain on weekdays to ensure staffing was sufficient; each of these visits would also be recorded on the Patients' clinical notes and an 'Elders' passport by Facilitators. To ensure the security of the building and safety is maintained, Elder's visits were facilitated via the standard visitation policy.

The visitation process was hampered by COVID-19, and subsequent public health measures within England to ensure infection control measures were maintained. Therefore, at the time of writing, the evaluation of the project was minimal due to visits only occurring for five weeks.

Reflections on organisational dynamics

Discussions on inclusivity and exclusivity were often a mainstay of the work, with Facilitators and allies often having to be mindful they were not perpetuating dynamics commonly associated with interventions focusing on diversity and difference. These discussions often can undermine the effectiveness of interventions. The project was hindered by discussions on which diverse characteristics should be included and why all diverse characteristics were not included. This is a recognised experience; in having these discussions, organisations can be stifled from making change as they engage in 'diversity Olympics', leading to inertia. Wilfred

Bion's (1961) work on the 'work group' is important here; this has been extended further by McRae and Short (2010) specifically focusing on racial and cultural dynamics in organisations.

During the process of recruitment, Facilitators were aware of the importance of focusing on the African–Caribbean community; however, they also recruited an Elder of South Asian (Pakistani) heritage. In Facilitator meetings, there was discussion on the importance of balancing inclusivity, with the specificity of the project, i.e., the African–Caribbean community. A possible understanding of this is the enactment of unprocessed anxiety that is projected into the work. During initial discussions, there had been concern by senior clinicians regarding the exclusivity of the project; there was a desire by the senior leadership team to ensure that everyone was 'treated the same and equally'. Extending the work of Wilfred Bion in groups and teams, Earl Hopper (2012) suggests traumatised organisations can aggregate or massify, leading to a rejection of difference (in this case racial difference). The fear that clinical practice may be structurally and institutionally racist, therefore bringing in the unacceptable and the subsequent fear of annihilation, the defensive response is to ensure everything is 'the same' (massify), therefore rejecting any difference. By including a South Asian Elder, it may also have addressed the anxiety of senior leaders that the project was being 'discriminatory' which also misunderstands the purpose and application of the UK Equality Act 2010.

This is emotional work, which can often be at odds with clinicians within a forensic environment who can separate themselves emotionally from the pain and distress of patients' lives and the pain patients have inflicted. Faced with uncovering structural inequalities along with reflection on one's role in maintaining such inequalities requires a compassionate approach. Often Facilitators found themselves containing the anxiety of the system and individuals; this is taxing work. When anxiety could not be contained, it resulted in various unconscious enactments, e.g., timely documentation not being sent out, poor communication between departments, and a lack of visible support for the project beyond the Facilitators. These enactments hinder progress towards change, ultimately responsibility being located in Facilitators alone as opposed to considering the organisational culture.

This project has also been affected by the social narrative within the world during 2020 and beyond. Ethnic inequalities have been in the spotlight due to the disproportional impact of COVID-19 on ethnic minorities in the United Kingdom and the scrutiny of statutory services as a consequence of high-profile deaths of Black men within the United Kingdom. Despite the project being proposed in 2017, it has been the recent shift in focus supported by the Chief Executive of the NHS Trust, that overt support and championing of the project has been felt by the Facilitators. There has also been a growing need for accountability as to what healthcare services are doing to meet the needs of ethnic minorities. The facilitators of the Elders Project welcome this, yet acknowledge the discomfort in being explicitly supported when the project is becoming valuable socio-politically, and not on the merits of the work to reduce inequalities related to ethnicity itself. To continue applying the project to a range of communities, the Facilitators hold hope that the interest generated goes further than accolades to a culture shift within the United Kingdom, incorporating cultural knowledge and strengths into mental health care.

Where do we go from here?

The process has been an important learning curve for the community and those involved. There are some key learning points for others who wish to take a similar approach forward.

Understand the communities we work with – Know that there are ethnic inequalities, be curious about why this is, and work towards partnerships with other departments, agencies, and the community. Forensic environments can be quite insular and support is needed from the outside.

Explore and critically appraise our work – Acknowledge the cultural and epistemological roots of the treatment, models, and interventions we deliver, and whether these fit with the multi-cultural communities that we live in.

Representation and connections matter – The Elders Project is built on representation and connection. The community values seeing people from its own community in professional roles and also values the bringing of self to these roles. It is hard work reflecting on what is natural to many members of ethnic minority communities; time is needed to connect with these experiences explicitly and to feel brave enough to share them.

Dialogue is crucial, ensure space for this is safeguarded – The Elders Project is shaped through conversations and based on relational trust. It can be difficult holding conversations that challenge one's professional and personal sense of self. There will be disagreements and discomfort; however, these are also spaces for growth and change.

The process can feel chaotic – Forensic services are familiar with being in control and the staff within them gain comfort from this. However, bringing the community in is a multi-layered and iterative process. Sometimes services may not know what will emerge through sharing ideas; senior clinicians should model 'not knowing' being compatible with collaborative learning.

Separating out interpersonal from institutional – The Elders Project addresses racial inequalities at an institutional level, which means moving beyond discussions of racism at an interpersonal level and thinking about institutional and structural practices that disadvantage African-Caribbean men and beyond.

Be open to innovation and creativity – Working with the community at a grassroots level means the goals may change midway through a project. The relational element is built through developing relationships in ways that work for the community, drawing on their ways of living, and what 'trust' looks like for the community, particularly when working with the impact of ethnic inequalities and socio-political histories of structural racism.

Be aware of generational and vicarious trauma – Undertaking a project to reduce ethnic inequalities can raise awareness in Facilitators and community members of traumatic experiences. These need to be considered and cared for. This experience is exacerbated and experienced as exploitative when support is explicitly provided only if the project gains broader positive feedback from quality assurance and good practice assessors.

Facilitators need space – The emotional work involved in a project such as that described in this chapter can connect with many experiences of oppression and racial trauma for the community and professionals. It is important that the project team also has a space to connect and work through challenges, separating what belongs where, and which emotions are projections that are being reacted to.

Support is key – For senior leadership staff, it is important to have curiosity, visibility, and presence within the project from start to finish. This can look like promoting the project, holding it in mind during meetings, and indicating that they are aware of the literature affecting Black men and women within mental health and forensic services. Crucially, staff should not wait for a member of the Black community to raise these issues.

Note

1. A Trust is an NHS healthcare organisation whose provision is defined either geographically or by specialisation.

References

Bhui, K., Halvorsrud, K., & Nazroo, J. (2018). Making a difference: Ethnic inequality and severe mental illness. *The British Journal of Psychiatry*, 574–578.

Bion, W. R. (1961). *Experience in groups*. New York: Brunner-Routledge.

Fernando, S. (2017). *Institutional racism in psychiatry and clinical psychology: Race matters in mental health*. Palgrave Macmillan.

Fryer, P. (2018). *Staying power: The history of black people in Britain*. Pluto Press.

Hinshelwood, R. D., & Skogstad, W. (2000). The dynamics of health care institutions. In R. D. Hinshelwood & W. Skogstad (Eds.), *Observing organisations: Anxiety, defence and culture in health care* (pp. 3–17). Routledge.

Hopper, E. (2012). Introduction: The theory of Incohesion: Aggregation/Massification as the fourth basic assumption in the unconscious life of groups and group-like social systems. In E. Hopper (Ed.), *Trauma and organizations* (pp. 1–xxxi). Routledge.

Kuhn, T. S. (1970). *The structure of scientific revolutions* (2nd ed.). University of Chicago Press Ltd.

Laugani, P. D. (2007). *Understanding cross-cultural psychology*. Sage.

Majors, R. (2020). Black mental health and the new millennium: Historical and current perspective on cultural trauma and 'everyday' racism in white mental health spaces – the impact on the psychological well-being of black mental health professionals. In R. Majors, K. Carberry, & T. S. Ransaw (Eds.), *The international handbook of black community mental health* (pp. 1–27). Emerald Publishing.

McRae, M. B., & Short, E. L. (2010). *Racial and cultural dynamics in group and organizational life: Crossing boundaries*. Sage.

Menzies-Lyth, I. ([1959] 1988). *Containing anxiety in institutions. Selected essays volume 1*. Free Association Books.

Nazroo, J. Y., Bhui, K. S., & Rhodes, J. (2019). Where next for understanding race/ethnic inequalities in severe mental illness? Structural, interpersonal and institutional racism. *Sociology of Health & Illness*, 262–276.

Olusoga, D. (2016). *Black and British: A forgotten history*. Picador.

Public Health England. (2018). *Health matters: Reducing health inequalities in mental illness*. UK Government.

Runnymede. (2021). *England civil society submission to the united nations committee on the elimination of racial discrimination*. Runnymede Trust.

Shannahan, C. (2013). *A theology of community organizing: Power to the people*. Routledge.

Chapter 14

Working in multicultural forensic settings

An integrated model of assessment

Stephane M. Shepherd and Mary O. Madu

Introduction

Forensic assessments are regularly carried out by clinical professionals at various stages of the criminal justice and forensic mental health systems. The forensic assessment process often employs a combination of tasks to gain an understanding of a client's prior and future behaviour. This process informs a diagnosis and management/intervention plan designed to provide positive outcomes for clients whose behaviour has led, or could lead, to serious offending (Ogloff et al., 2007). Forensic assessments can be requested for a variety of reasons including the determination of mental competency, violence risk, mental state, level of supervision required, and treatment needs (Kraus et al., 2011; Rogers et al., 2004).

In recent years, an increasing body of literature has underscored the need for clinical methods and approaches to be equally applicable to clients from different cultural backgrounds (Day et al., 2018; Hart, 2016; Shepherd & Lewis-Fernandez, 2016; Tamatea, 2016; Wilson & Gutierrez, 2014). Concerns have been raised that widely employed forensic assessment approaches are framed from western perspectives and patterns of behaviour, which may not reflect the norms, experiences, and worldviews of more diverse populations (Hart, 2016; Shepherd & Lewis-Fernandez, 2016).

This has led to broader discussions on the unique needs of consumers from minority and culturally and linguistically diverse (CALD) backgrounds, and how clinicians can work more effectively with individuals from these populations. In the Australian context, CALD often refers to migrant groups from non-English-speaking backgrounds. Australia has received CALD arrivals through humanitarian intake programmes over the past 15 years, including refugees from Sudan, Afghanistan, Iraq, Iran, Syria, and Myanmar (ABS, 2018). CALD communities are heterogeneous; they comprise people with diverse cultural norms, practices and traditions, languages, religions, family structures, pre- and post-migration challenges, and life experiences. This chapter will outline the literature on the varying cultural needs, presentations, and risk factors of CALD populations in the Australian context, the extent to which clinicians may need to consider these phenomena, and recommendations for culturally responsive forensic practice.

In Australia, almost half the population either are born overseas or have a parent born overseas (Australian Bureau of Statistics, 2016). Similar levels of diversity have been documented in other Western countries (i.e., United States, Canada, New Zealand, and England). This growing diversity is reflected in prison populations. For example, in Australia, more than 20% of the prison population were born overseas, with those from Sudanese, Pacific Islander, Vietnamese, and Lebanese backgrounds over-represented in custody (Australian Bureau of Statistics, 2017). Offending pathways for CALD populations are similar to those

DOI: 10.4324/9781003184768-18

of Anglo-Australian populations. Yet CALD groups also face a range of unique challenges including discrimination, family fragmentation, and social and economic marginalisation, which may lead to increased levels of social disconnection, frustration, and, in some cases, anti-social feelings and attitudes (Shepherd, 2016; Shepherd & Masuka, 2020). The combination of pre- and post-migration factors can also provide fertile grounds for established risk factors associated with offending to emerge.

Pathways to offending

There are a number of universal risk factors that have been shown to be associated with offending (Douglas et al., 1999; Loeber & Farrington, 2000; Andrews & Bonta, 2010). These include but are not limited to delinquent peers, social dysfunction, family breakdown, substance use, low educational achievement, unemployment, and anti-social attitudes. These factors are often embedded in correctional assessment and management frameworks such as the Risk-Need-Responsivity model (Andrews & Bonta, 2010). Common risk factors for offending likely extend to CALD populations. However, there may be additional challenges facing some CALD (sub)populations, which require articulation to better understand the broader contexts surrounding their involvement in the justice system.

The prevalence of mental health concerns appears to be similar across Anglo-Australian and CALD offenders (Rose et al., 2019, 2020). There is a paucity of research on the mental health of individuals from CALD backgrounds living in Australia (Minas et al., 2013); however, extant findings indicate generally similar levels of lifetime mental disorder between CALD and non-CALD individuals in Australia (Australian Institute of Health and Welfare [AIHW], 2011; Jatrana et al., 2017; Straiton et al., 2014). International research has identified ethnic disparities across rates of mental disorders. African Americans, Latino/Hispanic Americans, and Black, Asian, and Minority Ethnic populations have all been found to be diagnosed with psychotic disorders at higher rates than White Americans/Europeans (Cohen & Marino, 2013; Halvorsrud et al., 2019; Schwartz & Blankenship, 2014). Some evidence suggests findings in the opposite direction for personality disorders (McGilloway et al., 2010). Disparities in psychotic disorder diagnoses have been attributed to both social/environmental explanations and clinical misdiagnosis (Halvorsrud et al., 2019; Schwartz & Blankenship, 2014). The core characteristics of psychopathy appear to generalise cross-culturally (Latzman et al., 2015; Sullivan et al., 2006), and levels of psychopathy have been found to be similar for Black and White Americans (Skeem et al., 2004).

Mental disorder prevalence may be particularly high among particular CALD sub-groups. For example, humanitarian arrivals in Western countries are up to ten times more likely to have post-traumatic stress disorder (PTSD) than general populations (Fazel et al., 2005). Exposure to a range of traumatic circumstances (civil unrest, violence, and torture) is significantly associated with higher rates of PTSD (Breslau et al., 1999; Llamas, 2006; Shepherd, 2016). These experiences may be compounded by post-migration stressors including family fragmentation, language barriers, concerns over family members living overseas, social isolation, acculturative strain, family destabilisation, uncertainty about legal and asylum status, unstable housing and employment, and ostracism/discrimination (Queensland Government, 2010; Shepherd, 2016). The combination of resettlement pressures and any untreated mental health issues can lead to negative psychological health outcomes and susceptibility to negative behavioural outcomes (Shepherd, 2016).

The aforementioned challenges may be greater for those whose culture of origin differs widely from the host culture and in particular if sections of the host community are actively hostile towards the newly arrived population. Acculturation refers to cultural changes occurring when diverse groups of people encounter one another (Schwartz et al., 2010).

Acculturative stress may be heightened for groups who feel pressured to adapt quickly to the dominant culture, in particular for those wanting to hold onto their pre-existing cultural beliefs and practices (Berry, 1997). Typically, younger migrants integrate more rapidly than their older relatives and caregivers. This can result in familial tension and compromise inter-generational relationships as parents continue to hold onto traditional values with the expectation that their children will do the same. The balance between preserving their parents' culture and adopting mainstream values can cause younger people to feel as if they are caught between two cultures, resulting in decreased cohesion within families and increased levels of psychological distress. Moreover, caregivers who are often coping with family fragmentation, trauma, low English language proficiency and their own integration challenges are sometimes unable to provide the support and monitoring for younger relatives. For younger migrants, it may also prompt a loss of confidence in their parents' ability to manage the household and navigate the new social terrain.

Mental health

CALD populations may conceptualise mental health differently from mainstream medical frameworks. Cultural attributions for mental health concerns can impact symptom presentation and the course of treatment (Kirmayer, 1989; Kiropoulos et al., 2005; Gopalkrishnan, 2018). Western clinical practice has often focused on assessing, diagnosing, and treating individuals without a deep consideration of their wider socio-cultural and historical context (Deacon, 2013; Gopalkrishnan, 2018). For some CALD populations, the individual is inseparable from the community context, and as such, health is a wide-ranging phenomenon that includes socio-cultural connectedness, overall community well-being, and interconnected spiritual elements.

Evidence indicates that CALD populations underutilise mental health services (Davern et al., 2016; Francis & Cornfoot, 2007). This may be due to a lack of access to care, low mental health literacy, language barriers, a lack of culturally competent service provision, or the stigmatisation of mental health (Shepherd, 2016). In some CALD communities, mental health is often equated with being 'crazy' or demonstrating 'weakness' which can bring shame to the individual and their family (Colucci et al., 2014; Khawaja et al., 2014; Saunders et al., 2015). In some situations, mental illness is believed to have religious or supernatural causes (Colucci et al., 2014; Deng, 2016). These explanations and subsequent stigmas can impact help-seeking behaviours, in particular help sought from formal mental health services. Some CALD individuals may be resistant or show hostility in clinical settings because of previous injustices experienced in their countries of origin. Exposure to racism can also have a negative impact on the mental health of CALD groups (Ferdinand et al., 2013) which may impact their willingness to engage in clinical scenarios. Individuals from African and Muslim backgrounds report high rates of discrimination in Australia (Markus, 2016, 2018). This can contribute to feelings of social rejection, frustration and fear, and community disengagement. A breakdown in trust can take place in clinical settings if service professionals fail to consider the impact perceived discrimination may have on their client's well-being and behaviour.

Sub-groups within CALD communities may also possess attitudes and beliefs, which may prevent help-seeking and subsequent intervention. For example, reports on family violence in some CALD communities have pointed to trends of non-disclosure (Allimant & Ostapiej-Piatkowski, 2011; Chung et al., 2018; Queensland Government, 2010; Taylor & Putt, 2007) and, in some cases, indifference and or implicit endorsement (Taylor & Mouzos, 2006; Brewer, 2009; El-Murr, 2018). Family violence, or attitudes that validate family violence (in particular, multi-perpetrator family violence), may be culturally endorsed in some circumstances, justifying its continuation and precluding community intervention (Shepherd, 2016). Victim survivors may be threatened with community banishment and social ostracism if intending to report abuse to authorities (InTouch Multicultural Centre Against Family Violence, 2014). Additionally, some women and girls from CALD backgrounds have reportedly experienced forced marriage and dowry abuse (Royal Commission into Family Violence, 2016).

Cultural factors may also impact the presentation of symptoms (Alarcon, 2009; Lewis-Fernandez & Kirmayer, 2019). Across non-western cultures, mental and physical health are often closely intertwined (Lewis-Fernandez & Kirmayer, 2019). For instance, some may present with or refer to physical symptoms rather psychological symptoms (Chan & Parker, 2004; Chong et al., 2010; Lewis-Fernandez & Kirmayer, 2019). Particular groups may also exhibit culturally normative behaviours (i.e., religious fervour and bereavement-specific self-harm) that may mimic (or are difficult to discern from) mental health symptoms (Kirmyaer et al., 2011; Lewis-Fernandez et al., 2014). For example, religious/spiritual behaviours (speaking with the deceased or supernatural entities, assiduously adhering to regular rituals) may be mistaken for psychotic disorders or perhaps in the latter case, obsessive-compulsive disorder. There may also be cultural variance in emotional expression (Lim, 2016). Emotional suppression/stoicism may be emphasised or culturally expected within some populations.

While not all CALD individuals experience or subscribe to the aforementioned phenomena, the potential for justice involvement can escalate if these post-migratory challenges and cultural conceptualisations of mental health remain unaddressed or unconsidered. The extent to which clinicians need to identify and react to these issues will vary depending on the level of acculturation, preferred identity, and social context of the client. Several approaches for working carefully with CALD clients in criminal justice and forensic settings are outlined in the following.

Recommendations for practice

Multi-cultural communities possess varying degrees of acculturation and identity. As such, ethnocultural considerations may be of importance to some individuals; however, they may bear little significance, or relevance, to others. It is recommended to avoid having preconceived notions of an individual based on their supposed cultural background. It is perhaps more useful, and enlightening, to ascertain a client's 'personal' culture which may comprise several intersecting components ranging from peer group culture, professional culture, neighbourhood culture, school/employment culture, personal interest/hobby culture, political/religious culture, gender identity, and sexual orientation culture. All of these elements may interact with their ethnocultural background. In some cases, these intersecting factors may be more associated with behaviour than their ethno-culture, which may only be superficially held. There are also other personally idiosyncratic clinical concerns that impact an individual's behaviour including an individual's personality, temperament, cognitive ability, psychological state, and relationship stressors to name a few. This does not mean that exploring one's cultural background is unhelpful or misleading (it can be instructive); however, some caution is urged, given the varying levels of ethnocultural interest (and investment) and its relevance to offending behaviours. Nonetheless, some information (and steps to obtain that information) can be taken to ensure that useful cultural material is identified and incorporated into an assessment.

It is necessary to ascertain how long the client has been living in the country and any migration stressors they may have endured. Pre-migration trauma combined with post-settlement social challenges may have compromised the client's personal development, social interaction, help-seeking behaviours, and ability to engage in pro-social activities. Family acculturation challenges and language barriers may have precluded access to services to address their complex social and mental health needs. Family fragmentation may have diminished the support structures ordinarily expected for clients, which may leave some susceptible and exposed to negative experiences and influences. These concerns may be exacerbated for female clients. CALD women (in particular recent migrants and refugees) are more likely to be unemployed (due to lower levels of educational obtainment and child-rearing duties) and possess diminished support networks and a lack of knowledge regarding their legal rights (Commonwealth of Australia, 2015; InTouch Multicultural Centre Against Family Violence, 2010; Judicial Council on Cultural Diversity, 2016). For some, the absence of local family members and friends who can provide direct support, uncertainty around their immigration status (or fear of deportation), and a lack of financial autonomy means that they may be less likely to report violence (or leave an abusive relationship) due to fears of being isolated from their family or community (InTouch Multicultural Centre Against Family Violence, 2010; Judicial Council on Cultural Diversity, 2016). Interpreters may be required (even for those with some English language proficiency) to ensure that emotional nuances can be conveyed accurately. It may also be important to employ interpreters who understand psycho-legal terminology and court procedures.

It was noted earlier that particular groups may present with unique symptom reporting styles (i.e., somatisation and idiomatic metaphors) or exhibit culturally normative behaviours that may be difficult to discern from mental health symptoms. Health frameworks may include more holistic phenomena, including the centrality of family, religiosity/spirituality, gender role expectations, and culturally stoic responses to adversity. Some cultures do not share the same conceptualisation of family (non-nuclear). Therefore, episodes like family disruption, childhood supervision practices, parenting styles, caregiver separation, and intimate partner characterisations may require alternative interpretations (those that differ from Western explanations) when assessing individuals with large, connected family networks. There may also be challenges ascertaining the extent to which the client demonstrates empathy/remorse. For some CALD clients, feelings are often not explicitly discussed culturally (or within the family unit), nor are nuanced explanations as to why one may have transgressed (and how one may have felt). As such, some CALD clients may be unable to discuss their emotions liberally (possessing no script nor language). There are also cultural stigmas about sharing sensitive issues. The aforementioned dynamics may be transferred into clinical/justice settings, especially emotions that may be implicated in criminal behaviour, which may be perceived as shameful or humiliating.

A related issue often noted by clinicians and service providers is being able to read the presentations of particular CALD clients. There is a perception that some are more likely to present with flat or blunted affect. In cultures that value inter-connectedness, there appears to be a preference for emotional suppression as this reduces the risk of disrupting group harmony by mitigating the impact of negative emotional states on others. These cultural dynamics may not entirely be the case for younger clients or those who have spent more time in a Western country. Cultural and clinical (i.e., psychosis, PTSD, depression, and traumatic brain injury) exceptions aside, flat affect for younger clients may stem from social dynamics. For example, young CALD clients may be more likely to shut down when they feel threatened, insulted, patronised, or misunderstood. It could also be part of the offender façade – being guarded or not wanting to show emotion, weakness, or vulnerability (which may be heightened in an honour culture). Additionally, the affect may be a survival strategy. The young person may be so used to receiving negative judgement from the public and so they will present for some time with a blank façade. A client may persist with this expression or lack thereof until they perceive that the clinician is a safe person to work with.

An understanding of community stigmas pertaining to mental health is recommended. For some CALD groups, mental health concerns may be preferably handled 'in house' with notions of stigma and shame impeding individuals from seeking outside assistance. In a correctional environment, these barriers could prevent participation in programmes and an increased likelihood of violating institutional rules. For CALD individuals, their justice involvement or problem behaviours may engender ostracism from their own families and communities. This may impact their ability to seek help or draw on support for problems they may be having which in turn may have sustained or exacerbated problem behaviours. Confidentiality may need to be explicitly assured for some CALD clients who may be concerned that members of their community will discover their involvement in the justice system or discreet utilisation of legal and mental health services.

Experiences of racism should be acknowledged. Discrimination can contribute to feelings of social rejection, frustration, cynicism toward the criminal justice system, and feelings of ostracism. Experiences of racism can affect self-esteem, distress levels, cooperation with authority, adherence to clinical recommendations, threat perception, and feelings of safety. CALD clients may exhibit a level of resistance or hostility in medical or legal settings because of mistrust, fear, and/or perceived discrimination, perhaps stemming from past injustices experienced pre or during migration. It is important to examine the extent to which this is occurring for the client. There is evidence that CALD offenders are found to be more likely to minimise psychopathology compared to non-CALD offenders (Kenny et al., 2008).

Some CALD populations believe that they are treated differently in society which engenders a cynicism towards mainstream institutions and social relationships. This extends to the criminal justice system which imprisons particular CALD groups at higher rates. As such, some CALD clients will harbour a deep sense of social rejection and a susceptibility to feeling insulted very quickly. If these experiences are not understood well by a clinician, the client will perceive that they have been further invalidated and the clinical process to be an extension of the discrimination they already experience in society. The site of the clinical encounter (sterile office setting, clinic, prison) should also be acknowledged. The client may be functional in their community context but may be uncooperative, hyper-vigilant, and susceptible to distress and incivility in a foreign environment. Therefore, pushing for early disclosure of trauma and focusing on past experiences, past criminal actions, ahead of relationship building, trust, and current needs will be barriers to engagement. To minimise the non-disclosure of information and avoid triggering grievances and other internalised stigmas, a relational disposition and a commitment to rapport building are recommended. Moreover, possessing a clinical style that is open-minded, non-judgemental, and empathetic combined with a communication (and body language) approach that is warm, patient, and without condescension will be more receptive to a client who is guarded or reluctant to divulge personal information.

Obtaining cultural-specific information

A number of frameworks for working effectively cross-culturally and eliciting cultural-specific information in non-intrusive ways have been articulated in the literature. One notable framework, Cultural Humility (Tervalon & Murray-Garcia, 1998), comprises particular features that facilitate meaningful cross-cultural interaction in clinical encounters and empowers clients to determine the extent to which their culture is relevant to their presenting concern. The premise of Cultural Humility is that in most cases, clinicians will be unable to 'master' a client's culture (if markedly different from their own). As such, clinicians should allow a safe space (open-mindedness, non-judgement, awareness of power differentials) for the client to share with and educate them on cultural aspects that they deem relevant to the session. Within this larger framework, lines of questioning to identify cultural information can be employed. The DSM-5 Cultural Formulation Interview (CFI; Lewis-Fernandez et al., 2014) (and forensic iterations, Aggarwal, 2012) and other resources (Barber Rioja & Rosenfeld, 2018;

Khawaja, 2011) comprise a list of questions that gently probe cultural rationalisations for behaviours. Some examples are listed here:

- What is bothering you most about your current problem (legal/psychological matter)?
- What do you think are the causes of your current issues?
- What would your family/community describe as the causes of your current issues?
- How would your community/family members view your problem (legal or psychological matter)?
- How would you describe it to them?
- What kinds of support would make your current problems better?
- What has gotten in the way of you seeking help?
- Are people with these behaviours normally helped or punished in your community?
- Do you have any wishes for or concerns about treatment?
- What are your thoughts about medications or psychotherapy?
- Has anyone else you know ever had this problem?
- What activities have this problem stopped you from doing that you, your family, or your friends expect?
- Do your friends and family talk with lawyers/psychologists about problems like the one you have?
- Do you think your friends or family would be upset if you spoke to lawyers/psychologists about your problems?

Additional lines of questioning are encouraged to ascertain the level of acculturation or cultural attachment of the client:

- What is your ancestry?
- Have you or your parents lived in a different country?
- Was your life different from where you were living before you came here? Was your role in your family different before you came to Australia?
- Are there cultural differences between you and your parents?
- Did your parents/family have challenges or bad things happen to them/were treated badly before they came to Australia?
- How did this impact them and you?
- Do you feel a strong connection to any groups of people?
- How close do you feel towards your community?
- What are the most important aspects of your cultural background?
- Are there any aspects of your cultural backgrounds that can help with your problem or perhaps that are contributing to your problem?
- Does the client reside near their family/community or are they geographically isolated?

Last, specific questions can be employed to explore the extent to which the client's cultural background may have been implicated in social challenges:

- Have you been treated badly because of your race/ethnicity/religion?
- How did this impact you?
- Sometimes people misunderstand each other because they come from different backgrounds or have different expectations of each other. Has this been a concern for you?

The relevance of the information extracted from the aforementioned questions will then need to be established. Here, one can use frameworks like the Multi-cultural Assessment Procedure

(MAP; Ridley et al., 1998). The MAP is a process that helps clinicians ascertain the importance of cultural information by 'weighing up' this information with regard to other facets of their life and immediate social context. For example, could personal, clinical, or environmental phenomena more parsimoniously explain their behaviour than a cultural explanation? The aforementioned integrated model of cross-cultural assessment (Cultural Humility, DSM-V CFI-related questions, and the MAP) is a useful starting point for clinicians with little knowledge of their client's cultural background and can help avoid forwarding unnecessary pre-conceptions of clients based on their heritage.

Conclusion

With increasing levels of cultural diversity, it is important that mental health services are relevant, useful, and accessible to new populations. This chapter has provided an outline of the unique socio-cultural contexts of CALD populations and how these phenomena underpin behaviours prompting criminal justice system involvement. Directions were then offered for working with such populations in various psycho-legal contexts, and an integrated model of cross-cultural assessment was introduced to assist assessors working in forensic clinical scenarios. The model underscores the importance of the therapeutic alliance through the building of rapport and trust. Moreover, the framework is intended to be practically oriented. It is recommended that the proposed model is evaluated.

References

Aggarwal, N. K. (2012). Adapting the cultural formulation for clinical assessments in Forensic Psychiatry. *The Journal of the American Academy of Psychiatry and the Law, 40*(1), 113–118.

Alarcon, R. D. (2009). Culture, cultural factors and psychiatric diagnosis: Review and projections. *World Psychiatry, 8*(3), 131–139. doi:10.1002/j.2051.5545.2009.tb00233.x

Allimant, A., & Ostapiej-Piatkowski, B. (2011). *Supporting women from CALD backgrounds who are victim/survivors of sexual violence: Challenges and opportunities for practices* (No. 9). Australian Centre for the Study of Sexual Assault, Australian Institute of Family Studies.

Andrews, D. A., & Bonta, J. (2010). Rehabilitating criminal justice policy and practice. *Psychology, Public Policy, and Law, 16*, 39–55. doi:10.1037/a0018362

Australian Bureau of Statistics. (2016). *2071.0 – Census of population and housing: Reflecting Australia – Stories from the census.* Retrieved February 3, 2020, from www.abs.gov.au/ausstats/abs@.nsf/ Lookup/ by%20Subject/2071.0~2016~Main%20Features~Cultural%20Diversity%20 Data%20Summary~30

Australian Bureau of Statistics. (2017). *Prisoners in Australia, 2017.* www.abs.gov.au/AUSSTATS/abs@.nsf/ Lookup/4517.0Explanatory%20Notes12017?OpenDocument

Australian Bureau of Statistics. (2018). *3417.0 –Understanding migrant outcomes –Insights from the Australian census and migrants integrated dataset, Australia, 2016.* Retrieved from: https://www.abs.gov.au/AUSSTATS/ abs@.nsf/Lookup/3417.0Main+Features22016?OpenDocument

Australian Institute of Health and Welfare. (2011). *Comorbidity of mental disorders and physical conditions, 2007.* www.aihw.gov.au/getmedia/6a8b451c-8def-47b2-a41a-9bcf59c77e76/10953-20140807.pdf.aspx

Barber Rioja, V., & Rosenfeld, B. (2018). Addressing linguistic and cultural differences in the forensic interview. *International Journal of Forensic Mental Health, 17*(4), 377–386. doi:10.1080/14999013.2018. 1495280

Berry, J. W. (1997). Immigration, acculturation, and adaptation. *Applied Psychology, 46*, 5–34. doi:10.1111/j. 1464-0597.1997.tb01087.x

Breslau, N., Chilcoat, H. D., Kessler, R. C., & Davis, G. C. (1999). Previous exposure to trauma and PTSD effects of subsequent trauma: Results from the Detroit area survey of trauma. *American Journal of Psychiatry, 156*, 902–907.

Brewer, R. (2009). *Culturally and linguistically diverse women in the Australian capital territory. Enablers and barriers to achieving social connectedness.* ACT: Women's Centre for Health Matters

Chan, B., & Parker, G. (2004). Some recommendations to assess depression in Chinese people in Australasia. *Australian and New Zealand Journal of Psychiatry*, *38*(3), 141–147. doi:10.1080/j.1440-1614.2004.01321.x

Chong, J., Reinschmidt, K. M., & Moreno, F. A. (2010). Symptoms of depression in a Hispanic primary care population with and without chronic medical illnesses. Primary care companion to the *Journal of Clinical Psychiatry*, *12*(3). doi:0.4088/PCC.09m00 846blu

Chung, D., Fisher, C., Zufferey, C., & Thiara, R. (2018). *Young women from African backgrounds and sexual violence*. Australian Institute of Criminology.

Cohen, C. I., & Marino, L. (2013). Racial and Ethnic differences in the prevalence of psychotic symptoms in the general population. *Psychiatric Services*, *64*(11), 1103–1109.

Colucci, E., Minas, H., Szwarc, J., Paxton, G., & Guerra, C. (2014). *Barriers to and facilitators of utilisation of mental health services by young people of refugee background*. https://refugeehealthnetwork.org.au/wp-content/uploads/Barriers+and+facilitators+pdf+final.pdf

Commonwealth of Australia. (2015). *Hearing her voice. Kitchen table conversations on violence against culturally and linguistically diverse women and their children*. Department of Social Services, Commonwealth of Australia.

Davern, M., Warr, D., Block, K., La Brooy, C., Taylor, E., & Hosseini, A. (2016). *Humanitarian Arrivals in Melbourne: A spatial analysis of population distribution and health service needs*. Extended Report. University of Melbourne.

Day, A., Tamatea, A. J., Casey, S., & Geia, L. (2018). Assessing violence risk with Aboriginal and Torres Strait Islander offenders: Considerations for forensic practice. *Psychiatry, Psychology and Law*, *25*(3), 452–464.

Deacon, B. J. (2013). The biomedical model of mental disorder: A critical analysis of its validity, utility, and effects on psychotherapy research. *Clinical Psychology Review*, *33*, 846–861. doi:10.1016/j.cpr.2012.09.007

Deng, S. A. (2016). *South Sudanese youth acculturation and intergenerational challenges*. Proceedings of the 39th African Studies Association of Australasia and the Pacific (AFSAAP) Annual Conference, December 5–7, 2016, The University of Western Australia.

Douglas, K. S., Cox, D. N., & Webster, C. D. (1999). Violence risk assessment: Science and practice. *Legal and Criminological Psychology*, *4*, 149–184. doi:10.1348/1355325 99167824

El-Murr, A. (2018). *Intimate partner violence in Australian refugee communities: Scoping review of issues and service responses*. Retrieved from https://aifs.gov.au/cfca/publications/cfca-paper/intimate-partner-violence-australian-refugee-communities/scoping-review

Fazel, M., Wheeler, J., & Danesh, J. (2005). Prevalence of serious mental disorder in 7000 refugees resettled in western countries: A systematic review. *The Lancet*, *365*(9467), 1309–1314. doi:10.1016/S0140-6736(05)61027-6

Ferdinand, A., Kelaher, M., & Paradies, Y. (2013). *Mental health impacts of racial discrimination in Victorian culturally and linguistically diverse communities: Full report of the Localities Embracing and Accepting Diversity (LEAD) experiences of racism survey*. Victorian Health Promotion Foundation.

Francis, S., & Cornfoot, S. (2007). *Working with multicultural youth: Programs, strategies and future direction*. Australian Research Alliance for Children & Youth.

Gopalkrishnan, N. (2018). Cultural diversity and mental health: Considerations for policy and practice. *Frontiers in Public Health*, *6*. doi:10.3389/fpubh.2018.00179

Halvorsrud, K., Nazroo, J., Otis, M., Hajdukova, E. B., & Bhui, K. (2019). Ethnic inequalities in the incidence of diagnosis of severe mental illness in England: A systematic review and new meta-analyses for non-affective and affective psychoses. *Social Psychiatry and Psychiatric Epidemiology*, *54*, 1311–1323. doi:10.1007/s00127-019-01758-y

Hart, S. D. (2016). Culture and violence risk assessment: The case of Ewert v. Canada. *Journal of Threat Assessment and Management*, *3*(2), 76–96. doi.org/10.1037/tam0000068

InTouch Multicultural Centre Against Family Violence. (2010). *Barriers to the justice system faced by CALD women experiencing family violence*. https://aija.org.au/wp-content/uploads/2017/06/Avdibegovic.pdf

InTouch Multicultural Centre Against Family Violence. (2014). *Domestic violence in Australia* (Submission 138). Submission to Senate Standing Committee on Finance and Public Administration Inquiry into Domestic Violence in Australia.

Jatrana, S., Richardson, K., & Samba, S. R. A. (2017). Investigating the dynamics of migration and health in Australia: A longitudinal study. *European Journal of Population*. doi:org/10.1007/s10680-017-9439-z

Judicial Council on Cultural Diversity. (2016). *The path to justice: Migrant and refugee women's experience of the courts*. Canberra, ACT.

Kenny, D. T., Lennings, C. J., & Nelson, P. K. (2008). The mental health of young offenders serving orders in the community. *Journal of Offender Rehabilitation, 45*(1), 123–148. doi:10.1300/J076v45n01_10

Khawaja, N. G. (2011). Effective interviewing of culturally and linguistically diverse clients. *InPsych, 33*(3). www.psychology.org.au/effective-interviewing-culturally-linguistically-diverse-clients

Khawaja, N. G., McCarthy, R., Braddock, V., & Dunne, M. (2014). Characteristics of culturally and linguistically diverse mental health clients. *Advances in Mental Health, 11*(2). doi:10.5172/jamh.2013.11.2.172

Kirmayer, L. J. (1989). Cultural variations in the response to psychiatric disorders and emotional distress. *Social Science & Medicine, 29*, 327–339. doi:10.1016/0277-9536(89)90281-5

Kirmyaer, L. J., Narasiah, L., Munoz, M., Rashid, M., Ryder, A. G., Guzder, J., Hassan, G., Rousseau, C., & Pottie, K. (2011). Common mental health problems in immigrants and refugees: General approach in primary care. *CMAJ, 183*(12), E959–E967. doi:10.1503/cmaj.090292

Kiropoulos, L. A., Blashki, G., & Klimidis, S. (2005). Managing mental illness in patients from CALD backgrounds. *Australian Family Physician, 34*, 259–264.

Kraus, L. J., Thomas, C. R., Bukstein, O. G., Walter, H. J., Benson, R. S., Chrisman, A., . . . Medicus, J. (2011). Practice parameter for child and adolescent forensic evaluations. *Journal of American Academy Child and Adolescent Psychiatry, 50*, 1299–1312. doi:10.1016/j.jaac.2011.09.020

Latzman, R. D., Megraya, A. M., Hecht, L. K., Miller, J. D., Winiarski, D. A., & Lilienfeld, S. O. (2015). Self-reported psychopathy in the middle east: A cross-national comparison across Egypt, Saudi Arabia, and the United States. *BMC Psychology, 3*(37). doi:10.1186/s40359-015-

Lewis-Fernandez, R., Aggarwal, N. K., Baarnhielm, S., Rohlof, H., Kirmayer, L. J., Weiss, M. G., Jadhav, S., Hinton, L., . . . Lu, F. (2014). Culture and psychiatric evaluation: Operationalizing cultural formulation for DSM-5. *Psychiatry, 77*(2), 130–154. doi:10.1521/psyc.2014.77.2.130

Lewis-Fernandez, R., & Kirmayer, L. J. (2019). Cultural concepts of distress and psychiatric disorders: Understanding symptom experience and expression in context. *Transcultural Psychiatry, 56*(4), 786–803. doi:10.1177/1363461519861795

Lim, N. (2016). Cultural differences in emotion: Differences in emotional arousal level between the East and the West. *Integrative Medicine Research, 5*(2), 105–109. doi:10.1016/j.imr.2016.03.004

Llamas, J. (2006). Trauma and posttraumatic st Llamas, J. (2006). Trauma and posttraumatic stress disorder in ethnic minorities. *American Psychological Association, 6*, 337–344.

Loeber, R., & Farrington, D. P. (2000). Young children who commit crime: Epidemiology, developmental origins, risk factors, early interventions, and policy implications. *Development and Psychopathology, 12*, 737–762. doi:10.1017/S095 4579400004107

Markus, A. (2016). *Australian's today.* https://scanlonfoundation.org.au/wp-content/uploads/2018/10/Australians-Today-1.pdf

Markus, A. (2018). *Mapping social cohesion – The Scanlon Foundation surveys 2018.* https://scanlonfoundation.org.au/wp-content/uploads/2018/12/Social-Cohesion-2018-report-26-Nov.pdf

McGilloway, A., Hall, R. E., Lee, T., & Bhui, K. S. (2010). A systematic review of personality disorder, race and ethnicity: Prevalence, aetiology and treatment. *BMC Psychiatry, 10*(33). doi:10.1186/1471-244X-10-33

Minas, H., Kakuma, R., Too, L. S., Vayani, H., Orapeleng, S., Prasad-Ildes, R., Turner, G., Procter, N., & Oehm, D. (2013). Mental health research and evaluation in multicultural Australia: Developing a culture of inclusion. *International Journal of Mental Health Systems, 7*(23), 1–25.

Ogloff, J. R. P., Davis, M., Rivers, G., & Ross, S. (2007). *The identification of mental disorders in the criminal justice system.* https://aic.gov.au/publications/tandi/tandi334

Queensland Government. (2010). *Working with people from culturally and linguistically diverse backgrounds.* www.communities.qld.gov.au/resources/ childsafety/practice-manual/prac-paper-working-cald.pdf

Ridley, C. R., Li, L. C., & Hill, C. L. (1998). Multicultural assessment: Reexamination, reconceptualization, and practical application. *Journal of Counselling Psychology, 26*, 827–910.

Rogers, R., Heilbrun, K., & Otto, R. (2004). Forensic assessment: Current status and future directions. *Mental Health Law & Policy Faculty Publications, 314.* https://scholarcommons.usf.edu/mhlp_facpub/314

Rose, A., Shepherd, S. M., & Ogloff, J. R. P. (2020). The mental health of culturally and linguistically diverse offenders – What do we know? *Australasian Psychiatry.* doi:10.1177/1039856220924315

Rose, A., Trounson, J., Skues, J., Daffern, M., Shepherd, S. M., Pfeifer, J. E., & Ogloff, J. R. P. (2019). Psychological wellbeing, distress and coping in Australian Indigenous and multicultural prisoners: A mixed methods analysis. *Psychiatry, Psychology and Law.* doi:10.1080/13218719.2019.1642259

Royal Commission into Family Violence. (2016, March). *Summary and recommendations 2016*. State Government, Victoria.

Saunders, V., Roche, S., McArthur, M., Arney, F., & Ziaian, T. (2015). *Refugee communities intercultural dialogue: Building relationships, building communities*. Institute of Child Protection Studies, Australian Catholic University.

Schwartz, R. C., & Blankenship, D. M. (2014). Racial disparities in psychotic disorder diagnosis: A review of empirical literature. *World Journal of Psychiatry, 4*, 133–140. http://dx.doi.org/10.5498/wjp.v4.i4.133

Schwartz, S. J., Unger, J. B., Zamboanga, B. L., & Szapocznik, J. (2010). Rethinking the concept of acculturation: Implications for theory and research. *American Psychologist, 65*, 237–251. doi:10.1037/a0019330

Shepherd, S. M. (2016). Criminal engagement and Australian culturally and linguistically diverse populations: Challenges and implications for forensic risk assessment. *Psychiatry, Psychology and Law, 23*(2), 256–274. doi: 10.1080/13218719.2015.1053164

Shepherd, S. M., & Lewis-Fernandez, R. (2016). Forensic risk assessment and cultural diversity: Contemporary challenges and future directions. *Psychology, Public Policy, and Law, 22*(4), 427–438. https://doi.org/10.1037/law0000102

Shepherd, S. M., & Masuka, G. (2020). Working with at-risk culturally and linguistically diverse young people in Australia – risk factors, programming and service delivery. *Criminal Justice Policy Review* (Advance Online Publication). doi:10.1177/0887403420929416

Skeem, J. L., Edens, J. F., Camp, J., & Colwell, L. H. (2004). Are there ethnic differences in levels of psychopathy? *Law and Human Behavior, 28*, 505–527.

Straiton, M., Grant, J. F., Winefiled, H. R., & Taylor, A. (2014). Mental health in immigrant men and women in Australia: The North West Adelaide health study. *BMC Public Health, 14*. doi:10.1186/1471-2458-14-1111

Sullivan, E. A., Abramowitz, C. S., Lopez, M., & Kosson, D. S. (2006). Reliability and construct validity of the psychopathy checklist – revised for Latino, European American, and African American male inmates. *Psychological Assessment, 18*(4), 382–392. doi:10.1037/1040-3590

Tamatea, A. J. (2016). Culture is our business: Issues and challenges for forensic and correctional psychologists. *Australian Journal of Forensic Sciences, 49*(5), 564–578. doi.org/10.1080/00450618.2016.1237549

Taylor, N., & Mouzos, M. (2006). *Community attitudes to violence against women survey 2006: A full technical report*. Australian Institute of Criminology.

Taylor, N., & Putt, J. (2007). *Adult sexual violence in Indigenous and culturally and linguistically diverse communities in Australia (Trends & Issues in Crime and Criminal Justice No. 345)*. Australian Institute of Criminology.

Tervalon, M., & Murray-Garcia, J. (1998). Cultural humility versus cultural competence: A critical distinction in defining physician training outcomes in multicultural education. *Journal of Health Care Poor Underserved. 9*, 117–125.

Wilson, H. A., & Gutierrez, L. (2014). Does one size fit all? A meta-analysis examining the predictive ability of the Level of Service Inventory (LSI) with Aboriginal offenders. *Criminal Justice & Behavior, 41*(2), 196–219. https://doi.org/10.1177/0093854813500958

Part 5

Communicating with marginalised groups

Chapter 15

The individual as a marginalised cohort in secure and forensic mental health inpatient settings in the United Kingdom

Sarah Markham

Introduction

To marginalise someone is to make somebody feel as if they are not important and cannot influence decisions or events; to put somebody in a position in which they have no power (OALD, 2020). The historical marginalisation of those deemed to be mentally disordered is well recognised (Crighton et al., 2017). The association between mental disorder and compromised cognition and risk is embedded in both our culture and mental health legislation (Foucault, 2006). This chapter explores distinct types of marginalisation, primarily through an epistemic lens. It argues that patient involvement in risk assessment and treatment decision-making are crucial ways to mitigate the epistemic marginalisation of forensic mental health patients.

Epistemic marginalisation

An individual's self-concept is a collection of beliefs they hold regarding themselves (Leflot et al., 2010). Self-concept is made up of self-schemas; one's past, present, and future selves and interacts with self-esteem, self-knowledge, and the social self to form the self as a whole. Patients in forensic mental health settings subjected to disproportionate levels of restriction may experience difficulties in re-developing and expressing an adaptive sense of self or self-concept potentially leading to them becoming institutionalised, bored, hopeless, lonely, or lethargic (Hörberg et al., 2012).

One of the principal psychological harms to self-concept which patients may experience in risk-averse settings is epistemic injustice; a phenomenon in which a person is wronged in their capacity as a knower due to prejudice, and thus transmission of knowledge via testimony is impaired (Fricker, 2008). There are specific representations of those with mental health conditions, especially mentally disordered offenders that render them vulnerable to negative prejudices and stereotypes, which exacerbate their vulnerability to epistemic injustice (Bhugra et al., 2017). There have been reported instances of clinicians dismissing their patients' subjective accounts leading to one author remarking that clinicians wanted patients to be 'seen but not heard' (Hagen & Nixon, 2011, p. 54).

It is important for clinicians to be aware of the phenomenon of epistemic injustice to counter their own predisposition to commit such harm against their patients (Sanati & Kyratsous, 2015). In addition to the formal medico-legal discourse that renders a mentally disordered offender vulnerable to the denial of their epistemic capacity and agency, their criminal histories may also cause a patient to be viewed as undeserving of any platform for dissent. Such suppression and reconfiguration of freedom of expression constitute a form of ontological

DOI: 10.4324/9781003184768-20

violence in which dominant clinical ideologies interpret patients in a manner that 'determines (their) very being and social existence' (Žižek, 2008).

Fricker defined two forms of dysfunction in epistemic practice which harm individuals by disregarding their capacity as knowers and their human status: testimonial injustice and hermeneutic injustice (Fricker, 2008). *Testimonial injustice* presents when bias leads to a hearer attaching a diminished degree of credibility to an individual's self-report (Fricker, 2008). Patient testimonies are sought as sources of information but the testimony about the lived experience of illness, which may challenge clinical perspectives, may often be excluded or play no formal role in decision-making. Faulkner (2012) proposes that the organisational norm of credibility within mental healthcare services is biased against patients. This means that regardless of the conscientiousness of individual practitioners in giving due regard to their patients' views and requests, the wider service may function to suppress a patient's input in decision-making regarding their care and increase the epistemic marginalisation of the patient. Epistemic disregard and contempt can be creeping contagions; if one person in authority is seen to silence or disregard a patient's testimony or self-report, this may encourage others to follow suit.

Hermeneutic injustice pertains to social circumstances in which an individual's ability to make sense of their experience is compromised due to a paucity of conceptual and interpretative resources (Fricker, 2008). For instance, an over-emphasis within therapeutic relationships and dialogues on the biomedical as opposed to the psycho-emotional or social determinants of mental health may occlude patients' access to appreciation of their own experiential learning when developing an understanding of their illness. Hermeneutical injustice is principally structural and not agential, arising from specific contingent features of a social environment, such as its educational practices and authoritative hierarchy, rather than the actions of specific individuals. It may also result from epistemic isolation; circumstances in which someone lacks the knowledge of, or means of access to, information; for instance, because of living within the locked confines of a secure psychiatric ward with minimal access to the outside world or internet. The lived experience literature provides extensive examples of the consequential harms of epistemic injustice including isolation, threats to self-concept, and the perpetuation of stigma (Lee, 2013). Although patients may experience an increasing degree of involvement in service design and development, they continue to be subject to epistemic marginalisation in terms of decision-making regarding their own lives (Stacey et al., 2016).

Although the admissibility of testimony by individuals with mental disorders in courts might be thought to protect against testimonial injustice, the First-Tier Tribunal process via which patients are able to appeal against continued detention under the Mental Health Act, 1983 (MHA) has been criticised from a hermeneutic perspective as patients may not be familiar with the legal terminology used in such proceedings, and not be able to challenge evidence as it is presented (Dolan et al., 1999).

Epistemic hegemony

Mental health professionals enjoy significant epistemic regard, afforded by their clinical training, and enshrined in the MHA (1983). They are the ones with whom the epistemic hegemony sits (Pohlhaus, 2012), and as such, their judgement is privileged in determining the competency, relevance, and value of patients' testimonies (Carel & Kidd, 2014). When a clinical opinion is presented, it is accepted to be the authoritative one despite current awareness of the limitations of psychiatry as a medical discipline (Wardrope, 2015). Epistemic hegemony does not necessarily equate to or translate into epistemic expertise. Psychiatry has been criticised for being a discipline lacking precision; characterised by suboptimal treatment efficacy with a paucity of biomedical evidence to support current nosological frameworks

(Paulus, 2017). The imbalance between extreme authority on the one hand and suboptimal knowledge and expertise on the other have led to questionable practice and public and patient concern regarding the care and treatment of those detained in psychiatric settings. There also exist recorded instances in which clinicians have claimed that as trained professionals they invariably know best and that mentally disordered offenders have insufficient decision-making competence to participate in meaningful ways (Grim, 2019).

The negative consequences of the obstacles patients encounter in attempting to have their opinions on care heard have been well documented, including impoverished clinical knowledge regarding patient well-being and worse health outcomes for service users (Miller Tate, 2019). A patient may also be epistemically marginalised regarding how their daily lives, especially their behaviour and interactions with staff are documented. Clinical records can be read as pejoratively distorted reductive narratives and construct patients as inferior and innately flawed risk entities who need regular monitoring and intervention to correct their aberrant behaviour and symptoms (Parrott, 2010). Patients have reported that the opinions and concerns of staff invariably take precedence over their own understandings of their situation and that they have little or no influence or control over how their problems are conceptualised and documented (Farber, 1993). Patients have described how they have self-edited their communication with professionals to reduce the chance of misinterpretations and associated negative consequences (Holley & Gillard, 2018).

It has been reported that clinicians regard the extent of alignment between their own views and those of their patients as a significant aid to their clinical and risk assessments (Langan, 2008). Once a patient has been labelled as resistant or non-compliant and this has been recorded in their clinical notes, it may be difficult to convince future care and treatment decision-makers that this is not an accurate representation. A patient's expression of legitimate dissent or disagreement with a clinical view may be reconstructed as indicative of a lack of insight, non-compliance, and further evidence of psychiatric symptomatology, thereby exposing them to denial of their personhood, sense of self, and social existence (Liegghio, 2013). This may exert a considerable pressure on them to forfeit their opinions and agency to appear compliant and deserving of the reinstatement of their liberty (Fabris & Aubrecht, 2014).

Procedural marginalisation

Procedural justice in the context of secure and forensic care involves ensuring patients are treated fairly by receiving competent treatment delivered in a manner that preserves their dignity and considers their preferences and experiential learning. It is recognised that for mentally disordered offenders, the process of developing trusting therapeutic relationships may be extremely problematic due to the restrictive nature of the physical environment of the secure ward and associated security-focused protocols and practices (Ruszczynski, 2010). This underlines the need for procedurally just care and treatment. However, research indicates that the experience of procedural injustice remains a widespread reality for patients. Some studies have recorded patients claiming that they had to demand attention or even beg staff to get anything on the ward they needed (To et al., 2015; Ireland et al., 2014). Patients have reported that they may avoid expressing to staff how they feel because of fear of punishment or loss of privileges (Hörberg et al., 2012).

Coercive practices, whilst seen as necessary in some situations, can have physical and psychological consequences for the patient and are viewed as adverse events. Patients have voiced an especial concern regarding the use of coercive interventions as a first-line strategy, reporting feelings of powerlessness and re-traumatisation (Heumann et al., 2017). A 2019 study found that informal forms of coercion such as persuasion, inter-personal leverage, and inducements, e.g., the offer of escorted leave (with the possible potential to pass into emotional blackmail in certain situations), threats, cheating, e.g., giving patients medication without their knowledge, using a disciplinary style, and referencing rules and routines, have been evidenced in mental health settings (Pelto-Piri et al., 2019). It also reported that if persuasion or negotiation fails to induce a patient to comply, then staff may immediately turn to threats, for example, forced medication (Pelto-Piri et al., 2019).

It remains a perplexing characteristic of the legal authority endowed by the Mental Health Act that whilst restrictive practices and treatment without consent are in theory only used to maintain safety, in the context of staff's inevitably subjective and imprecise perceptions of risk of harm to self or others, they have significant implications for a patient's sense of ontological security, self, and autonomy. Patients may feel compelled to gain the trust of care team members by presenting as compliant regardless of any conflict between their own views and those of their team (Holley & Gillard, 2018). This may seem to them to be the only means by which they will be granted more freedom and allowed to take more responsibility for themselves. Thus, the degree to which patients are deemed to make progress in their recovery may be less an indicator of their wellness and level of adaptive functioning and more a marker of their overt alignment to the positions taken by their formal carers (Askola et al., 2017; Gildberg et al., 2012).

Forensic psychiatry and the management of risk

The aim of forensic psychiatry is the evaluation, care, and treatment of mentally disordered offenders and of others who need equivalent care. Risk assessment, formulation, and management, together with the prevention of further offending are key organisational and structural concepts (Nedopil et al., 2012). Mentally disordered offenders constitute a heterogeneous group with respect to diagnosis, clinical need, offending history, and risk (Edworthy et al., 2016). Risk is contextualised in mental health settings as the possibility of a patient engaging in abusive, harmful, or antisocial behaviours with respect to others or themselves (Morgan, 2007). Forensic populations are perceived as posing an especial risk to the public and therefore forensic psychiatry places significant weight on an association between past violence committed by a patient and their potential for future violence (Wilkie et al., 2014). Accordingly, minimisation of a patient's perceived risk regarding others and themselves and reduction of the likelihood of recidivism are viewed as the overarching goals of a patient's treatment in secure hospital settings and community forensic services.

It has been suggested that clinicians and mental health services hold substantial anxiety regarding risk management and that staff use defensive practice such as over-medication and delayed approval or augmentation of a patient's use of S17 leave, to deal with this (Menzies Lyth, 1960). This was recently echoed in the final report of the Independent Review of the MHA (DHSC, 2018). The Care Quality Commission (CQC) has also warned that the more positive recommendations from national mental health policy such as a shift towards more collaborative decision-making and risk assessment are in effect ignored by services characterised by compulsion, coercion, containment, and control (CQC, 2015). This rise in risk aversion and increased focus on the management of perceived risk is reflected more widely in society, as acknowledged in some key sociological texts (Beck, 1992).

Shared decision-making and collaborative risk assessment

Medical practice is reported to be moving away from a paternalistic compliance model to more person-centred and evidence-based medicine (Deegan & Drake, 2006). According to policy and other directives, shared decision making (SDM) is to become paradigmatic in health care, including mental health services. The National Health Service (NHS) Long-Term Plan has directed services in England and Wales to place greater emphasis on patient engagement, autonomy, and choice; for clinicians and patients to make decisions together using the best available evidence about the benefits and harms of each option, and for patients to be supported to arrive at clinically informed preferences (DHSC, 2019).

In the context of mental health, SDM is both a rational epistemic (knowledge-based) process and a relational one, with the balance between allowing the patient autonomy and imposing restrictions commensurate with the perceived vulnerability and capacity of the patient (Van Heijst, 2011).

There is a clear rationale for integrating an individual's self-insight, experiential learning, and other forms of knowledge, into decision-making in mental health. The patient possesses lived experience of their disorder in addition to self-derived expertise regarding its management. A patient's unique access to their own internal mental states may be crucial to optimising the quality and efficacy of clinical assessment and intervention processes (Vazire & Mehl, 2008). In assessing their own treatment and associated intervention needs, patients are empowered to engage in and take responsibility for their own actions. This process is a motivator for change (Ryan & Deci, 2008), and psychological research has provided evidence that an individual will make a greater commitment to progress if there is a keen sense of engagement and responsibility (Janis, 1984).

A key aim of patient-centred care is to help patients make and contribute to informed decisions about their care. In theory, this is protective against epistemic injustice, i.e., having one's knowledge or perspective unfairly discounted; however, in practice, implementation appears to be sub-optimal. There is evidence that SDM is not reliably implemented in mental health settings and that SDM training for staff is often unavailable (Stiggelbout et al., 2015). An essential element of being effectively involved in decisions regarding care and treatment is access to appropriate information. Mental health service patients have reported examples of lack of choice, of decisions imposed, or care plans drafted with little input from themselves (Coffey et al., 2019). Furthermore, clinicians and patients may present with conflicting assumptions, values, and goals (Coles, 2012) which may further hinder the SDM process.

Patient involvement in risk assessment and the creation of risk management strategies may encourage the development of a greater sense of ownership of their behaviour and responsibility in monitoring and controlling the factors that relate to any risk of harm they may pose (Kroner, 2012). Risk may be dynamic and complex and encompass several life domains and factors specific to the individual concerned which may be missed by assessment tools or assessors, such as self-concept and sense of self-determination. Exclusion or poor representation of the diverse forms of knowledge and understanding held by patients may compromise the validity and the value and efficacy of assessment and decision-making processes.

Research indicates that although some patients may be involved in their care planning and risk management, there is little continued engagement or understanding of how to actualise those plans (Haines et al., 2018). There exists little literature concerning patients' views and experiences of these processes. One observational study found that patients 'attempted to understand the system of assessment and sought to affect and reduce their risk status by engaging in overt, compliant behaviours' (Reynolds et al., 2014). Another study claimed that the 'risk assessment process is subverted by the restriction of the flow of information, and patients are left with frustrations that they must contain and manage' (Langan, 2008).

However, a 2019 review of the literature to explore models of patients' involvement in risk assessment and the impact on outcomes in forensic mental health care found encouraging evidence of the predictive validity of self-rated risk alongside staff-rated risk assessment (Ray & Simpson, 2019). It is therefore crucial that patients are involved collaboratively in treatment and risk assessment and safety planning, not merely in terms of their own treatment and care but also in the wider context of development and revision of service security and other risk-based policies and practice.

Discussion

It can be argued that disproportionate risk aversion and consequent harm to patients are embedded within the mental health system; that they are 'business as usual', banal. The Independent Review of the MHA 2018 acknowledged that patients are perceived and treated primarily as risk entities, rather than as human beings in need of compassionate care and treatment and that professionals place far too little gravity on removing an individual's liberty (DHSC, 2018).

How can we instil within secure and forensic services a sense that uncertainty and the unknown don't necessarily mean there exists a potential for harm? How can we encourage uncertainty to be perceived and experienced as an opportunity for positive learning and development rather than a precursor of danger? The paradoxical nature of the presumption within secure and forensic services that the goal of providing care and treatment which improve a patient's health is in tension with the goal to provide security has not been fully examined (Caplan, 1993). This tension can lead to the imposition of interventions that can be classified as controlling and potentially harmful regarding the recipient's mental well-being (Gildberg et al., 2010). Yet research has found that increasing a mentally disordered offender's level of autonomy doesn't necessarily lead to an increase in violence or other misdemeanours (Urheim et al., 2011). There remains much scope and potential for change.

The value of subjective lived experience and associated experiential knowledge is increasingly recognised in mental healthcare policy and recovery-related literature. The development by mentally disordered offenders of their own risk narratives may enhance self-awareness and insight and enable them to make better sense of their life experiences. This may also help them to begin to reposition themselves in society. According to Felton and Stickley, 'the opportunity for new narratives and interpretations are important in terms of risk, particularly in relation to historical incidents of harm caused by or to an individual' (Felton & Stickley, 2018: 57). The reinterpretation of events provides scope for an individual to come to terms and move on in accordance with the principles of recovery. Engaging with a patient's own interpretations also enables professionals to consider the meaning of such events in the context of said individual's current circumstances and can facilitate the development of shared understanding and epistemic trust between clinicians and patients (Felton & Stickley, 2018).

There is a need for both structural and relational support and change if the value of patients' experiential learning and epistemic agency are to be recognised and marginalisation countered (Treichler & Spaulding, 2017). Personal narratives are a critical means via which self-concept and identity are shaped and mentally disordered offenders become intelligible to both the clinical community and wider society (Gergen, 1994).

Conclusion

Attempts to extend therapeutic ways of working to include increased patient collaboration in discussion and decision-making can be experienced as threatening by clinicians and services. Changes in practice and the many ways of working carry with them uncertainties that professionals may emotionally experience as unsettling and psychologically construe as indicative of risk. Mental health legislation sanctions epistemological and other power disparities between patients and their statutory carers, privileging professional opinions and epistemological frameworks. Clinicians and services may be culpable of taking and maintaining unjustified and unjust epistemic stances that tacitly incorporate presumptions regarding the capabilities of patients to possess, process, and provide clinically relevant knowledge. There is a clear need to challenge the psychiatric hegemony and non-evidence-based professional discourses within mental health settings.

An individual's perceived epistemic capacity is intrinsic to their human value, and it remains important for practitioners to acknowledge and accept the potential for experiential learning to liberate patients from past maladaptive attitudes and behaviours. The reification of epistemic injustice in secure and forensic settings via evaluation of the quality of deliberative processes and associated decision making, especially in the context of patients seeking to negotiate the provision of their care and treatment needs, has the potential to provide valuable insights and ways to improve practice. Resolving such oppression in forensic psychiatry will necessitate clinicians being able to enter interdependent epistemic relationships with their patients in addition to giving them due regard with respect to their self-report, lived experience, and experiential learning. The value of enhancing the self-concept and reducing the marginalisation of mentally disordered offenders and of supporting them to change their personal narratives, the stories they tell of themselves about who they are, and what they are worth should never be underestimated.

References

Askola, R., Nikkonen, M., Putkonen, H., Kylmä, J., & Louheranta, O. (2017). The therapeutic approach to a patient's criminal offense in a forensic mental health nurse-patient relationship – the nurses' perspectives. *Perspectives in Psychiatric Care*, *53*(3), 164–174.

Beck, U. (1992). *Risk society*. Sage.

Bhugra, D., Tasman, A., Pathare, S., Priebe, S., Smith, S., Torous, J., et al. (2017). The WPA-lancet psychiatry commission on the future of psychiatry. *The Lancet Psychiatry*, *4*.

Caplan, C. A. (1993). Nursing staff and patient perceptions of the ward atmosphere in a maximum security forensic hospital. *Archives of Psychiatric Nursing*, *7*(1), 23–29.

Care Quality Commission. (2015). *Monitoring the mental health act in 2013/14*. CQC.

Carel, H., & Kidd, I. J. (2014). Epistemic injustice in healthcare: A philosophical analysis. *Medicine, Health Care and Philosophy*, *17*, 529–540.

Coffey, M., Hannigan, B., Meudell, A., Jones, M., Hunt, J., & Fitzsimmons, D. (2019). Quality of life, recovery and decision-making: A mixed methods study of mental health recovery in social care. *Soc Psychiatry Psychiatr Epidemiol*, *54*(6), 715–723.

Coles, S. (2012). Collaborative decision making. *Clinical Psychology Bite-Size*, *36*.

Crichton, P., Carel, H., & Kidd, I. J. (2017). Epistemic injustice in psychiatry. *BJPsych Bulletin*, *41*(2), 65–70.

Deegan, P. E., & Drake, R. E. (2006). Shared decision making and medication management in the recovery process. *Psychiatric Services*, *57*(11), 1636–1639.

Department of Health and Social Care. (2018). *Modernising the mental health act – final report from the independent review*, Published 6 December 2018 Last updated February 14, 2019. Department of Health and Social Care Publications.

Department of Health and Social Care. (2019). *The NHS long term plan*. Department of Health and Social Care Publications.

Dolan, M., Gibb, R., & Coorey, P. (1999). Mental health review tribunals: A survey of special hospital patients' opinions. *Journal of Forensic Psychiatry*, *10*, 264–275.

Edworthy, R., Sampson, S., & Vollm, B. (2016). Inpatient forensic-psychiatric care: Legal frameworks and service provision in three European countries. *International Journal of Law Psychiatry*, *47*, 18–27.

Fabris, E., & Aubrecht, K. (2014). *Chemical constraint: Experiences of psychiatric coercion, restraint, and detention as carceratory techniques*. In Book: Disability Incarcerated.

Farber, S. (1993). *Madness, heresy, and the rumor of angels: The revolt against the mental health system*. Open Court.

Faulkner, P. (2012). Trust and the assessment of credibility. *Social Epistemology Review and Reply Collective*, *1*, 1–6.

Felton, A., & Stickley, T. (2018). Rethinking risk: A narrative approach. *Journal of Mental Health Training, Education and Practice*, *13*(1), 54–62.

Foucault, M. (2006). *History of madness* (J. Khalfa, Ed. and J. Murphy, Trans.). Routledge.

Fricker, M. (2008). *Forum on Miranda Fricker's epistemic injustice: Power and the ethics of knowing: Precis.* Theoria.

Gergen, K. J. (1994). *Realities and relationships: Soundings in social construction.* Harvard University Press.

Gildberg, F. A., Bradley, S. K., Fristed, P., & Hounsgaard, L. (2012). Reconstructing normality: Characteristics of staff interactions with forensic mental health inpatients. *International Journal of Mental Health Nursing, 21*(2), 103–113.

Gildberg, F. A., Elverdam, B., & Hounsgaard, L. (2010). Forensic psychiatric nursing: A literature review and thematic analysis of staff – patient interaction. *Journal of Psychiatric and Mental Health Nursing, 17*, 359–368.

Grim, K. (2019). Legitimizing the knowledge of mental health service users in shared decision making. Promoting participation through a web-based decision support tool (Dalarna Doctoral Dissertations in Health Sciences 1). Dalarna University. ISBN 978-91-88679-01-7.

Hagen, B., & Nixon, G. (2011). Spider in a jar: Women who have recovered from psychosis and their experience of the mental health care system. *Ethical Human Psychology and Psychiatry, 13*, 47–63.

Haines, A., Perkins, E., Evans, E. A., & McCabe, R. (2018). Multidisciplinary team functioning and decision making within forensic mental health. *Mental Health Review Journal, 23*(3), 185–196. Emerald Publishing Limited, ISSN 1361–9322.

Heumann, K., Bock, T., & Lincoln, T. M. (2017). Please do something – no matter what! A nationwide online survey of mental health service users about the use of alternatives to coercive measures. *Psychiatr Prax, 44*, 85–92.

Holley, J. R., & Gillard, S. (2018). Developing and using vignettes to explore the relationship between risk management practice and recovery-oriented care in mental health services. *Qualitative Health Research, 28*(3), 371–380.

Hörberg, U., Sjögren, R., & Dahlberg, K. (2012). To be strategically struggling against resignation: The lived experience of being cared for in forensic psychiatric care. *Issues in Mental Health Nursing, 33*(11), 743–775.

Ireland, C. A., Halpin, L., & Sullivan, C. (2014). Critical incidents in a forensic psychiatric population: An exploratory study of motivational factors. *Journal of Forensic Psychiatry & Psychology, 25*(6), 714–732.

Janis, I. L. (1984). The patient as decision maker. In W. D. Gentry (Ed.), *Handbook of behavioural medicine.* (pp. 326–368). Guilford Press.

Kroner, D. G. (2012). *Service user involvement in risk assessment and management: The transition inventory.* Criminal Behaviour and Mental Health.

Langan, J. (2008). Involving mental health service users considered to pose a risk to other people in risk assessment. *Journal of Mental Health, 17*(5), 471–481.

Lee, J. E. (2013). Mad as hell: The objectifying experience of symbolic violence. In B. A. LeFrançois, R. Menzies, & G. Reaume (Eds.), *Mad matters: A critical reader in Canadian mad studies* (pp. 105–121). Canadian Scholars' Press.

Leflot, G., Onghena, P., & Colpin, H. (2010). Teacher–child interactions: Relations with children's self-concept in second grade. *Infant and Child Development, 19*(4), 385–405.

Liegghio, M. (2013). A denial of being: Psychiatrization as epistemic violence. In B. A. LeFrançois, R. Menzies, & G. Reaume (Eds.), *Mad matters: A critical reader in Canadian mad studies* (p. 122). Canadian Scholars' Press.

Mental Health Act. (1983). *UK Public General Acts.* The Stationary Office.

Menzies Lyth, I. (1960). A case-study of the functioning of social systems as a defence against anxiety: A report on a study of the nursing service of a general hospital. *Human Relations, 13*, 95–121.

Miller Tate, A. J. (2019). Contributory injustice in psychiatry. *Journal of Medical Ethics, 45*, 97–100.

Morgan, J. F. (2007). *Giving up the culture of blame: Risk assessment and risk management in psychiatric practice.* Royal College of Psychiatrists.

Nedopil, N., Gunn, J., & Thomson, L. (2012). Teaching forensic psychiatry in Europe. *Criminal Behaviour and Mental Health, 22*, 238–246.

OALD. (2020). *Definition of marginalise verb from the Oxford advanced learner's dictionary.* www.oxfordlearnersdic tionaries.com/definition/english/marginalize

Parrott, F. R. (2010). Real relationships: Sociable interaction, material culture and imprisonment in a secure psychiatric unit. *Culture, Medicine and Psychiatry, 34*(4), 555–570.

Paulus, M. P. (2017). Evidence-based pragmatic psychiatry – a call to action. *JAMA Psychiatry, 74*(12), 1185–1186.

Pelto-Piri, V., Kjellin, L., Hylén, U., Valenti, E., & Priebe, S. (2019). *Different forms of informal coercion in psychiatry: A qualitative study.* BMC Research Notes.

Pohlhaus, G., Jr. (2012). Relational knowing and epistemic injustice: Toward a theory of willful hermeneutical ignorance. *Hypatia, 27,* 715–735. https://doi.org/10.1111/j.1527-2001.2011.01222.x

Ray, I., & Simpson, A. I. F. (2019). Shared risk formulation in forensic psychiatry. *The Journal of the American Academy of Psychiatry and the Law, 47*(1). doi:10.29158/JAAPL.00381319

Reynolds, L. M., Jones, J. C., Davies, J., Freeth, D., & Heyman, B. (2014). Playing the game: Service users' management of risk status in a UK medium secure forensic mental health service. *Health, Risk and Society, 3,* 199–209.

Ruszczynski, S. (2010), Becoming neglected: A perverse relationship to care. *British Journal of Psychotherapy, 26,* 22–32. https://doi.org/10.1111/j.1752-0118.2009.01153.x

Ryan, R. M., & Deci, E. L. (2008). A self-determination theory approach to psychotherapy: The motivational basis for effective change. *Canadian Psychology, 49,* 186–193.

Sanati, A., & Kyratsous, M. (2015). Epistemic injustice in assessment of delusions. *Journal of Evaluation in Clinical Practice, 21*(3), 479–485.

Stacey, G., Felton, A., Morgan, A., Stickley, T., Willis, M., Diamond, B., & Dumenya, J. (2016). A critical narrative analysis of shared decision-making in acute inpatient mental health care. *Journal of Interprofessional Care, 30*(1), 35–41.

Stiggelbout, A. M., Pieterse, A. H., & De Haes, J. C. J. M. (2015). Shared decision making: Concepts, evidence, and practice. *Patient Education and Counseling, 98*(10), 1172–1179.

To, W. T., Vanheule, S., De Smet, S., & Vandevelde, S. (2015, December). The treatment perspectives of mentally ill offenders in medium- and high-secure forensic settings in flanders. *International Journal of Offender Therapy and Comparative Criminology, 59*(14), 1605–1622. doi:10.1177/0306624X14566355. Epub 2015 Jan 12. PMID: 25583981.

Treichler, E. B., & Spaulding, W. D. (2017). Beyond shared decision-making: Collaboration in the age of recovery from serious mental illness. *American Journal of Orthopsychiatry, 87*(5), 567–574.

Urheim, R., Rypdal, K., Palmstierna, T., & Mykletun, A. (2011). Patient autonomy versus risk management: A case study of change in a high security forensic psychiatric ward. *The International Journal of Forensic Mental Health, 10*(1), 41–51.

Van Heijst, A. (2011). *Professional loving care. An ethical view of the health care Sector.* Peeters.

Vazire, S., & Mehl, M. R. (2008). Knowing me, knowing you: The accuracy and unique predictive validity of self-ratings and other-ratings of daily behavior. *Journal of Personality and Social Psychology, 95,* 1202–1216.

Wardrope, A. (2015). Medicalization and epistemic injustice. *Medicine, Health Care and Philosophy, 18*(3), 341–352.

Wilkie, T., Penney, S. R., Fernane, S., & Simpson, A. (2014). Characteristics and motivations of absconders from forensic mental health services: A case-control study. *BMC Psychiatry, 14*(1), 1–13.

Žižek, S. (2008). *Violence: Six sideways reflections* (p. 62). Profile Books.

Chapter 16

Including older forensic service users in research

Renske Visser, Janet Parrott, Fiona Houben and Douglas MacInnes

Introduction

With populations ageing worldwide, it is not surprising to observe an increase in the number of older patients in secure mental health facilities. The proportion of people over 50 in forensic mental health services is rising, although older adults remain a minority in forensic mental health care overall (Parrott et al., 2019). Older adults may be placed in specialist older adult forensic settings or in forensic mental health services that accommodate service users of widely differing age. Due to the small numbers of women in forensic settings, and the lack of specialist services, older women are most likely to use generic forensic services. To date, little is known about the similarities and differences between older women and men in forensic mental health. The ageing population poses many interesting questions regarding the purpose of these types of facilities and whether they can meet the needs of older forensic service users. Additionally, assumptions about the characteristics of 'older people' and 'forensic service users' are challenged by the presence of older service users in forensic wards. For example, forensic service users are stereotypically envisioned to be 'young' people, and 'older people' are often depicted as 'vulnerable' and not as serious offenders (Yorston, 2013).

In our research, we were interested in understanding the lived experience of growing older in secure forensic settings, as it is important to understand ageing experiences from the perspective of older service users themselves. To this end, we conducted ethnographic research that consisted of both interviews and observations to explore the everyday lived reality of older people in a secure hospital. Studies involving older forensic service users have used age thresholds ranging from 50 to 65 years and above (De Smet et al., 2010). In our study, we used the lower age threshold of 50, following the most common age threshold used in ageing research in secure environments (Merkt et al., 2020). This was also deliberate to be able to include as many people as possible in this research.

In this chapter, we will describe our research. Fifteen older men and women aged 50–71 years in a low- and medium-secure unit in the southeast of England participated. In this study, service users expressed themselves in their own words and shared aspects of their everyday lives. Data were combined to analyse the impact of being an older adult in a forensic mental health setting, providing key insights into the visibility and marginalisation of their needs and wishes.

Terminology used to describe people with severe mental health problems or older people matters, as it can shape the way these groups are perceived in wider society. In this chapter, we deliberately use the word 'older' and not 'old' to describe older forensic service users. Referring to 'the old' or 'elderly' is stigmatising and invokes images of frail people (Avers et al., 2011); these terms do not account for the diversity and the range of lived experience

DOI: 10.4324/9781003184768-21

older people may have (Degnen, 2012). Terms like 'the elderly' point to the negative attitude people have towards ageing and later life and reinforce ageist assumptions. Importantly, it is not a term that older people use to describe themselves (Kaufman, 1986; Avers et al., 2011; Degnen, 2012). While the terminology used to describe older people is changing, concepts like 'elderly' are still part of a needs assessment for older people: e.g., the Camberwell Assessment Needs for the Elderly (see Di Lorito et al., 2017). Intentional or not, these terms frame older age in a negative way and imply dependency and frailty.

There are many categories to distinguish people in younger life, such as toddlers, teens, tweens, young adults, etc., yet there is a paucity of categories to account for the diversity in later life (Hockey & James, 2003; Degnen, 2007).

> Being old has come to be associated with predominantly negative stereotypes – decline, loss, and disease. Because all of the assumed losses – reduced sensory awareness, deaths among relatives and friends, lowered economic status due to retirement, for example – aging is often viewed as negative and problematic.
>
> (Kaufman, 1986, p. 4)

The experience of later life is much more complex than just a series of losses. 'Old age' is relational and dependent on other people as there can only be 'older' people if 'younger' people exist (Degnen, 2012). In our study, this relationality particularly came to the fore in one of the women's wards, where one service user was in her 70s whereas the other service users were teenagers or 20-somethings. The stark difference in chronological age made her 'older', yet, hypothetically, if she would have been living in a nursing home, she would have been considered 'young'.

The majority of older forensic service users in in-patient settings have entered care as a 'younger' person (i.e., < 50) and become 'older' (i.e., age 50 and over) while residing in secure mental health care with long lengths of stay and chronic of mental health needs. A small group of older service users have become mentally ill and offended for the first time in older age, however (O'Sullivan & Chesterman, 2007).

Who are older service users?

Chronological age as a measure of 'oldness' has been critiqued for a long time in disciplines such as gerontology and anthropology, as it does not adequately capture the range of experiences people with the same chronological age have (Degnen, 2012; Bytheway, 2005; Conway & Hockey, 1998). In the census of the United Kingdom, someone aged 65 and over is considered an 'older person' (ONS, 2013). In prison and secure forensic care, the age threshold is considerably lower as someone is considered 'older' aged 50 and over (Public Health England, 2017).

There are several reasons for this lower age threshold. First, it has been suggested that people with severe mental health problems have a life expectancy that is 15–20 years lower compared with the general public (Ilyas et al., 2017; Public Health England, 2017). One of the reasons for this is that people with severe mental health problems are already at a greater risk of developing cardiovascular problems and some antipsychotics increase this risk (Ilyas et al., 2017). Second, it has been suggested that people in secure environments experience so-called 'accelerated ageing'. Jewkes (2018, p. 230) has noted that custodial environments are very stressful places and can affect the process of ageing: 'So severe can be the effects of these stressors that serving a long-term custodial sentence has not only been shown to accelerate the ageing process but has been analogously compared to being diagnosed with a chronic or terminal illness'. Cipriani et al. (2017) argue that issues preceding imprisonment such as low economic status and poor health-seeking behaviour as well as being in a secure environment all add to the disparity between chronological and biological age for people in secure environments.

Research on older forensic service users

Research on older forensic service users has been concerned with whether services available are appropriate (De Smet et al., 2015; Di Lorito et al., 2017; Di Lorito et al., 2018), whether specialist services need to be developed for this group (Nnatu et al., 2005; Tomar et al., 2005; Shah, 2008; Yorston, 1999; Natarajan & Mulvana, 2017). Additionally, some studies have been interested in the lived experience of older forensic service users (De Smet et al., 2015; Di Lorito et al., 2018; Visser et al., 2019). In prison research, it has been suggested that the needs of older people are not being met because of so-called 'institutional thoughtlessness' (Crawley, 2005). In other words, prisons are not designed with the needs of older people in mind. Prisons follow certain regimes, and these can negatively impact the experience of older people in prison in unique ways. There is a paucity of research concerned with exploring institutional thoughtlessness in forensic secure environments, yet the concept of institutional thoughtlessness can similarly be applied within secure mental health as it is important to understand to what extent secure mental health facilities are, intentionally or not, thoughtless towards older service users. Similar to prisons, secure forensic units are often designed with younger bodies in mind.

There have been several retrospective studies conducted to explore the demographic, psychiatric, and criminological characteristics of older forensic service users (Coid et al., 2002; O'Sullivan & Chesterman, 2007; Das et al., 2011; Curtice et al., 2003). These studies tell us little about the individual lived experience of older forensic service users. To understand the complexity and the diversity of experiences of older forensic service users, it is important to include these voices in research.

A small number of qualitative studies examined the experience of older forensic service users. A study conducted in a high secure hospital in England consisted of interviews with twelve service users aged 60 and over and 21 members of staff (Graeme Yorston & Taylor, 2009). This research suggests that older forensic service users have different needs compared to younger service users in terms of physical health and quality of life needs. Furthermore, older service users mentioned that their lived experience of being in a secure mental health hospital was unique compared to older people living in the community:

> It would be difficult to reminisce with people of the same age outside – I've always been inside, so I haven't got the normal life experiences. . .. I like to keep mentally active. I wouldn't want to mix with older people in the community, they sit around and reminisce about the war. (Hugh, patient)
>
> (Graeme Yorston & Taylor, 2009, p. 264).

A Belgian study, based on interviews with eight older forensic service users, showed the complexity of the trajectories of this group (De Smet et al., 2015). Participants revealed complicated life stories with periods of being in prison, in secure mental healthcare, and independent living. The movement and various living circumstances of older forensic service users are important to take into account; while there might be people who grow older within an institutional environment, equally there are people who experience the revolving door of community and institutional living.

Another English study with fifteen older service users (aged 50 and over) showed the complexity and diversity of ageing in secure environments. When asked about developing services specifically for older service users, answers were mixed. Some welcomed this:

> I imagine it'd be a lot quieter. And I can see better conversation, rather than shouting all over the place.
>
> (Participant in: Di Lorito et al., 2018, p. 949)

Whereas others noted:

> I think wards need to be like a community, and in a community, you get people of all ages.
>
> (Participant in: Di Lorito et al., 2018, p. 949)

This difference was also found in our study. Participants, in principle, were in favour of wards for older people but when asked if they would want to move on to an older age-specific ward, some people noted that those wards would be good for 'other people' and not for them. Based on their study, Di Lorito et al. (2018, p. 953) suggest four areas for the development of services for older service users, highlighting the need for 'age-sensitive' approaches:

1) Age-inclusive educational, occupational, vocational, recreational, and social activities
2) Age-relevant treatment and therapy (e.g., cognitive stimulation therapy, speech and language therapy, and arts therapy)
3) Improved accessibility, including modifications to environments (e.g., shower chairs and handrails) and flexible regimes (e.g., dedicated hours for phone calls)
4) Personalised packages (e.g., for discharge, social care, and sexual expression).

These suggestions point to where the ongoing development of services should be for older forensic service users. Furthermore, these qualitative studies all reveal there is no singular 'older forensic service user'. Services and care provisions need to be tailored to individuals and not necessarily to specific age groups.

Our study

We conducted a qualitative service evaluation in a medium- and low-secure hospital in a National Health Service (NHS) trust (healthcare provider) in the South of England. Twenty-five per cent of inpatients (40 of a total of 163) detained at the Trust between April 2017 and April 2018 were aged 50 years and over. Our research was ethnographic in nature, and 15 service users (aged 50–71) took part in semi-structured interviews and were asked to pick an activity that would be typical for their week, so that researcher Renske Visser could accompany them. Ethical approval was obtained from the Health Research Authority (Project number 844).

To get a broader sense of the lived experience of service users, Renske Visser attended both hospital-wide and individual ward community meetings as well as various hospital-wide activities such as a talent show and a food festival. Observational data and interview data formed the basis of our findings. We identified five themes in our research data: 1) age-related identities, 2) ward environments and age balance, 3) participation in activities, 4) management of physical health, and 5) aspirations for the future (Visser et al., 2019). We will consider these five themes.

Age-related identities

Most participants rejected the label of being older and were reluctant to be considered an older person. Some, like John, felt that coping with a mental illness and being on strong medication accelerated their physical ageing:

> I don't feel old in my mind. But I am in my body sometimes. I think it's not just about my age or anything I think it's for decades and decades of taking this medication because it's strong stuff (John, 50s).

(Visser et al., 2019, p. 3)

Our study also highlights the limits of chronological age as a marker of oldness. Patricia (50s), chronologically one of the youngest participants identified most strongly with being an older person, repeatedly stating she 'felt like an old woman'. Keith (70s), on the other hand, while chronologically one of the oldest participants did not think himself to be old. The individual lived experience of older forensic service users, similar to other studies in the general public, challenges assumptions about who is 'old', while chronological age is a commonly used marker for 'oldness' older people themselves might not adopt this identity of an 'older person'. The acceptance and rejection of the label of 'older person' are closely linked to wider societal trends of oldness being portrayed as negative and something to stave off and reject at all costs.

Ward environments and age balance

The social environment of the wards played an important role in the formation of friendships and feelings of social isolation. Ward composition varied widely and mattered for the development of social relationships. Particularly, on the two women wards, there were big age gaps between younger and older service users. One of the men's wards, over the past years, had evolved to be the ward for longer-term service users and thus housed many participants aged 50 and over. Some older service users felt they connected more with some of the staff, as they were chronologically closer to their age. They felt that they could have better conversations with staff members and some reported they 'did not understand these kids' sense of humour'.

Participation in activities

Five of the older service users had been in secure services for 20 years or more. They were the least likely to participate in ward activities and expressed strong feelings of boredom. The reasons for not participating were manifold; on the one hand, these service users expressed that they had 'done them all'; on the other hand, they felt some activities were 'childish'. Importantly, older forensic service users reported ambivalence about the way the hospital was able to cope with their increasing physical health problems. As one participant noted: 'There were a few teething problems because it is not a physical hospital, is it? It's a mental hospital'. There were sometimes tensions between service users and staff and the way physical health problems were being managed.

Management of physical health

Secure forensic hospitals are specialised in mental health. Older service users can have multiple physical health problems in addition to their mental health problems. This can be challenging for healthcare staff to manage, as one of our participants noted 'It is not a physical hospital is it, it is a mental hospital'. Keith (70s), chronologically the oldest participant, mentioned that he experienced several falls. Keith found that staff were panicking and overzealous in trying to manage the potential of him falling. Keith felt staff were overreacting, as the occasional tumble was just part of his everyday life. As a consequence, Keith was reluctant to report any physical health problems to staff as they would 'worry too much' and would try to micro-manage his movements

Aspirations for the future

Older service users face additional worries about growing older in relation to care pathways and their futures. The older people in our study had aspirations for the future that follows typical transitions as experienced by people living in the community. For example, people spoke about finding jobs or retiring once they would leave the secure unit. Hypothesising about the future was difficult as service users were uncertain if and when they would leave the unit and what their lives would look like beyond the walls of the unit.

Our study highlights the importance of acknowledging the diversity between older service users and how they experience life in a secure unit. Importantly, many of the participants had similar aspirations and worries about the future when compared to older people living in the community, such as worries about their own ageing body and ageing family members such as siblings and parents. While their lives are very much shaped by the environment of a secure ward, it is important to highlight and acknowledge these similarities.

Including older forensic service users in research

Our research with older service users showed the importance of *trust* and *time*. As we noted elsewhere; 'a multi-year research strategy, in which the researcher has time to build rapport and trust with participants, may be helpful in increasing participation' (Visser et al., 2019, p. 6). We interviewed and observed 15 service users. We had limited time and resources to conduct the research. While we were able to build relationships with a large proportion of the older service users, but for a small group of service users, there was not enough time to develop a relationship of trust. More time would have been needed to include them in the research. Relationship building tends to happen in shared spaces and attending community events such as a hospital-wide talent show, food events, and individual ward meetings helped to establish trust. Some older service users were sceptical of research in general; some were interested in taking part in an interview but would refuse to be interviewed on the scheduled date.

While researcher Renske Visser had several informal conversations with older service users not included in the results, signing consent forms was a real barrier to including them. Their voices were captured in some of the fieldnotes, but as these people had not given written consent, these notes were not included in the analysis. During the observational periods of the study, the presence of Renske Visser was appreciated by service users as she 'did not want anything' from the older service users beyond spending time together. Participants were aware that this spending time together was part of the research but did not experience this as such. Future researchers might build these moments of spending time together into their research methodology to break down barriers between older service users and researchers.

That it takes time to develop relationships with participants is not unique to older service users but still important to take into account (Völlm et al., 2017). Service users had seen many people (both staff and other service users) come and go, and they had knowledge of various initiatives that had started and subsequently disappeared. This research project was again a temporal thing, that some did not see the point to invest in. Furthermore, some older service users were difficult to reach as their daily routine did not match the routine of the researcher. As our inclusion criterion was age-based, this caused a division as well, as various younger service users were very keen to be included in the research and very disappointed that they were perceived to be 'too young'.

Collaboration with older service users

One way to overcome the barrier of lack of engagement with research or distrust in researchers would be to involve older service users in the design and conduct of studies. Involving people with lived experience is increasingly a priority both in healthcare research (Hovén et al., 2020; Brett et al., 2014) as well as research in custodial settings (Buck et al., 2020). The involvement of forensic service users in the design, conduct, analysis, and dissemination of research to date is limited (MacInnes et al., 2011; Coffey, 2006; Völlm et al., 2017). There are particular challenges in including forensic service users in research, including practical considerations in terms of reaching participants, complex power relationships that occur within secure settings, and issues around confidentiality and communication (Völlm et al., 2017). In our study, we invited two older service users to comment on our information sheets and interview schedule.

While in policy service users aged 50 and over are labelled 'older', this might not correspond with the subjective lived experience of service users themselves. Thus, it is important to not only bring in service users as advisors on research projects but include them in the design of studies as well. Some people in our study personally did not identify as being 'older' but were made 'older' by us as they fit in our research criteria. The service users were consulted to advise, but future research might benefit from a more collaborative or participatory approach throughout all stages of research. Many of the reflections of the research team revolved around how to engage some of the older service users reluctant to take part in this study. Involving service users in these conversations and potentially in the collection of data could be a way to build rapport. Involvement in research can be a powerful and empowering activity for service users which can bring fulfilment and could potentially elevate the boredom expressed by some service users. Some of our participants expressed being 'experts in their own mental health'. Being part of research could be an avenue to use this expertise for personal growth.

Conclusion

Older people in secure forensic settings are considered 'older' at a much younger chronological age compared to those people living in the community. This labelling might not match the lived experience of older service users themselves. This chapter has focused on the importance of qualitative research in understanding what it is like to grow older in a secure environment. It has also been suggested that including the experience of older service users in research as their lived experience challenges popular notions around who is considered 'older' and what a forensic service user looks like. We propose that the longer-term research and the involvement of older forensic service users in every stage of research can be a powerful way to reach participants that would otherwise not engage with research. More research is needed to unpack the complexities and overlap of mental health, ageing, and secure environments. It can be challenging and time-consuming to try to engage older forensic service users in research, but our research has shown that listening to the voices of those with lived experience can both be very meaningful and challenge stereotypical understandings of what it means to be an 'older service user'.

References

Avers, D., Brown, M., Chui, K. K., Wong, R. A., & Lusardi, M. (2011). Use of the term 'elderly.' *Journal of Geriatric Physical Therapy, 34*(4), 153–154. https://doi.org/10.1519/JPT.0b013e31823ab7ec.

Brett, J, Staniszewska, S., Mockford, C., Herron-Marx, S., Hughes, J., Tysall, C., Suleman, R., et al. (2014). A systematic review of the impact of patient and public involvement on service users, researchers and communities. *Patient, 7*, 387–395. https://doi.org/10.1007/s40271-014-0065-0.

Buck, G., Harriot, P., Ryan, K., Ryan, N., & Tomczak, P. (2020). All our justice: People with convictions and 'participatory' criminal justice. In *The Routledge handbook of service user involvement in human services research and education* (pp. 285–295). Routledge.

Bytheway, B. (2005). Ageism and age categorization. *Journal of Social Issues, 61*(2), 361–374. http://doi.wiley.com/10.1002/psp.1994.

Cipriani, G., Danti, S., Carlesi, C., & Di Fiorino, M. (2017). Old and dangerous: Prison and dementia. *Journal of Forensic and Legal Medicine, 51*, 40–44. https://doi.org/10.1016/j.jflm.2017.07.004.

Coffey, M. (2006). Researching service user views in forensic mental health: A literature review. *Journal of Forensic Psychiatry & Psychology, 17*(1), 73–107. https://doi.org/10.1080/14789940500431544.

Coid, J., Fazel, S., & Kahtan, N. (2002). Elderly patients admitted to secure forensic psychiatry services. *Journal of Forensic Psychiatry, 13*(2), 416–427. https://doi.org/10.1080/09585180210154470.

Conway, S., & Hockey, J. (1998). Resisting the 'mask' of old age? The social meaning of lay health beliefs in later life. *Ageing and Society, 18*, 469–494.

Crawley, E. (2005). Institutional thoughtlessness in prisons and its impacts on the day-to-day prison lives of elderly men. *Journal of Contemporary Criminal Justice, 21*(4), 350–363. https://doi.org/10.1177/1043986205282018.

Curtice, M., Parker, J., Schembri Wismayer, F., & Tomison, A. (2003). The elderly offender: An 11-year survey of referrals to a regional forensic psychiatric service. *Journal of Forensic Psychiatry and Psychology, 14*(2), 253–265. https://doi.org/10.1080/1478994031000077989.

Das, K., Murray, K., Driscoll, R., & Rao Nimmagadda, S. (2011). A comparative study of healthcare and placement needs among older forensic patients in a high secure versus medium/low secure hospital setting. *International Psychogeriatrics, 23*(5), 847–848. https://doi.org/10.1017/S1041610210002231.

Degnen, C. (2007). Minding the gap: The construction of old age and oldness amongst peers. *Journal of Aging Studies, 21*(1), 69–80.

Degnen, C. (2012). *Ageing selves and the everyday life in the North of England. Years in the making.* Manchester University Press.

De Smet, S., Vandevelde, S., Verté, D., & Broekaert, E. (2010). What is currently known about older mentally ill offenders in forensic contexts: Results from a literature review. *International Journal of Social Sciences and Humanity Studies, 2*(1), 127–135.

De Smet, S., Van Hecke, N., Verté, D., Broekaert, E., Ryan, D., & Vandevelde, S. (2015). Treatment and control: A qualitative study of older mentally ill offenders perceptions on their detention and care trajectory. *International Journal of Offender Therapy and Comparative Criminology, 59*, 964–985.

Hockey, J., & James, A. (2003). *Social identities across the life course.* Palgrave Macmillan.

Hovén, E., Eriksson, L., Månsson D'Souza, A., Sörensen, J., Hill, D., Viklund, C., Wettergren, L., & Lampic, C. (2020). What makes it work? Exploring experiences of patient research partners and researchers involved in a long-term co-creative research collaboration. *Research Involvement and Engagement, 6*(1), 1–12. https://doi.org/10.1186/s40900-020-00207-4.

Ilyas, A., Chesney, E., & Patel, R. (2017). Improving life expectancy in people with serious mental illness: Should we place more emphasis on primary prevention? *The British Journal of Psychiatry : The Journal of Mental Science, 211*(4), 194–197. https://doi.org/10.1192/bjp.bp.117.203240.

Jewkes, Y. (2018). Just design: Healthy prisons and the architecture of hope. *Australian and New Zealand Journal of Criminology, 51*(3), 319–338. https://doi.org/10.1177/0004865818766768

Kaufman, S. (1986). *The ageless self. Sources of meaning in late life.* University of Wisconsin Press.

Lorito, C. Di, Castelletti, L., Tripi, G., Gloria Gandellini, M., Dening, T., & Völlm, B. (2017). The individual experience of aging patients and the current service provision in the context of Italian forensic psychiatry: A case study. *Journal of Forensic Nursing, 13*(3), 118–125. https://doi.org/10.1097/JFN.0000000000000163

Lorito, C. Di, Dening, T., & Völlm, B. (2018). Ageing in forensic psychiatric secure settings: The voice of older patients. *Journal of Forensic Psychiatry and Psychology*, *29*(6), 934–960. https://doi.org/10.1080/1478 9949.2018.1513545.

MacInnes, D., Beer, D., Keeble, P., Rees, D., & Reid, L. 2011. "Service-user involvement in forensic mental health care research: Areas to consider when developing a collaborative study. *Journal of Mental Health*, *20*(5), 464–472. https://doi.org/10.3109/09638231003728109.

Merkt, H., Haesen, S., Meyer, L., Kressig, R. W., Elger, B. S., & Wangmo, T. (2020). Defining an age cut-off for older offenders: A systematic review of literature. *International Journal of Prisoner Health*. Emerald Group Publishing Ltd. https://doi.org/10.1108/IJPH-11-2019-0060

Natarajan, M., & Mulvana, S. (2017). New horizons: Forensic mental health services for older people, *23*, 44–53. https://doi.org/10.1192/apt.bp.113.012021

Nnatu, I. O., Mahomed, F., & Shah, A. (2005). Is there a need for elderly forensic psychiatric services ? *Medicine, Science and the Law*, *45*(2), 154–160.

O'Sullivan, P. C. J., & Chesterman, L. P. (2007). Older adult patients subject to restriction orders in England and Wales: A cross-sectional survey. *Journal of Forensic Psychiatry and Psychology*, *18*(2), 204–220. https://doi.org/10.1080/14789940601110906

ONS. (2013). *What does the 2011 census tell us about older people?* Department of Health.

Parrott, J. M., Houben, F. R., Visser, R. C., & Macinnes, D. L. (2019). Mental health and offending in older people: Future directions for research. *Journal of Criminal Behaviour and Mental Health*, *29*(4), 218–226.

Public Health England. (2017). *Health and social care needs assessments of the older prison population a guidance document about public health England*. Public Health England.

Shah, A. (2008). Can a case be made for developing specialist forensic geriatric psychiatry services ? *The Open Law Journal*, *1*, 1–5. https://doi.org/10.2174/1874950X00801010001

Smet, S. De, Van Hecke, N., Verté, D., Broekaert, E., Ryan, D., & Vandevelde, S. (2015). Treatment and control: A qualitative study of older mentally ill offenders perceptions on their detention and care trajectory. *International Journal of Offender Therapy and Comparative Criminology*, *59*(9), 964–985. https://doi.org/10.1177/0306624X14521129

Tomar, R., Treasaden, I. H., & Shah, A. K. (2005). Is there a case for a specialist forensic psychiatry service for the elderly? *International Journal of Geriatric Psychiatry*, *20*(1), 51–56. https://doi.org/10.1002/gps.1247

Visser, R. C., MacInnes, D., Parrott, J., & Houben, F. (2019). Growing older in secure mental health care: The user experience. *Journal of Mental Health* Online Fir. https://doi.org/10.1080/09638237.2019.1630722

Völlm, B., Foster, S., Bates, P., & Huband, N. (2017). How best to engage users of forensic services in research: Literature review and recommendations. *International Journal of Forensic Mental Health*, *16*(2), 183–195. https://doi.org/10.1080/14999013.2016.1255282

Yorston, G. (1999). Aged and dangerous: Old age forensic psychiatry. *British Journal of Psychiatry*, *174*(3), 193–195.

Yorston, G. (2013). Crime, mental illness, and older people. In T. Dening & A. Thomas (Eds.), *Oxford textbook of old age psychiatry* (pp. 785–797). Oxford University Press.

Yorston, G., & Taylor, P. J. (2009). Older patients in an English high security hospital: A qualitative study of the experiences and attitudes of patients aged 60 and over and their care staff in Broadmoor Hospital. *Journal of Forensic Psychiatry & Psychology*, *20*(2), 255–267. https://doi.org/10.1080/14789940802327259

Chapter 17

Men in 'Limbo'

Masculinities in medium-secure care in Scotland

Christine Haddow

Introduction

Since their inception, medium-secure settings have garnered modest research interest. Yet, in spite of their position as a steppingstone from in-patient care to the community, accounts of the lived experience of those detained in this setting are lacking. This chapter will present the case for a criminological approach to deepen understanding of secure forensic care. Findings from qualitative, biographical interviews with male patients in a medium-secure forensic psychiatric hospital in Scotland will provide insights through the lens of masculinity. In doing so, it will illuminate how masculinities are constructed and operate within this setting, arguing that medium security undermines and marginalises pre-institutional masculinities, which were often synonymous with violence. The chapter will therefore give a voice to a marginalised population – men in medium-secure care in Scotland – and provide insights for practice based on their accounts while evidencing the utility of qualitative approaches to psychiatric research contexts.

Medium-secure care in Scotland

The Forensic Mental Health Services Managed Care Network's *Matrix of Security* (2004) defined standards across high-, medium-, and low-secure settings in Scotland (Crichton, 2009). High security is 'the level of security necessary only for those patients who pose a grave and immediate risk to others if at large' (Forensic Mental Health Services Managed Care Network, 2004, p. 21) and, in Scotland, is provided by the State Hospital at Carstairs. Medium-secure units emerged from a need to provide treatment settings for those who pose an insufficient risk for high-secure conditions but require restrictions beyond low-secure or open wards. Until the late 90s, a consensus remained that local medium-secure units were unnecessary in Scotland, leaving the nation comparatively slower than England and Wales to establish these units (Gow et al., 2010; Nelson, 2003). The first of three such facilities, the Orchard Clinic in Edinburgh, opened in 2000. The Mental Health (Care and Treatment) (Scotland) Act 2003 created a right of appeal against excessive security, establishing the principle that individuals should be detained in the least restrictive setting possible. Of the first 100 appeals, 44% were decided in the patient's favour, further cementing the need for medium-secure services (Bennett et al., 2013).

There are approximately 140 medium-secure forensic beds available across the three Scottish units, a relatively small patient population. Gow et al. (2010) provided a demographic overview of the Orchard Clinic during its first five years, highlighting that the population was overwhelmingly male (87.2%), in line with the wider secure forensic population in the

DOI: 10.4324/9781003184768-22

United Kingdom (Hill et al., 2019). Patients were generally referred directly from court or high-secure settings, and reasons for admission were primarily related to violence in the community or in a hospital context. Further patient characteristics included violence (perpetration and victimisation), substance misuse, past institutional care, poor interpersonal relationships, and low educational attainment. A two-year follow-up of patients discharged from medium-secure care into the community, other hospital settings, or prison found that 4.2% committed serious violent offences during this period, with a further 40% committing more than 100 minor offences (Ho et al., 2009). Overall, medium-secure settings are tasked with the care of a cohort of men with histories of violence who may pose an ongoing risk, yet who have also experienced multiple forms of deprivation and marginalisation across the life course.

The *Matrix of Security* (Forensic Mental Health Services Managed Care Network, 2004) identifies three forms of security in forensic settings: environmental security, involving physical measures; procedural security, pertaining to practices in place to ensure the effective functioning of the unit and its physical security; and relational security, concerning the quality of care. Medium-secure units are characterised by their decreased physical and procedural security, for example, the lack of a perimeter fence, while still requiring high standards of relational security between staff and patients. Also central is embeddedness in the community, with all three Scottish sites sitting within the grounds of existing hospitals which serve the local area. There is an increased emphasis on 'testing out', via a system of escorted visits and leave from the hospital, with medium security acting as a final step in many patients' recovery before return to the community.

The inception of medium-secure hospitals has therefore created an arguably unique environment, with patients existing between secure care and the community. This state of existence between spaces and, crucially, identities is often described as 'liminality' (Turner, 1967). This concept has been applied to consider the particularities of the lived experiences of criminal justice institutions (Jewkes, 2011; Wooff & Skinns, 2017). Within this chapter, the concept of liminality will be drawn upon to illustrate aspects of life in secure care and the particular ways in which being in 'limbo' in this setting shapes masculine identities.

Experiences of secure care

While the development and characteristics of medium-secure settings are relatively well documented, studies have also examined risk assessment approaches, length of stay, violence, and recidivism in this context (Coid et al., 2001, 2007; Edworthy & Völlm, 2016; Hinsby & Baker, 2004; Khiroya et al., 2009; Shah et al., 2011). Where attention has turned to the service user experience in forensic and other inpatient settings, the literature suggests relationships with staff, autonomy, and being informed about care arrangements are central to a positive experience (Hanson, 2003; Hopkins et al., 2009; Howard et al., 2003; Kuosmanen et al., 2006).

It is perhaps unsurprising, given the histories of violence which are common among patients in this setting, that some attention has alighted on responses to aggression and how these are experienced in secure care. Seclusion and manual restraint for the purpose of administering medication are not unique to forensic settings but are often used there (Stewart et al., 2009). For patients, this can result in increased distress, embarrassment, anger, and vulnerability, which may lead to resistance and disassociation from the event itself (Macpherson et al., 2005; Wynn, 2004).

While the earlier provides some insight into how patients experience secure care, emphasising the significance of the emotional impact of this setting and regime, contextualised accounts of life in secure care remain scarce. There is a lack of qualitative research to give a voice to this population. The remainder of this chapter will make a case for a criminological perspective in forensic secure care and provide insight from a study that adopted such an approach, to illustrate the lived experiences of men in medium-secure care in Scotland and masculinities in this context.

The need for a criminological perspective

Calls have been made for the inclusion of criminological and sociological approaches in forensic psychiatry. Silver (2006) proposed that research has focused too singularly on the relationship between mental illness and violence:

> A research framework is needed that looks beyond mental disorder as the primary cause of and solution to the problem of violence. Instead, we need research aimed at understanding both the clinical *and criminological* risk factors.
>
> (p. 689).

While Silver refers to the capacity of criminology to provide a more nuanced understanding of the intricate associations between mental disorder and violence, the discipline also has more to offer in the context of secure care. As a field of study which brings together diverse perspectives from sociology, psychology, law, and beyond, to address problems of crime, criminology can provide an integrative approach to addressing questions that arise in this setting. A well-established body of work within criminology charts the sociology of penal institutions and their populations, citing the impact of these establishments on identity, power structures that operate within, and how these are adapted to and navigated (Cohen & Taylor, 1972; Crewe, 2009; Goffman, 1968; Sykes, 1958). While Goffman's (1968) seminal work *Asylums* examined power and institutionalisation within the psychiatric hospital and other 'total institutions', a more recent sociology of secure forensic care remains absent from the literature. Moreover, criminology's tradition of critical enquiry, which explores 'hidden' populations and challenges traditional narratives about crime (Scraton, 2007), and the innovative methodological approaches that have developed through the discipline leave it well suited to an exploration of the experience of marginalised groups in secure care.

Masculinities in secure care

The research that forms the basis of this chapter advances from the aforementioned assertions. It has focused on a concept that has gained prominence in criminological literature – masculinity – as a means to better understand the experiences and identities of men in secure forensic care.

Criminology has long acknowledged gender differences in the perpetration of crime, in particular that violence 'always has been highly gendered behaviour' (Wiener, 2006, p. 2). Frameworks of gender have shifted from reductive notions of two oppositional sex roles based on biological categorisation, to position masculinity as an identity that is constructed and achieved through interaction (West & Zimmerman, 1987). One model, Connell's 'hegemonic masculinity' (Connell, 1987, 2005; Connell & Messerschmidt, 2005) has gained particular prominence within the field and forms the conceptual basis of the present study. The theory adopts a hierarchical model, acknowledging multiple masculinities within society, with hegemonic masculinity at its peak, typically characterised by dominance, physical strength and normative heterosexuality. These characteristics imply violence as part of this package, which Connell illustrates more explicitly:

> The relationship of men to hegemonic masculinity is often fraught, the enactment partial, contested and capable of shifting into violence.
>
> (Connell, 2002, p. 94)

Thus, violence becomes a way to 'do' masculinity in the absence of other means. While the nature of the association between aggression and maleness is contested, masculinity remains at the centre of criminology's attempts to better understand violence (Brookman, 2003; Gadd & Jefferson, 2011; Messerschmidt, 1993, 1995, 2000; Polk, 1994).

As a concept, masculinity has gained less traction in forensic psychiatry research. Variations have been noted between genders in their presentation of mental illness or perpetration of violence, yet this has rarely been explored in depth. For example, Teasdale et al. (2006) posit that 'fight or flight' stress coping mechanisms employed by males during acute psychosis explain increased violence in these circumstances, yet ultimately lacked the data to explore these 'mediating mechanisms' (ibid., p. 656) in greater detail. Searle et al.'s (2018, 2019) recent examination of masculinity among men with psychosis found that they tend not to aspire to hegemonic masculine norms such as power, dominance, and normative heterosexuality. Their research posits that psychological support while in secure care can foster openness and the development of supportive networks, resulting in more heterogeneous, pro-social masculine identities which may benefit the recovery process.

Masculinity is also a lens through which experiences within institutions of punishment, particularly the prison, have been examined. Prison masculinities are shaped by institutional power structures and constituted through interactions with staff and other inmates (Crewe, 2009; Evans & Wallace, 2008; Maycock & Hunt, 2018; Ricciardelli et al., 2015). Similarly, hegemonic masculinity has been cited as the foundation of hierarchical structures between prisoners, as males who conform to these ideals are dominant while those who do not are subordinated. Sim (1994) notes how this positions violence in prison as 'part of the normal routine which is sustained and legitimated by the wider culture of masculinity: the culture that condemns some acts of male violence but condones the majority of others' (p. 105). Equivalent sociological accounts of the secure hospital are scarce, and the same can be said of masculinity, in spite of the overwhelmingly male population (Gow, 2010).

Ultimately, a developed account of masculinities in secure care, and how they operate within and are constructed through this setting, appears warranted. If we consider defining features of the secure forensic care experience, such as dependence on others for basic needs or resources, being physically overpowered, and restriction of liberty, these are at stark odds with Connell's account of hegemonic masculinity. The negative experiences of these settings identified in the service user experience literature – such as feeling disempowered, uninformed, vulnerable, and unable to express anger – may reflect this. This study adopts a criminological approach to explore these issues, through qualitative research with men in medium-secure care in Scotland.

An empirical study of the lived experiences of men in forensic hospitals

Methods

The remainder of this chapter will draw on data from biographical interviews with 10 male forensic inpatients. Narrative interviews explored their life histories and institutional experiences, aiming to extract the interviewee's understanding of the experiences comprising their life – their 'narrative' – from their recounting of these events (Bamberg, 2011). The level of depth and flexibility in eliciting stories afforded by this method was crucial in this project and is well documented in criminological enquiry (Presser, 2009). The flexibility of this methodology was suited to the vulnerable sample, allowing interviews to be tailored to accommodate participants' needs. There is a potential for data to be limited by participants' recall, and a reliance on subjective, co-constructed accounts of the past which emerge through interviews (Slembrouck, 2015). Information provided in interviews was triangulated through a review of all participants' clinical notes, and attendance at clinical team meetings which provided further context about their experiences.

Participants were purposively recruited from one medium-secure unit in Scotland. Diagnoses among the sample included: schizophrenia (6); bipolar disorder (2); mood disorder (1); and schizophreniform disorder (1). Further inclusion criteria were being male, aged over 18, with a history of violence. Offending histories among the final sample varied and included a wide range of violence such as assault, fire raising, sexual violence, homicide, attempted murder, and breach of the peace.

Using a thematic analysis approach (Braun & Clarke, 2006), interview transcripts were carefully read, coded, and sorted into themes. This approach is interpretivist in nature, offering theoretical rather than statistical generalisation which may be transferable beyond the immediate sample (Flick, 2018). Samples of this size are not uncommon for qualitative studies and the data collected meets Dibley's (2011) standard of thematic saturation being both 'rich' in terms of the nuance and quality of the data, and 'thick' in terms of the quantity of narrative accounts generated.

Life in 'Limbo': the liminality of medium-secure care

Patients' accounts of life in medium-secure care and their adaptation to this setting provided insight into masculinities. All participants were subject to measures such as a Compulsion Order, which mandates detention in hospital indefinitely for the purpose of treatment under the Criminal Procedure (Scotland) Act and 1995 and the Mental Health (Care and Treatment) Scotland Act 2003. Their reflections therefore focused on indeterminacy and comments about the uncertainty stemming from having no anticipated date of discharge were common:

> It is a bit in limbo . . . It's hard for me to sort of really see how long that piece of string is.
>
> (E., 49)

> I had so much time before I was going to get out, I didn't know [when], it was a problem, it was depressing me.
>
> (C., 34)

In this sense, patients reaffirmed the suggestion made earlier in this chapter that the medium-secure setting is a liminal environment, where they existed between secure care and freedom for an undefined amount of time. Within this setting, participants cited increased freedoms and opportunities to lead a more 'normal' life:

> It's just like bein' in here, you take advantage of what you have, like privileges and things like that. Like, you can go away on passes. . . . It's like you try your best.
>
> (A., 54)

'Pass', as mentioned here, is a leave of absence into the community to test patients' readiness to return to this setting. This is not unique to medium security but is more routine here than in high secure hospitals, where any absence requires a minimum of two escorting staff (Forensic Mental Health Managed Care Network, 2004, p. 31). Some participants highlighted that they were often out of the unit for as much as eight hours per day. Patients often had one foot in the community and one in the hospital setting, and this liminality was a defining feature of life in secure care. Moreover, existing in this ongoing state of transition constrained the ways in which patients were able to do masculinity in this setting, as will be demonstrated in subsequent sections.

Identities in Secure Care: Diagnosis and Masculinity

As participants reflected on their life histories, their comments revealed their self-narratives. Prior to hospitalisation and in line with what is known about forensic patient populations (Gow et al., 2010), participants often recounted chaotic lives characterised by drug and alcohol misuse, fractured relationships with families and partners, and low educational attainment. For many, their identities in the community had been contingent upon violence:

> I jumped up and grabbed him and hit his head off a car . . .. At the time I was more . . . markin' out my territory sort of thing, tryin' to make a name for myself.
>
> (C., 34)

> I built up a reputation, then people were wary of me and never bothered me.
>
> (A., 54)

In line with criminological accounts, aggression and physical confrontation were a means of doing masculinity in the community for patients where other resources (e.g., socio–economic status and successful heterosexual relationships) failed (Messerschmidt, 1993).

A key factor shaping identities in the present context of secure care was the acceptance or denial of mental disorder. Of the interviewed patients, half accepted their diagnosis and an additional two patients suggested that, while they did not perceive themselves to suffer from a major mental illness, they had experienced at least one psychotic episode preceding their hospitalisation. For most patients, this period was the time when felt most unwell and their accounts often conveyed symptoms of active psychosis:

> I kept goin' on about the devil, god, that I was supposed tae do it and that, and that I can't remember doin' it, I was forced tae do [commit the offence]. . . . I just was that unwell.
>
> (A., 54)

Research documents the significant distress which accompanies acute psychotic episodes as outlined earlier (Appelbaum et al., 2000; Swanson et al., 2006). At the time of hospitalisation, most patients had also recently committed a serious violent offence, further adding to this:

> I have to say it was probably one of the worst times of my life . . . I was just overwhelmed with disgust at my actions and what I did, but then having that [illness] on top of my own disgust.
>
> (F., 32)

Conversely, three participants stated that they did not agree with the diagnoses made by clinicians. They asserted that the interpretation of past behaviour as symptomatic of mental illness was inaccurate, or represented an isolated incident:

> I've been consistent in this all the way through, I didn't really think I was delusional, how I acted – all I was trying to do was to highlight my grievances.
>
> (E., 49)

> I can't say it's an illness because I've only had one psychotic episode.
>
> (I., 19)

Individuals may be unaccepting of mental health diagnoses for varying reasons, including shame and stigma (Jones & Crossley, 2008; Saks, 2009). Speaking more directly about the issue of identity, one patient posited that his denial of mental illness was a conscious decision due to the expectations of his peers:

> If I was to fully accept that I'm a psychiatric patient. . . . I don't do that because it's not part of the character that my friends would know.
>
> (C., 34)

These comments also represent the affront that an admission of mental illness poses to masculinity. As Matza (1964) suggests, 'The idea of being sick or mixed up seems incongruous with the delinquent's traditional self-image of manly toughness and precocious independence' (p. 83). This is particularly significant when we consider the wealth of literature that posits an association between masculine attitudes and a lack of help-seeking behaviour in relation to mental health (McCusker & Galupo, 2011; Yousaf et al., 2015). A criminological perspective here helps us to understand how denial of mental illness is also an attempt to conform more closely to hegemonic ideals.

Doing masculinity in secure care: compliance and control

Patients adapted to this liminal environment and constructed masculine identities in the face of their diagnoses in two key ways: compliance with and rebellion against the institutional regime. These responses were consistent with their acceptance or denial of mental disorder. The 'accepters' tended to engage with treatment and therapeutic activities, understanding this as 'making the most' of their situation:

> I like to try to get as much quality as I can in a place.
>
> (A., 54)

> You can get involved in things when you want and how you want. You're living a more normal life and that's the best way, it relieves a lot of the tension.
>
> (E., 49)

The second comment here acknowledges an element of flexibility in medium security. While it was acknowledged that 'some guys just prefer to sleep all day' (A., 54), actively engaging in recovery was a means of taking ownership of life in secure care:

> It's kind of like you shape your own destiny here because the onus is on you.
>
> (F., 32)

For these patients, masculinities were constructed through a sense of agency in being the master of their own journey through recovery. Power and autonomy, central to hegemonic masculinities (Connell, 1987), are enacted in medium-secure care through a pro-active approach to recovery. This is not to suggest this agency is absolute. While on the surface, there is flexibility in the decision to comply, there was a pervasive undercurrent of scrutiny from various angles and a sense that freedoms were given or 'earned':

> They do individual self assessments for people and they say 'Right okay, this can happen and that can happen, you can have a laptop.
>
> (F., 32)

> They're trusting me to go out 15 minutes a day on my own.
>
> (H., 49)

The aforementioned experience echoes Crewe's (2011) account of the sociology of the prison, which cites 'tightness' as a relatively new penal pain. This soft yet coercive form of power, enacted through indeterminacy and increased monitoring and assessment, incites those within an institution to comply. It is particularly pronounced in the liminality of medium-secure care, where a lack of compliance is likely to prevent progression to the community. In relation to masculinities and how these are constructed within the medium-secure space, this process of subtle control serves to infantilise patients and marginalise hegemonic masculinities. The perception of self-determination within a coercive regime allows patients to 'do' masculinity in a way that is compliant, yet ultimately subject to concerns about gaining permission from staff members and the institution.

Doing masculinity in secure care: rebellion and violence

Patients who denied their mental illness diagnoses tended to – perhaps unsurprisingly – feel that their hospitalisation was not legitimate. They were less inclined to engage with treatment and comply with the conditions of medium security, holding a negative view of the institution:

INTERVIEWER: Is there anything you think is good about [hospital]?
D. (49): Not really, no. It's not a life, you're best being out of the hospital, in the community.

While disengagement with treatment is common in a hospital setting where individuals are acutely unwell, it can serve another purpose. Rebelling against the 'tightness' of the institution and the infantilisation process outlined earlier can be understood as an attempt to cling to pre-institutional masculine identities, of which autonomy was a key feature.

In its most serious form, this rebellion was enacted through violence. Disorder as a means of challenging an institution is well documented in criminological accounts of the prison (Sparks & Bottoms, 1995) and five participants had histories of such incidents in the hospital. Due to the closed nature of this environment, victims tended to be other patients or hospital staff. Violence between patients was generally accepted as a product of the volatility which often characterises mental illness and its symptoms:

> When I went into the State Hospital there was a guy – he was quite unwell – he sort of attacked me a couple of times. . . . I think it was just unfortunate that I was there at that time, you know.
>
> (E., 49)

In two incidents of violence perpetration described by patients, the victims were clinical staff members. Both incidents occurred in the context of patients' unhappiness with institutional management. Rather than resulting from acute illness, violence in these cases was employed as a response to unhappiness with procedures within the secure unit:

G. (39): It just aboot came tae a head. All ae the inmates and that, all the patients faced up tae the staff. . . . They were pinnin' folk doon and injectin' them

INTERVIEWER: So that was the restraint procedures, you weren't happy with them?

G.: Aye.

Although restraint is often necessary for the instance that a patient poses a risk to the safety of themselves or others, it is likely to be experienced as an act of hard power, and, as noted earlier in this chapter, elicit negative emotions. The loss of autonomy and physical domination which the procedure involves were highlighted as motivating factors for violence:

> They said 'we're going to inject you, we're going to do it', it wasn't 'you can have it if you want' . . . and that's why I went against them.
>
> (H., 49)

While power and physical strength are central features of hegemonic masculinity, the experiences outlined earlier are in direct opposition to these attributes. Violence in hospitals therefore appears to be a means of regaining the independence and control which is denied through such measures. Through a return to pre-institutional masculinities which were characterised by and constructed through violence, participants seek to reclaim a sense of power through this rebellion.

Power and hierarchy in the secure hospital

While the aforementioned sections outline the performance of masculinity in relation to the power of the institution, relationships and social structures between peers in medium security also warrant attention. As noted previously in this chapter, a wealth of literature outlines the social order and moral codes present among those in prison (Sykes, 1958; Sykes & Messinger, 1960; Crewe, 2009). These in turn reflect the hierarchical nature of the hegemonic masculinity framework, which posits dominant and subordinate masculinities. Within the medium-secure unit, participants' accounts suggested that they shared some of the views traditionally held by prisoners which can underpin the structuring of social life. This was evidenced in one patient's comments on his experiences of interacting with patients with convictions for sexual offences:

> I would call them [men with histories of sexual violence perpetration] lowlives, because it's a terrible thing to put a female through or a child through . . . I just, like, stayed out of their way and never really bothered them.
>
> (F., 32)

While F shared the negative attitudes towards this group, and this stigma is well documented within prison settings (Ievins & Crewe, 2015; Mann, 2012; van den Berg et al., 2018), there was no expectation of violence perpetration towards them or overt enforcement of these attitudes, as is common in prisons.

Instead, social structures between patients appeared to be less rigid than has been documented in the prison setting and reflected the challenge of living with others who are acutely unwell. Patients described particular individuals within the unit as having lower social status, rather than sub-populations or categories of patients:

A patient the other night, he was sitting shouting his mouth off at us all that somebody has been in his room slashing his CDs and that . . . I says 'Who the hell's going to go into your room and touch your CDs? It's all in your mind'. I ended up frustrated. (A., 54)

> It was just a petition that somebody wanted to put together . . . because people were strongly against the behaviours of this individual patient . . . I thought it was the right way to go about it, his behaviours were absolutely atrocious. . . . But you just have to tolerate it you know, but it's difficult when you're living in such a close environment with guys twenty-four-seven.
>
> (F., 32)

As reflected earlier, those with lower social status were generally acutely unwell and, as a result, had behaved disruptively within the secure unit. It is significant that in both of the incidents outlined earlier, violence was not employed as a tool to resolve conflict, and more formal measures were instead adapted to appeal to the institution. This is a divergence from masculine peer relations which characterised patients' pre-institutional lives, in which violence was a means of resolving conflicts.

Overall, the social structure outlined here diverges from traditional accounts of institutional power and signifies a move away from typically masculine peer relations. Aspects of 'the inmate code' (Sykes, 1958; Sykes & Messinger, 1960) may also exist in the secure hospital, yet a rigid hierarchy characterised by violence was not in evidence or enforced those in this setting. The continuous monitoring present within the hospital again appears to dissuade many within from aggressive behaviour and undermine these more typically masculine interactions between peers. The liminal nature of the hospital setting is likely a further contributing factor here, leading patients to enforce social norms in non-violent ways so as to avoid damaging their own progression out of secure care.

Conclusion

Through the application of a criminological approach that employed qualitative interview techniques, and by viewing the lived experience of medium-secure care through the lens of Connell's (1987, 2005) hegemonic masculinity, this chapter has illustrated key features of life in this setting. It has shed light on the impact of this liminal setting on identities, demonstrating how pre-institutional masculinities, often characterised by violence, are marginalised here. The 'soft power' of secure care which aligns with Crewe's (2009) concept of tightness, a feeling of monitoring and restriction from all sides, plays a role here. Through ongoing risk assessment and a system of permissions and perceived privileges, such as pass (leave) out of the unit, patients find themselves in a space that feels 'betwixt and between' (1967) secure care and the community. For many, the result is compliance with this coercion, in order to progress through the forensic secure care system. This results in the development of a masculine identity that prizes ownership of and dedication to recovery from mental disorder. For others, rebellion is an adaptation to this attempt to undermine features of hegemonic masculinity which are at odds with life in secure care, such as power and physical strength, and to reassert more subtle aspects such as autonomy. This often takes the form of violence as a means to 'do' masculinity in this setting in the absence of other resources. These active and agentic 'masculine' behaviours can be contrasted with other forms of behaviour that are not described by Connell as masculine, e.g., inactivity or a passive receipt of care. These adaptations are also in evidence when considering social structures between patients, which appear less hierarchical as a result of these restricted masculinities.

There are implications of this work for clinical practice. A heightened awareness of the implications of institutionalisation for traditional masculine identities can provide practitioners with an understanding of patients' adaptations to these settings. Clinicians should be made aware of how hospitalisation and particular practices, for example, restraint procedures, are perceived as challenges to masculinity. These insights leave practitioners better equipped to negotiate potentially volatile situations which could lead to violence, for example, through the development of de-escalation techniques that are cognisant not to undermine hegemonic traits. Similarly, masculinity could be capitalised on to support patients to engage with care and treatment, by framing engagement as resilience and ownership, rather than weakness. This approach has gained purchase in other contexts. For example, exploring the 'depleted masculinities' of refugee men in Canada, Affleck et al. (2018) highlight the need of this group to rebuild masculinities to support mental health and resilience, and how this can be achieved through activities such as community leadership. Similar principles apply in forensic settings and opportunities to do masculinity in these more pro-social contexts could be fostered.

This chapter has evidenced the capacity of criminology to provide new perspectives in secure forensic care. Further research that applies criminological and sociological concepts, such as gender and the sociology of the prison, to key issues in forensic psychiatry is needed. In addition, there is a need for further application of methodologies, such as qualitative interviewing and ethnographic approaches, which allow for contextualised understandings of the lived experience of mental disorder and secure care. Above all, research and practice in this area must remain cognisant that 'An illness and its symptoms do not occur in a vacuum' (Taylor et al., 1998, p. 224).

References

Affleck, W., Thamotharampillai, U., Jeyakumar, J., & Whitley, R. (2018). "If one does not fulfil his duties, he must not be a man": Masculinity, mental health and resilience amongst Sri Lankan Tamil refugee men in Canada. *Culture, Medicine & Psychiatry*, *42*(4), 840–861. https://doi-org.ezproxy.napier.ac.uk/10.1007/s11013-018-9592-9

Appelbaum, P. S., Robbins, P. C., & Monahan, J. (2000). Violence and delusions: Data from the Mac-arthur violence risk assessment study. *The American Journal of Psychiatry*, *157*(4), 566–572. https://doi.org/10.1176/appi.ajp.157.4.566

Bamberg, M. (2011). Who am I? Narration and its contribution to self and identity. *Theory & Psychology*, *21*(1), 3–24. https://doi.org/10.1177/0959354309355852

Bennett, D., Skilling, G., Brown, K., & Thomson, L. (2013). Appeals against detention in conditions of excessive security in Scotland. *The Journal of Forensic Psychiatry & Psychology*, *24*(3), 386–402. https://doi.org/10.1080/14789949.2013.795240

Braun, V., & Clarke, V. (2006). Using thematic analysis in psychology. *Qualitative Research in Psychology*, *3*(2), 77–101. https://doi.org/10.1191/1478088706qp063oa

Brookman, F. (2003). Confrontational and revenge homicides among men in England and Wales. *Australian & New Zealand Journal of Criminology*, *36*(1), 34–59. https://doi.org/10.1375/000486503764805275

Cohen, S., & Taylor, L. (1972). *Psychological survival: The experience of long-term imprisonment*. Penguin Books.

Coid, J., Hickey, N., Kahtan, N., Zhang, T., & Yang, M. (2007). Patients discharged from medium secure forensic psychiatry services: Reconvictions and risk factors. *British Journal of Psychiatry*, *190*(3), 223–229. https://doi.org/10.1192/bjp.bp.105.018788

Coid, J., Kahtan, N., Gault, S., Cook, A., & Jarman, B. (2001). Medium secure forensic psychiatry services: Comparison of seven English health regions. *British Journal of Psychiatry*, *178*(1), 55–61. https://doi.org/10.1192/bjp.178.1.55

Connell, R. W. (1987). *Gender and power: Society, the person and sexual politics*. Allen & Unwin.

Connell, R. W. (2002). On hegemonic masculinity and violence: Response to Jefferson and hall. *Theoretical Criminology*, *6*(1), 89–99. https://doi.org/10.1177/136248060200600104

Connell, R. W. (2005). *Masculinities* (2nd ed.). Polity.

Connell, R. W., & Messerschmidt, J. W. (2005). Hegemonic masculinity: Rethinking the concept. *Gender & Society*, *19*(6), 829–859. https://doi.org/10.1177/0891243205278639

Crewe, B. (2009). *The prisoner society power, adaptation, and social life in an English prison*. Oxford University Press.

Crewe, B. (2011). Depth, weight, tightness: Revisiting the pains of imprisonment. *Punishment & Society*, *13*(5), 509–529. https://doi.org/10.1177/1462474511422172

Crichton, J. (2009). Defining high, medium, and low security in forensic mental healthcare: The development of the matrix of security in Scotland. *The Journal of Forensic Psychiatry & Psychology*, *20*(3), 333–353. https://doi.org/10.1080/14789940802542808

Dibley, L. (2011). Analyzing narrative data using McCormack's lenses. *Nurse Researcher*, *18*(3), 13–19. http://nurseresearcher.rcnpublishing.co.uk/news-andopinion/commentary/analysing-qualitative-data

Edworthy, R., & Völlm, B. (2016). Long-stay in high and medium secure forensic psychiatric care – prevalence, patient characteristics and pathways in England. *European Psychiatry*, *33*(S1), S180–S180. https://doi.org/10.1016/j.eurpsy.2016.01.38

Evans, T., & Wallace, P. (2008). A prison within a prison?: The masculinity narratives of male prisoners. *Men and Masculinities*, *10*(4), 484–507. https://doi.org/10.1177/1097184X06291903

Flick, U. (2018). *Managing quality in qualitative research* (2nd ed.). SAGE Publications.

Forensic Mental Health Services Managed Care Network. (2004). *Definition of security levels in psychiatric inpatient facilities in Scotland*. www.forensicnetwork.scot.nhs.uk/documents/previous_reports/LevelsofSecurityReport.pdf

Gadd, D., & Jefferson, T. (2011). *Psychosocial criminology: An introduction*. VLeBooks.

Goffman, E. (1968). *Asylums: Essays on the social situation of mental patients and other inmates* (Penguin Books ed.). Penguin Books.

Gow, R., Choo, M., Darjee, R., Gould, S., & Steele, J. (2010). A demographic study of the orchard clinic: Scotland's first medium secure unit. *The Journal of Forensic Psychiatry & Psychology*, *21*(1), 139–155. https://doi.org/10.1080/14789940903188956

Hanson, M. (2003). Evaluating user experience of an NHS mental health service. *International Journal of Healthcare Quality Assurance*, *16*(7), 342–346. https://doi.org/10.1108/09526860310500005

Hill, S. A., Riordan-Eva, E., & Hosking, A. (2019). Trends in the number of restricted patients in England and Wales 2003–2016: Implications for forensic psychiatry services. *Medicine, Science and the Law*, *59*(1), 42–48. https://doi.org/10.1177/0025802419825596

Hinsby, K., & Baker, M. (2004). Patient and nurse accounts of violent incidents in a medium secure unit. *Journal of Psychiatric and Mental Health Nursing*, *11*, 341–347. https://doi.org/10.1111/j.1365-2850.2004.00736.x

Ho, H., Thomson, L., & Darjee, R. (2009). Violence risk assessment: The use of the PCL-SV, HCR-20, and VRAG to predict violence in mentally disordered offenders discharged from a medium secure unit in Scotland. *The Journal of Forensic Psychiatry & Psychology*, *20*(4), 523–541. https://doi.org/10.1080/14789940802638358

Hopkins, J., Loeb, S., & Fick, D. (2009). Beyond satisfaction, what service users expect of inpatient mental health care: A literature review. *Journal of Psychiatric and Mental Health Nursing*, *16*(10), 927–937. https://doi.org/10.1111/j.1365-2850.2009.01501.

Howard, P., El-Mallakh, P., Kay Rayens, M., & Clark, J. (2003). Consumer perspectives on quality of inpatient mental health services. *Archives of Psychiatric Nursing*, *17*(5), 205–217. https://doi.org/10.1016/S0883-9417(03)00096-7

Ievins, A., & Crewe, B. (2015). "Nobody's better than you, nobody's worse than you": Moral community among prisoners convicted of sexual offences. *Punishment & Society*, *17*(4), 482–501. https://doi.org/10.1177/1462474515603803

Jewkes, Y. (2011). Loss, liminality and the life course sentence: Managing identity through a disrupted life-course. In A. Liebling & S. Maruna (Eds.), *The effects of imprisonment*. Routledge, pp. 366–390.

Jones, A., & Crossley, D. (2008). "In the mind of another" shame and acute psychiatric inpatient care: An exploratory study. A report on phase one: Service users. *Journal of Psychiatric and Mental Health Nursing*, *15*(9), 749–757. https://doi.org/10.1111/j.1365-2850.2008.01316.x

Khiroya, R., Weaver, T., & Maden, T. (2009). Use and perceived utility of structured violence risk assessments in English medium secure forensic units. *Psychiatric Bulletin, 33*, 129–132. https://doi.org/10.1192/pb.bp.108.019810

Kuosmanen, L., Hätönen, H., Jyrkinen, A., Katajisto, J., & Välimäki, M. (2006). Patient satisfaction with psychiatric inpatient care. *Journal of Advanced Nursing, 55*(6), 655–663. https://doi.org/10.1111/j.1365-2648.2006.03957.x

Macpherson, R., Dix, R., & Morgan, S. (2005). A growing evidence base for management guidelines: Revisiting guidelines for the management of acutely disturbed psychiatric patients. *Advances in Psychiatric Treatment: The Royal College of Psychiatrists' Journal of Continuing Professional Development, 11*(6), 404–415. https://doi.org/10.1192/apt.11.6.404

Mann, N. (2012). Ageing child sex offenders in prison: Denial, manipulation and community. *The Howard Journal of Criminal Justice, 51*(4), 345–358. https://doi.org/10.1111/j.1468-2311.2012.00705.x

Matza, D. (1964). *Delinquency and Drift.* Wiley & Sons.

Maycock, M., & Hunt, K. (2018). *New perspectives on prison masculinities.* Springer International Publishing. https://doi.org/10.1007/978-3-319-65654-0

McCusker, M. G., & Galupo, M. P. (2011). The impact of men seeking help for depression on perceptions of masculine and feminine characteristics. *Psychology of Men & Masculinity, 12*, 275–284. doi:10.1037/a0021071

Messerschmidt, J. W. (1993). *Masculinities and crime: Critique and reconceptualization of theory.* Rowan and Littlefield.

Messerschmidt, J. W. (1995). Schooling, masculinities and youth crime by white boys. In T. Newburn & E. Stanko (Eds.), *Men, masculinities and crime: Just boys doing the business.* Routledge.

Messerschmidt, J. W. (2000). *Nine lives: Adolescent masculinities, the body and violence.* Westview Press Inc.

Nelson, D. (2003). Service innovations: The orchard clinic: Scotland's first medium secure unit. *Psychiatric Bulletin of the Royal College of Psychiatrists, 27*(3), 105–107. https://doi.org/10.1192/pb.27.3.105

Polk, K. (1994). *When men kill: Scenarios of masculine violence.* Cambridge University Press.

Presser, L. (2009). The narratives of offenders. *Theoretical Criminology, 13*(2), 177–200. https://doi.org/10.1177/1362480609102878

Ricciardelli, R., Maier, K., & Hannah-Moffat, K. (2015). Strategic masculinities: Vulnerabilities, risk and the production of prison masculinities. *Theoretical Criminology, 19*(4), 491–513. https://doi.org/10.1177/1362480614565849

Saks, E. R. (2009). Some thoughts on denial of mental illness. *American Journal of Psychiatry, 166*(9), 972–973. https://doi.org/10.1176/appi.ajp.2009.09030409

Scraton, P. (2007). *Power, conflict and criminalisation.* Routledge.

Searle, R., Hare, D., Davies, B., & Morgan, S. (2018). The impact of masculinity upon men with psychosis who reside in secure forensic settings. *Journal of Forensic Practice, 20*(2), 69–80. https://doi.org/10.1108/JFP-05-2017-0014

Searle, R., Hare, D., Davies, B. et al. (2019). A systematic review of adherence to masculinity in men with psychosis. *Mental Health Practice.* https://doi.org/10.7748/mhp.2019.e1303

Shah, A., Waldron, G., Boast, N., Coid, J. W., & Ullrich, S. (2011). Factors associated with length of admission at a medium secure forensic psychiatric unit. *The Journal of Forensic Psychiatry & Psychology, 22*(4), 496–512. https://doi.org/10.1080/14789949.2011.594902

Silver, E. (2006). Understanding the relationship between mental disorder and violence: The need for a criminological perspective. *Law and Human Behaviour, 30*(6), 685–706. https://doi.org/10.1007/s10979-006-9018-z

Sim, J. (1994). Tougher than the rest? Men in prison. In T. Newburn & E. A. Stanko (Eds.), *Just boys doing business?: Men, masculinities and crime.* Routledge.

Slembrouck, S. (2015). The role of the researcher in interview narratives. In A. De Fina & A. Georgakopoulou (Eds.), *The handbook of narrative analysis.* Wiley.

Sparks, J., & Bottoms, A. (1995). Legitimacy and order in prisons. *The British Journal of Sociology, 46*(1), 45–62. doi:10.2307/591622

Stewart, D., Bowers, L., Simpson, A., Ryan, C., & Tziggili, M. (2009). Manual restraint of adult psychiatric inpatients: A literature review. *Journal of Psychiatric and Mental Health Nursing, 16*(8), 749–757. https://doi.org/10.1111/j.1365-2850.2009.01475.x

Swanson, J. W., et al. (2006). A national study of violent behaviour in persons with schizophrenia. *Archives of General Psychiatry, 63*(5), 490–499.

Sykes, G. M. (1958). *The society of captives: A study of a maximum security prison.* Princeton University Press.

Sykes, G., & Messinger, S. (1960). The inmate social system. In R. A. Cloward, D. R. Cressey, G. H. Grosser, R. McCleery, L. E. Ohlin, G. M. Sykes, & S. L. Messinger (Eds.), *Theoretical studies in social organization of the prison* (pp. 5–19). Social Science Research Council.

Taylor, P. J., Leese, M., Williams, D., Butwell, M., Daly, R., & Larkin, E. (1998). Mental disorder and violence. A special (high security) hospital study. *The British Journal of Psychiatry: The Journal of Mental Science, 172,* 218–226. https://doi.org/10.1192/bjp.172.3.218

Teasdale, B., Silver, E., & Monahan, J. (2006). Gender, threat/control-override delusions and violence. *Law and Human Behavior, 30*(6), 649–658. https://doi.org/10.1007/s10979-006-9044-x

Turner, V. (1967). *Betwixt and between: The liminal period in rites de passage.* Cornell University Press.

van den Berg, C., Beijersbergen, K., Nieuwbeerta, P., & Dirkzwager, A. (2018). Sex offenders in prison: Are they socially isolated? *Sexual Abuse, 30*(7), 828–845. https://doi.org/10.1177/1079063217700884

West, C., & Zimmerman, D. H. (1987). Doing gender. *Gender and Society, 1*(2), 121–151.

Wiener, M. J. (2006). *Men of blood: Violence, manliness and criminal justice in Victorian England.* Cambridge University Press.

Wooff, A., & Skinns, L. (2018). The role of emotion, space and place in police custody in England: Towards a geography of police custody. *Punishment & Society, 20*(5), 562–579. https://doi.org/10.1177/1462474517722176

Wynn, R. (2004). Psychiatric inpatients' experiences with restraint. *The Journal of Forensic Psychiatry & Psychology, 15*(1), 124–144. https://doi.org/10.1080/14789940410001655187

Yousaf, O., Popat, A., & Hunter, M. S. (2015). An investigation of masculinity attitudes, gender, and attitudes toward psychological help-seeking. *Psychology of Men & Masculinity, 16*(2), 234–237. https://doi.org/10.1037/a0036241

Chapter 18

Carers and forensic services

Towards carers' peer support

Karen Machin, Shelagh Musgrave, Karen Persaud, and Julie Ridley

Introduction

This chapter discusses the support needs for family and friend carers of people detained in secure care, with specific attention to the experiences of carers from racialised communities. Carers within secure care can feel marginalised and unheard. We suggest that the mutuality and reciprocity of peer support for and by carers may be a useful development to ensure that their support needs are heard, understood, and met.

This chapter has been co-authored by people with lived and academic experience in a caring role, including roles working with secure care services and with carers. It draws on the published work of two of the authors (Ridley and Machin) in forensic services who have reached out to carers who are often easy to ignore or seen as hard to reach. Musgrave and Persaud have written sections from a perspective of lived experience, and these are included throughout the chapter as quotes.

In this chapter, we want to step away from the service and from the service user and patient focus and put the spotlight on their family and friend carers. Interviewing carers has unique challenges: where we invite carers to speak about themselves, they often speak about the difficulties of the person they are supporting (Ridley et al., 2014). Their concerns are about the person who is in forensic services, rarely identifying needs and challenges that they face in their role and relationship to the person.

The importance of language

Most service users and patients, including those who have longer stays in medium- or high-secure settings, do have some contact with family and friends (Völlm et al., 2017), and these relationships need to be maintained and nurtured. But the word 'carers' in forensic mental health settings is often used synonymously with 'careworkers'; with staff viewing patients' relatives and friends as 'visitors', while these 'visitors' often identify by their relationship with the person, as 'mum', 'brother' or 'friend', or use 'carer' to show they have a particular role now in supporting the person in forensic services (Ridley et al., 2014).

There are slight variations in the definition of 'carer', related to the specific legislative contexts in the different countries of the United Kingdom. In summary of the legal definitions used within the United Kingdom, the common activity is about providing, or intending to provide, care for an adult. Care for young people in services is considered separately, apart from in Wales where the Social Services and Wellbeing Act 2014 is also inclusive of care for disabled children. In Northern Ireland, there is still no legislated definition of carer.

DOI: 10.4324/9781003184768-23

However, assumptions about the notion of a 'carer', as someone 'providing or intending to provide care' on a day-to-day or regular basis, can feel confusing for people whose relative or friend is detained for a lengthy period in a hospital and who may feel that this definition excludes them because care and support is now being provided by the hospital system. Some people may thus accept a new identity as 'visitor', or 'Nearest Relative' or 'Nominated Person', terms from mental health legislation which imply specific responsibilities which feel distant from their previously intimate relationship. But carers still provide emotional and financial support and may need to take responsibility for a wide range of personal matters including liaison with solicitors. Some carers suggest that terms such as 'nearest relative' feel cold and clinical.

Additionally, these definitions all focus on one individual, a primary carer, whereas the reality for most families is of shared caring responsibilities. The situation may also be further complicated when a move to forensic care has been precipitated by an act of violence within the family which may have shaken the foundations of these relationships. The word 'carer', therefore, may not feel like an appropriate term for many reasons. Yet it is the term for an identity or label which is key to accessing support.

Throughout this chapter, we refer to 'carers' as family and friends, in the broadest sense of a network of supporters and allies, who offer support and care to the person. Additionally, we specifically discuss carers of people who are detained within the secure care mental health system called forensic services. Many people will have had a journey that will include other mental health services, including being detained in an acute or general psychiatric ward or using prison mental health services. Family and friends may have faced similar experiences and challenges in having their needs recognised with all these services and this may influence their experience of forensic care.

Additionally, we recognise the variety of terms used for the people supported by family and friend carers, including patient, service user, client, resident, consumer, survivor, and, in the carers' literature, relative, friend, and loved one. We acknowledge the challenge of finding a word that is suitable in all situations (NSUN, 2015). We refer to 'people', although in some places for clarity, we have used 'patient' for a person detained in a hospital, and 'relative' for 'people they support'. We mean 'relative' to include both family members and friends, recognising that most carers in secure care are relatives.

Carers and mental health services: potential for partnerships

In their concern for their relative or friend, carers may offer suggestions on how services might be improved (Giacco et al., 2017), both on a personal level and on a more strategic level, about improvements for local or national services (NHSE/UCLan, 2018). They focus on the quality of services, taking a view that if services were providing appropriate care, then, as carers, they would experience less stress and be able to rebuild their own lives, returning to a role defined by their relationships, as parents, partners, siblings, or friends. A level of involvement with services is to be welcomed, especially where services pay meaningful regard to principles of involvement and co-production (Faulkner et al., 2014; Slay & Stephens, 2013), but it can have unintended consequences for carers.

> As carers, we are a valuable source of information about the person we are supporting – both in terms of who that person is as well as how their illness has impacted upon them, and we will share that information gladly as we know it will help to shape their care. However, as we tend to be viewed as this, it becomes how we see ourselves, our purpose if you like, further adding to the loss of self that we experience in our care-giving role.

The valuing of carers' contributions to services needs to be balanced with an equal value for the support needs of the carers themselves. Within mental health services in general, these support needs have often been overlooked, leading to the development of guidelines such as the Triangle of Care (Mitchell & Hannan, 2015; Worthington & Rooney, 2010), and the Secure Carers Toolkit (NHSE/UCLan, 2018), the foreword of which notes 'Carers will still be there when secure services are no longer required and it is vital for them to be supported from the word go as valued partners in care' (p. 3). The experience of carers, however, is still that their own support needs are often overlooked and go unrecognised by services and even by themselves:

> When in a caring role it is easy to lose sight of the person that we are as we become consumed with the care of the person we love/are supporting. We advocate for them, we fight against their demons which try to take over our lives as well as theirs, we turn away from the painful emotions that we are faced with time and again, we manage multiple crises, incidents of self-harm, suicidal thoughts and behaviour. We wake up with a feeling of dread as to what this particular day is going to bring us, we go to bed exhausted but relieved to have got through the day, whilst knowing that we will have to do it all again tomorrow. We wonder where we will get the strength to do so but we do, because we have to – experience has taught us that whilst we may be able to reach out to professionals for additional input for the service user, resources are stretched so thin that to get it, when they, and we, need it, is rare.

The aforementioned description could apply to any carer of someone experiencing mental health challenges (Sief et al., 2021 *pre-print*). In this chapter, we demonstrate that 'forensic carers' are even further marginalised.

The impact of being a carer

All mental health carers experience stresses related to the caring role (Cleary et al., 2020), especially at points of crisis (Albert & Simpson, 2015; Stuart et al., 2019). At the same time as trying to negotiate services and support for their relative, carers are also trying to maintain their own daily lives, which may include employment and family responsibilities.

Although there is limited research on the experiences of carers of people in secure care, the authors acknowledge there are additional stresses in relation to the offences which brought someone into forensic services, which might include experiences of violence (Paradis-Gagné et al., 2020), negative experiences with both police and mental health services (Brennan et al., 2016), and challenges in navigating mental health systems (Chemerynska et al., 2021). A literature review conducted as part of a study of forensic carers in Scotland (Ridley et al., 2014) established key issues specific to these carers which we expand on here:

- Increased stress compared with carers of non-forensic service users including fear of violence and damage to property, with the embarrassment of being classified as a victim and the ensuing links with social services
- Stress related to an index offence including treatment by the police, courts, and media, and including fear of abuse towards their relative from a range of sources, and including the potential for injury and death within the mental health care system
- The impact and effect on troubled family relationships
- Stigma of mental health and of offending
- Guilt and self-blame
- Physical separation in visiting institutions some distance from home

- Stress in relation to services including security regimes
- Needs for information, including in future preparation for discharge, while being excluded because of confidentiality or a lack of communication
- Uncertainties about the mental health experiences of their relative or friend.

For many families, these challenging experiences are further magnified by intersectionality with other forms of discrimination such as sexism or racism. Within England, Black and Black British patients, and consequently their family carers, are overrepresented in secure care, with longer lengths of stay and are more likely to have a primary diagnosis of psychosis (Bignall et al., 2019). In work related to the development of the Forensic Mental Health Community Service Model, patients described being unaware they were experiencing a mental health problem until contact with statutory services, which may have involved an abrupt and escalating confrontation. Their experiences of services included cultural stereotyping and a tolerance of racially abusive language, including from other patients, and they wanted to speak with people who had a shared cultural understanding. Family and friends are acutely aware of such difficulties:

> For Black and Brown skinned people the colour of your skin is like having a target on you that you can't disguise or remove. We are not the same, but we're placed in one pot like a stew. Imagine waking up every day knowing that the system is against you just because of how you look? You can be restrained or even worse, killed just because of the colour of your skin.
>
> Every day the fear, despair and emotional strains faced by people 'of colour' is reported on. The daily news compounds this: George Floyd, Breonna Taylor, Black Lives Matter. Roger Sylvester, Sean Rigg, Olaseni Lewis, Rocky Bennett, Kingsley Burrell, Kevin Clarke, Leon Briggs . . . the list goes on and on and we, the minority, see the pattern of discrimination replicated in social, judicial and mental health services. Patients/Service Users feel powerless but can't show the emotional pain for fear of punitive measures being taken against them. Meanwhile carers also suffer emotional pain and distress as well as a sense of responsibility for the plight of their dependant.

There is a lot for a family or friend carer to make sense of, yet they may feel isolated from others, bound by a culture of confidentiality not to speak about their situation, and not knowing where to turn for help. For some, it can feel like their life is on hold, including their relationship with their relative (Robinson et al., 2017). But despite this list of issues that might imply clear practical and emotional support needs, carers still feel excluded and unheard:

> Any support tends to focus on carers supporting the service user as opposed to supporting themselves. In the current climate, carers are so unused to being offered support that they don't believe they need it.

Barriers to being heard

Too often, family and friend carers' experiences are of not being heard when raising concerns of deteriorating mental health or threatening behaviour, or worse, feeling marginalised in an 'illusion of inclusion' (Sampson et al., 2019, p. 309) where a triangle of care feels like 'a three-legged stool with two long legs and one half leg, which is the carer's'. Carers in such a situation are unsurprisingly unlikely to enquire about support for themselves. In this common scenario, being a carer can feel like constantly having to battle with services to be recognised and to be heard.

> Being heard is critical. You get a release, otherwise it becomes an internal dialogue and rotating thought which impacts your mental health. Staff need to be trained and supported with this. Working collaboratively with carers can help staff get a better understanding and work more effectively. It fits well with Triangle of Care quality.

As a first step to being heard and getting their own support needs met, carers have to be able to describe their needs and they may need help to be able to do this. They need to be able to communicate openly and honestly, knowing that they will be listened to in a non-judgemental space. But stuck in someone else's crisis (the patient's), carers can find it difficult to articulate their own independent needs and instead may frame it as the need to look after themselves so they can better look after their relative:

> Somewhere along the way we realise that not only have we turned off the painful emotions, we have turned off **all** emotion because it is impossible to turn off only those which cause us pain. Somewhere along the way we may realise that the sense of dread has become a permanent feeling. Somewhere along the way we may realise that our responses have become trauma responses – we may recognise that this is unhealthy, but we are at a loss as to what to do about it. If we are lucky, we may have an understanding GP [General Practitioner] or there may be a mental health professional who is supportive of carer health and wellbeing to whom we can talk, but more often, there is nobody suggesting to us that looking after our own health and wellbeing is essential if we want to continue to look after somebody else.

Confidentiality has been a long-standing barrier to being heard as a carer (Wynaden & Orb, 2005), which can leave carers further isolated and not involved in discussions:

> A service user may request that carers are not involved in their care. This tends to be heard as a blanket message of 'you cannot have contact with my carers' as opposed to the message 'I do not want to have my carers involved in my care'. These are **very** different messages but the former offers a get-out clause to under-resourced professionals in terms of responsibility to carers. This is often where we start to see the issue of confidentiality come into play – the service user has requested their carer not be involved in their care, therefore I cannot be in touch with their carer as there is potentially a confidentiality conflict issue.

These two main potential barriers to finding the words and confidentiality prevent carers' needs from being heard so that they can access the support they need for themselves. But something as relatively simple as feeling that you are being heard can itself have a profound effect. Carers' feelings about being heard are reflected in some qualitative research studies which note that the carers they interviewed valued being able to speak with someone about their experience, with examples provided in Finlay-Carruthers et al. (2018) and also in the following quote from our Scottish study:

> It's absolutely amazing getting to chat to you and explain my side of the story.
> (carer in Ridley et al., 2014, p. 28)

Family and friend carers have a fundamental need to have someone listen in a non-judgemental way, with time and respect, to their experiences and perspective. Some services are developing the role of Carer Peer Supporter, a paid role, to use listening skills, familiarity with well-being, and knowledge of services, to support family and friends.

Peer support within secure care

Peer support for service users has become a key element of recovery-focused mental health services supported by national policy. Based on relationships of mutuality and reciprocity, support from someone who has faced similar challenges has been shown to have a range of positive outcomes including increased confidence and hope as well as satisfaction with services (Davidson et al., 2012) including within secure services (Shaw, 2014). Within England, a recent innovative programme of work to develop specialist community forensic teams and women's secure blended services has included the development of peer-based approaches within these settings. Peer support for service users by current or former service users is a key element of these models, and is particularly welcomed by carers where the 'peer-ness' is seen to extend beyond specific experiences of mental health challenges and services to include shared cultural and political understandings:

> As a carer, for your own mental well-being as much as for the person you care for, you need a break from the 'wrap around' service you provide. You want someone who understands the needs of your loved one, can relate to their experiences, share their interests and embrace their spiritual perspective, to provide that social interaction and support beyond that of a carer.
>
> As a Caribbean with a distinct experience of what it is to be black and the daily prejudices black people face, I'd particularly like commonality in a peer for my dependent. Someone culturally representative with an understanding and empathy towards his worldview. An independent social support with whom he wouldn't have to explain himself or his experiences.

Carers peer support

Carers seek a similar support for themselves from each other in carers groups, recognising the value of shared understanding:

> There is a shorthand in communication which is missing when talking with professionals – our situations may be different, but our experiences are frequently shared.

Some services have extended this notion of mutual support to paid peer support roles for carers. Carers' peer support is support provided by another carer, someone who has been through a similar experience. Within carers' peer support in general, there are complexities about how the 'peer-ness' is defined, including whether it is related to the carer, for example, by their relationship to the person they support, as parent or sibling, or whether it is related to the person being supported, for example, by their diagnosis or service use (Machin et al., 2019). Within secure care, experience of the unique additional stresses listed earlier seems to be sufficient for this group of carers to develop mutual trust.

> Recognition from both parties builds up a trust quickly, for the person being supported they know that they don't have to find the words, it is just known by the peer without the

need for description. As one carer put it – 'I was made to feel at ease about my situation, I wasn't in any way different to the peer support worker, she had lived it too, and "got it", not many people do, even the professionals who care for my daughter. They are treating an illness and can walk away at the end of a shift'.

A qualitative study in Australia suggested that such support should be tailored to the needs of individual carers, varying according to their culture, years of caring experience, and previous experiences with mental health services, with some carers feeling that they did not need such support (Visa & Harvey, 2019). However, while carers may value peer support, there may still be the same barriers to implementation as faced by any peer support programme, with challenges of culture and role clarity creating uncertainty within teams (Byrne et al., 2021). The introduction of carers' peer support demands that the whole team reflects on the inclusion of both a lived experience workforce and carers, two potentially counter-cultural topics within secure care.

> My own experience as a carer peer support worker was a challenging one, it was made challenging by the culture of the mental health team into which I was placed. My role was a trail blazing one and at the outset, I felt confident that within a small team I could make a difference to the way the team worked with families and carers.
>
> Individually, many professionals recognised that more needed to be done, but as a team they were unable to make the changes that were needed to move to proactive, ongoing communications with carers that was focused on their health and wellbeing. I meanwhile engaged with carers proactively and on an ongoing basis simply by picking up the phone and building a relationship – it wasn't complicated and many of the team's perceived barriers just didn't exist.
>
> At the end of my time in role I realised that one person alone cannot change a long-ingrained culture, particularly on a short-term contract. It was a missed opportunity for the team and a demoralising personal experience.
>
> But, for the carers I supported, through perseverance and open and honest conversations, they realised their own needs are important, that it is okay to express anger and despair alongside hope, and they could do that in a safe space alongside someone who 'just knows'.

Carers peer supporters understand the boundaries of confidentiality and work within them, without seeing them as a barrier to working with the family:

> We very rarely talked about anything that would have taken us into an area where I couldn't share information. In short, confidentiality when engaging with carers was not the issue that it tends to be blown up into. I made the boundaries clear from the outset – I am here to support your health and wellbeing, I can answer generalised questions about mental illness, but I cannot provide specific information. Confidentiality was certainly never a barrier to my engagement with carers.

Carers peer support workers can provide unique emotional and practical support for family and friends, based on their shared experiences and learning. Just as for all peer support workers, the benefits are likely to be multiple, with positive impacts on the care team and organisation as well as all family members including the patient (Visa & Harvey, 2019). However, at the time of writing, carers' peer support work is a relatively new development, and further research on implementation processes and outcomes is required, with specific attention to cultural differences and the range of settings for secure care.

Conclusion

One author reflects on her personal experience to connect with the issues throughout the chapter.

As a new mother, I felt nervous welcoming my baby. A little unsure of myself and how I'd cope but I had family, friends and a medical service that provided ante and post-natal care and mother and baby clubs where we could share experiences, provide support and much needed social interaction. As a carer of someone with mental health issues, this wasn't available to me. I was totally unprepared, unsupported, ignorant and because of the stigma, isolated and lonely. The mental health issue wasn't acknowledged or supported by family, friends. Within my community, poor mental health wasn't a 'thing', or so I thought.

The sense of isolation and helplessness was only impounded by my experience of trying to access information and support via the mental health teams. Communication was the first hurdle, no one reached out to me, I had to bang on doors to get a response and was often met with disregard or treated as an irritant. However, I'd persist and being reasonably intelligent and with a good grasp of English, I could persist. I could only imagine how difficult this is for people who speak little or no English because the system is a maze and not easy to navigate and interact with for any of us. So, having communications hurdles would be a significant hurdle.

The time was the darkest I'd ever experienced so I frantically spent every spare hour researching mental health alongside work, being a mother and juggling my caring role. Every day was a mental, emotional, and physical challenge. I lost contact with friends and family and withdrew more and more until inevitably, I burnt out. It was on my road to recovery I met other carers; simple things like attending walks, coffee mornings, having non-judgemental space to share mutuality all helped to build me up. It was through these interactions I learnt much more than I ever did through the mental health services. Some experiences I could learn from, some I could empathise with, some gave me hope and some gave me strength. However, I still didn't feel confident to be open about my experiences, so I was still fragile.

I found an event that spoke of inequality and listened intently as the speaker, a black woman, told her story and it impacted me greatly. I felt emotional hearing about her experiences as they reflected mine too. She echoed the worry I internalised. The additional burden you have of knowing that black males are the ones most likely to have negative outcomes, more likely to be restrained, over medicated and even killed, in the service. I was finally able to connect with someone who understood me.

It was through these interactions that I was truly able to grow. It was informal peer support and not readily available. I reflected on how different my experience would have been had I had a safe space to talk, be listened to, and be supported. These connections were the most valuable to me, they reinforced my sense of me, they reassured me that I wasn't alone in my experience and that it wasn't my fault, they helped me recognise the importance of looking after yourself firstly in order to be able to look after others. They were and continue to be the safe space for me as a carer, empowering, highlighting my personal strengths, and making me an equal.

Providing support for carers must include carers peer support workers and training for staff delivered by carers. Only with this input can a service truly be responsive to the needs of the people they serve. We live with the impact of mental ill health 24/7, there is no end of shift. When a person is discharged, if they have a carer, it's the carer that will take up the reigns. It stands to reason that if a carer is well empowered with the right skills, knowledge, access to resources, and is able to influence service delivery, there will be a profound effect on whether a person is able to sustain recovery or not.

I'm fortunate now to be working in a Trust [healthcare provider] to develop this aspect of provision and truly hope that others are doing the same too because this small investment would have profound impact if done correctly. One moment can change a day, one day can change a life and one life can change the world.

References

Albert, R., & Simpson, A. (2015). Double deprivation: A phenomenological study into the experience of being a carer during a mental health crisis. *Journal of Advanced Nursing*, *71*(12), 2753–2762. https://doi.org/10.1111/jan.12742

Bignall, T., Jeraj, S., Helsby, E., & Butt, J. (2019). *Racial disparities in mental health*. Race Equality Foundation.

Brennan, A., Warren, N., Peterson, V., Hollander, Y., Boscarato, K., & Lee, S. (2016). Collaboration in crisis: Carer perspectives on police and mental health professional's responses to mental health crises: Collaboration in Crisis. *International Journal of Mental Health Nursing*, *25*(5), 452–461. https://doi.org/10.1111/inm.12233

Byrne, L., Roennfeldt, H., Wolf, J., Linfoot, A., Foglesong, D., Davidson, L., & Bellamy, C. (2021). Effective peer employment within multidisciplinary organizations: Model for best practice. *Administration and Policy in Mental Health and Mental Health Services Research*. https://doi.org/10.1007/s10488-021-01162-2

Chemerynska, N., Arsuffi, L., & Holdsworth, E. (2021). Ascertaining the needs of carers of forensic psychiatric inpatients through their experience of navigating mental health services: Guidance for service providers. *Journal of Forensic Psychology Research and Practice*, *21*(3), 230–248. https://doi.org/10.1080/24732850.2020.1851546

Cleary, M., West, S., Hunt, G. E., McLean, L., & Kornhaber, R. (2020). A qualitative systematic review of caregivers' experiences of caring for family diagnosed with schizophrenia. *Issues in Mental Health Nursing*, *41*(8), 667–683. https://doi.org/10.1080/01612840.2019.1710012

Davidson, L., Bellamy, C., Guy, K., & Miller, R. (2012). Peer support among persons with severe mental illnesses: A review of evidence and experience. *World Psychiatry*, *11*(2), 123–128.

Faulkner, A., Yiannoullou, S., Kalathil, J., Crepaz-Keay, D., Singer, F., James, N., Griffiths, R., Perry, E., Forde, D., & Kallevik, J. (2014). *National involvement partnership: 4PI standards for involvement*. NSUN. www.nsun.org.uk/4pi-involvement-standards

Finlay-Carruthers, G., Davies, J., Ferguson, J., & Browne, K. (2018). Taking parents seriously: The experiences of parents with a son or daughter in adult medium secure forensic mental health care. *International Journal of Mental Health Nursing*, *27*(5), 1535–1545. https://doi.org/10.1111/inm.12455

Giacco, D., Dirik, A., Kaselionyte, J., & Priebe, S. (2017). How to make carer involvement in mental health inpatient units happen: A focus group study with patients, carers and clinicians. *BMC Psychiatry*, *17*(1), 101. https://doi.org/10.1186/s12888-017-1259-5

Machin, K., Meddings, S., & Clarke-Mapp, J. (2019). Peer support for family and friends: Carers supporting each other. In E. Watson & S. Meddings (Eds.), *Peer support in mental health*. Palgrave Macmillan.

Mitchell, A., & Hannan, R. (2015). *The triangle of care for young carers and young adult carers: A guide for mental health professionals*. Carers Trust.

NHS England/University of Central Lancashire. (2018). *Carer support and involvement in secure mental health services*. NHSE/UCLan. www.england.nhs.uk/wp-content/uploads/2018/05/secure-carers-toolkit-v2.pdf

NSUN. (2015). *The language of mental wellbeing*. NSUN.

Paradis-Gagné, E., Holmes, D., & Perron, A. (2020). Experiences of family violence committed by relatives with severe mental illness: A grounded theory. *Journal of Forensic Nursing*, *16*(2), 108–117. https://doi.org/10.1097/JFN.0000000000000272

Ridley, J., McKeown, M., Machin, K., Rosengard, A., Little, S., Briggs, S., Jones, F., & Deypurkaystha, M. (2014). *Exploring family carer involvement in forensic mental health services*. Support in Mind Scotland.

Robinson, L., Haskayne, D., & Larkin, M. (2017). How do carers view their relationship with forensic mental health services? *Journal of Forensic Psychology Research and Practice*, *17*(4), 232–248. https://doi.org/10.1080/24732850.2017.1326804

Sampson, S., Foster, S., Majid, S., & Völlm, B. (2019). Carers of long-stay patients' perspectives of secure forensic care: An exploratory qualitative study. *International Journal of Forensic Mental Health*. doi:10.1080/14999013.2018.1552635

Shaw, C. (2014). *Peer support in secure services*. Together.

Sief, N. A., Wood, L., & Morant, N. (2021). *Invisible experts: A systematic review & thematic synthesis of informal carer experiences of inpatient mental health care* [Preprint]. In Review. https://doi.org/10.21203/rs.3.rs-647106/v1

Slay, J., & Stephens, L. (2013). *Co-production in mental health: A literature review*. New Economics Foundation.

Stuart, R., Akther, S. F., Machin, K., Persaud, K., Simpson, A., Johnson, S., & Oram, S. (2020). Carers' experiences of involuntary admission under mental health legislation: Systematic review and qualitative meta-synthesis. *British Journal of Psychiatry Open*, 6(2), e19. https://doi.org/10.1192/bjo.2019.101

Visa, B., & Harvey, C. (2019). Mental health carers' experiences of an Australian carer peer support program: Tailoring supports to carers' needs. *Health & Social Care in the Community*, 27(3), 729–739. https://doi.org/10.1111/hsc.12689

Völlm, B., Edworthy, R., Holley, J., Talbot, E., Majid, S., Duggan, C., Weaver, T., & McDonald, T. (2017). A mixed-methods study exploring the characteristics and needs of long stay patients in high and medium secure settings in England: Implications for service organisation. *Health Services and Delivery Research*, 5(11), 268. https://doi.org/10.3310/hsdr05110

Worthington, A., & Rooney, P. (2010). *Triangle of care*. Carers Trust. https://professionals.carers.org/working-mental-health-carers/triangle-care-mental-health

Wynaden, D., & Orb, A. (2005). Impact of patient confidentiality on carers of people who have a mental disorder. *International Journal of Mental Health Nursing*, 14(3), 166–171. https://doi.org/10.1111/j.1440-0979.2005.00377.x

Part 6

Conclusion

Chapter 19

Conclusion

Pulling towards justice

Jack Tomlin and Birgit Völlm

Barack Obama repopularised the phrase: 'The arc of the moral universe is long, but it bends toward justice'. This exact wording in fact comes from Martin Luther King Jr. and is itself a paraphrasing of a speech given by a US abolitionist minister in 1853 named Theodore Parker. His version is more cautious, hinting at the uncertainties of pursuing justice: 'I do not pretend to understand the moral universe. The arc is a long one. My eye reaches but little ways. I cannot calculate the curve and complete the figure by the experience of sight. I can divine it by conscience. And from what I see I am sure it bends toward justice'. In 2016, US former Attorney General Eric Holder said of this in an interview that 'the arc bends toward justice, but it only bends toward justice because people pull it towards justice. It doesn't happen on its own'.

Whose justice, what this looks like, and how we get it is unclear. However, a recognition of injustices and inequalities within criminal justice and forensic mental health systems around the world motivated the writing of this book. Contributors identified a range of problems that need to be addressed in pursuit of more equitable and fairer experiences and outcomes. Authors – practitioners, researchers, people with lived experience – also offered ways forward, describing individual, group, and cultural undertakings and interventions intended to pull us towards something that looks more like justice.

The causes and correlates of disparities in the experiences of forensic mental health patients described in this book were myriad. Wells and Kavanaugh (chapter two) contextualised the US criminal justice system within its history of slavery, segregation and Jim Crow inspired laws old and current. This speaks to the analysis that current US criminal justice practices of mass incarceration and a lack of dedicated correctional mental health services pose a structural and perpetuating barrier to the full inclusion of marginalised groups in social, economic, and political life.

Such structural concerns were echoed by Shephard and Madu (Chapter 14), and Opitz-Welke et al. (Chapter 6). Both groups of authors implicated the importance of social inclusion, shared cultural values, common language, ethnically diverse communities, and representation in political life in the development of serious mental illnesses like psychosis (Morgan et al., 2019). The authors demonstrated how migrants who flee persecution, war, or economic hardship and arrive in countries with different cultural norms, languages, or prejudices are at higher risk of incarceration and detention in secure forensic settings.

Attitudes towards individuals from marginalised, vulnerable or minority groups produce and reinforce the differential experiences of criminal justice and forensic mental health care. Maclennan et al. (Chapter 4) wrote about the experiences of transgender inmates. The paucity of literature on the mental health needs and appropriate models of support for this group has no doubt been influenced by social and political debate. Spending millions to fund

DOI: 10.4324/9781003184768-25

transgender-specific services or research is harder to accomplish when some public discourse denies the ontological reality of trans-identities. Sadie and colleagues (Chapter 5) described how 'powerful social, political, and psychological factors' shape reforms in youth custody. They cite the death of James Bulgar at the hands of two 10-year-old boys in 1993 and the strong political and media reaction to this as demonstrative of the macro meeting the micro, crime and justice rhetoric meeting youth experiences in custody, still consequential three decades later.

Taylor and Walker (chapter three) made the case that for women forensic patients, socio-economic considerations – poverty, isolation, employment – interact with individual-level factors to increase women's vulnerability to victimisation and violence perpetration. These individual factors – domestic violence, childcare issues, eating disorders, and substance use – can be myriad and reinforcing, illustrating that patients can have multiple marginalised characteristics and backgrounds. Even when attempting to provide cultural, identity, gender, sex-specific, and responsive treatment, services may struggle to see patients as unique, located wholes with multiple and fluctuating identities. Understanding how (un)suited the criminal justice system and forensic services are for people with less-frequently diagnosed mental disorders like autism (Longfellow and Skelding, Chapter 8) and learning disability (Skelding and Longfellow, Chapter 9) is of utmost importance. So too is investigating the experiences of patients who do not progress through forensic services in a 'typical' way. For example, patients for whom progress takes much longer than the average, staying for ten or more years in some cases (Völlm, Chapter 11) or young patients who transition from child and adolescent services to adult care settings – a significant move at an important developmental phase (Livanou and Furtado, Chapter 10).

Any progress towards reformed forensic mental health services that are more equitable and just must include the voice of patients and their carers. This book aimed to capture the voices of people with lived experience of forensic services and how marginalised identities or characteristics, such as cultural and linguistic group, age, gender, sex, sexual orientation, ethnicity, and migration background, shaped their care and support. People with lived experiences of services co-authored chapters on youth custody (Sadie et al., Chapter 5), epistemic marginalisation (Markham, Chapter 15), and the marginalised experiences of carers of diverse patients (Machin et al., Chapter 18). This kind of involvement speaks to the expression 'Nothing about us, without us' and contemporary efforts to engage patients in their care as much as possible. Markham (Chapter 15) described different forms of epistemic marginalisation and exclusion faced by forensic patients, whilst Visser and colleagues (Chapter 16) argued for the increased involvement of older patients in research.

One barrier to effective communication in male forensic patients is the social construction of the masculine identity and its concomitant expectations relating to strength, stoicism, or violence as accepted forms of (non-)expression. Conceptions of masculinity that eschew vulnerability, shame, ageing, or regret as normal human experiences can discourage patients or inmates from engaging in care or seeking help in secure or correctional settings. Haddow (Chapter 17) explored masculinity in medium-secure settings and finds that some men reconceptualise agency and ownership in their recovery as masculine exercise of control. Morgan and her co-authors (Chapter 7) looked at fatherhood and proposed that it should be more widely and meaningfully considered in treatment plans.

We hope this book encourages people to ask 'What does 'pulling towards justice' look like?'. We think that the contributions in this book point to at least four domains where marginalisation-attenuating work needs to take place. These are described in brief, as a guide for further thought. The first of these is *orientation*. This refers to the way all individuals working and living in or alongside forensic mental health services conduct themselves on a daily basis. Are our approaches to thinking, problem-solving, and communicating sensitive to the myriad marginalised characteristics present in forensic settings? Do our actions, beliefs, and postures reinforce or mitigate disparities in experiences and outcomes based on arbitrary socially defined characteristics? Are staff 'culturally competent'?

The second is *intervention and treatment*. Here we refer to all aspects of the rehabilitative work undertaken proximal to forensic settings. Is care strength-based, individualised to the unique needs and skillset of each patient? Are group or individual therapeutic interventions sensitive to cultural, ethnic, or religious biographies of patients? Can a therapeutic culture be developed where carers and local communities are involved in recovery and reintegration? Are interventions available in a range of languages or modes of delivery? Recovery colleges, peer support workers, and culturally adapted models of care are important here.

Third, as researchers, we are convinced of the utility of *evidence-based care*. However, few studies — especially high-quality RCTs — are conducted in forensic settings and fewer still weight samples to produce findings suitably powered to speak to efficacy across minority groups. Further, myriad considerations need to be addressed in the design of research projects so that findings are representative of the population, reliable, valid, trustworthy, and disseminated appropriately. These considerations extend to the use of measurement instruments, language comprehension, sampling strategies, coding ethnicity or migration background variables in quantitative analyses, and exercising reflexivity to mitigate the extent to which personal biography and political orientation influence research conception and implementation. Peer researchers are an important element of such marginalisation-sensitive research.

Finally, *systemic changes* to the way individuals with mental disorders interact with criminal justice and forensic systems are needed. It has long been acknowledged that periods of deinstitutionalisation have resulted in much unmet mental health need, especially for complex forensic cases (Jansman-Hart et al., 2011; Prins, 2011). Inadequate community mental health provision serves to reinforce structural disparities in outcomes for the most marginalised groups. Radical reconceptualisations of the methods and aims of contemporary western criminal justice rehabilitative agencies such as restorative justice or (gender-specific) mental health and drug treatment courts are gaining increasing attention and evidence bases as successful alternatives to traditional criminal justice disposals (Sherman et al., 2014; Wittouck et al., 2013). Prisons exacerbate mental health needs and should only be used as a last resort and where there is appropriate mental health care provision *en par* with the best in the community (UN General Assembly, 2015). These alternatives should reflect the structural inequalities faced by most marginalised forensic mental health patients and accordingly adopt reintegrative, rehabilitation, human rights, and strength-based orientations.

We hope this book helps readers to think about their efforts to pull towards the provision of and research into a forensic mental system that is responsive and sensitive to the needs and strengths of a diverse patient population, especially those who experience multiple and intersecting marginalised characteristics.

References

Jansman-Hart, E. M., Seto, M. C., Crocker, A. G., Nicholls, T. L., & Côté, G. (2011). International trends in demand for forensic mental health services. *International Journal of Forensic Mental Health, 10*(4), 326–336. https://doi.org/10.1080/14999013.2011.625591

Morgan, C., Knowles, G., & Hutchinson, G. (2019). Migration, ethnicity and psychoses: Evidence, models and future directions. *World Psychiatry, 18*(3), 247–258. https://doi.org/10.1002/wps.20655

Prins, S. J. (2011). Does transinstitutionalization explain the overrepresentation of people with serious mental illnesses in the criminal justice system? *Community Mental Health Journal, 47*(6), 716–722. https://doi.org/10.1007/s10597-011-9420-y

Sherman, L. W., Strang, H., Mayo-Wilson, E., Woods, D. J., & Ariel, B. (2014). Are restorative justice conferences effective in reducing repeat offending? Findings from a Campbell systematic review. *Journal of Quantitative Criminology*, *31*(1), 1–24. https://doi.org/10.1007/S10940-014-9222-9

UN General Assembly. (2015). The united nations standard minimum rules for the treatment of prisoners (the Nelson Mandela Rules): General assembly resolution 70/175, annex, adopted on 17 December 2015.

Wittouck, C., Dekkers, A., de Ruyver, B., Vanderplasschen, W., & vander Laenen, F. (2013). The impact of drug treatment courts on recovery: A systematic review. *The Scientific World Journal*. https://doi.org/10.1155/2013/493679

Index

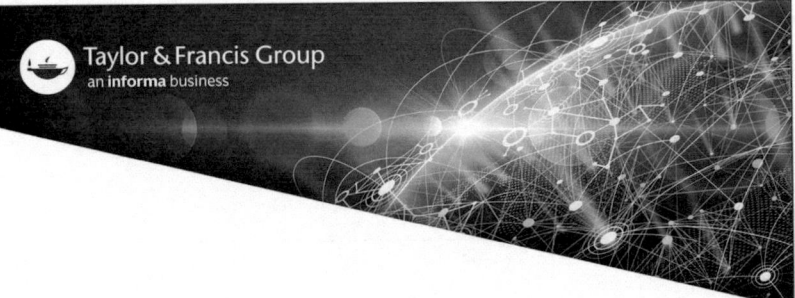
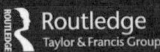
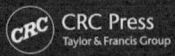